M. D. ANDERSON
CANCER CARE
SERIES

Series Editors

Aman U. Buzdar, MD   Ralph S. Freedman, MD, PhD

T0138080

Springer
New York
Berlin
Heidelberg
Hong Kong
London
Milan
Paris
Tokyo

M. D. ANDERSON CANCER CARE SERIES

Series Editors: Aman U. Buzdar, M.D., and
Ralph S. Freedman, M.D., Ph.D.

K.K. Hunt, G.L. Robb, E.A. Strom, and N.T. Ueno, Eds., *Breast Cancer*

Frank V. Fossella, MD, Ritsuko Komaki, MD, and Joe B. Putnam, Jr., MD

Editors

The University of Texas M. D. Anderson Cancer Center, Houston, Texas

Lung Cancer

Foreword by James D. Cox, MD, Waun Ki Hong, MD, and Jack A. Roth, MD

With 34 Illustrations

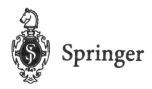 Springer

Frank V. Fossella, MD
Department of
   Thoracic/Head and
   Neck Medical Oncology
The University of Texas
   M. D. Anderson
   Cancer Center
Houston, TX 77030-4009
USA

Ritsuko Komaki, MD
Department of
   Radiation Oncology
The University of Texas
   M. D. Anderson
   Cancer Center
Houston, TX 77030-4009
USA

Joe B. Putnam, Jr., MD
Department of Thoracic
   and Cardiovascular
   Surgery
The University of Texas
   M. D. Anderson
   Cancer Center
Houston, TX 77030-4009
USA

Series Editors:
Aman U. Buzdar, MD
Department of Breast Medical
   Oncology
The University of Texas
   M. D. Anderson Cancer Center
Houston, TX 77030-4009
USA

Ralph S. Freedman, MD, PhD
Immunology/Molecular Biology
   Laboratory
Department of Gynecologic Oncology
The University of Texas
   M. D. Anderson Cancer Center
Houston, TX 77030-4009
USA

Cover illustration: © Fiona King/Images.com

Library of Congress Cataloging-in-Publication Data

Lung cancer / editors, Frank V. Fossella, Ritsuko Komaki, Joe B. Putnam.
      p. ; cm. — (M. D. Anderson cancer care series)
      Includes bibliographical references and index.
      ISBN 0-387-95507-0 (s/c : alk. paper)
      1. Lungs—Cancer. I. Fossella, Frank V. II. Komaki, Ritsuko III. Putnam, J. B. (Joe Billy),
   1953– IV. Series.
      [DNLM: 1. Lung Neoplasms—therapy. WF 658 L96063 2002]
   RC280.L8 L76533 2002
   616.99'424—dc21

                                                                                              2002070465

ISBN 0-387-95507-0   Printed on acid-free paper.

Printed in the United States of America.

9 8 7 6 5 4 3 2 1   SPIN 10879972

www.springer-ny.com

Springer-Verlag   New York Berlin Heidelberg
A member of BertelsmannSpringer Science+Business Media GmbH

FOREWORD

The care of patients with cancer has been a multidisciplinary effort throughout the 60-year history of M. D. Anderson Cancer Center. In the early years, cancer care at M. D. Anderson involved primarily the disciplines of diagnostic imaging, pathology, and a treatment modality. The complexity of these interrelationships has increased at a seemingly exponential rate, especially in the last decade. Technological advances, introduction of new drugs, improvements in supportive care, and exciting findings in basic and translational research have placed demands on the entire medical team for constant education and coordination.

Lung cancer is a leading cause of death from cancer throughout the world. It is by far the leading cause of death in all urbanized countries, and it has rapidly risen in importance in developing countries. An intensely committed group of physicians and laboratory investigators has been gathered at M. D. Anderson to treat lung cancer. Their understanding of the diseases involved and their commitment to thoughtful, carefully coordinated collaborations in the care of patients with lung cancer are reflected in this monograph, the second volume in the M. D. Anderson Cancer Care Series.

The subjects in this book are presented in much the order a patient might perceive events: symptoms and signs, diagnostic imaging, and biopsy and pathologic diagnosis, followed by differing sequences of treatment depending upon the particular disease. Surgical resection is the most successful treatment for early cancer of the lung, but efforts to enhance the benefit of surgery with chemotherapy and radiation therapy are also explored. Treatment of advanced cancer of the lung involves, at least, interactions between the medical oncologist and the radiation oncologist and often, in the case of non–small cell cancer of the lung, the thoracic surgeon. The distinction was made years ago between small cell carcinoma of the lung, a tumor strikingly responsive to chemotherapy and radiation therapy, and non–small cell carcinomas (including squamous cell carcinoma, adenocarcinoma, and large cell carcinoma), which are not very responsive to these treatments. Although the terms "small cell lung cancer"and "non–small cell lung cancer"are preserved for simplicity of expression, important differences in subcategories within these categories are recognized and play a role in treatment decisions.

The commitment to patient care occurring in the setting of clinical investigations is implied throughout the chapters in this book. With every patient seen, the goal is definitive treatment with curative intent if at all possible. Since the results of current standard treatments are not as successful as they could be, developments from the laboratory, new approaches to focusing radiations, new drugs, and therapeutic agents derived from research in molecular cell biology are an important part of therapeutic considerations for individual patients. Clinical research is essential if progress is to be made. By agreeing to enrollment in a protocol, a patient may become a collaborator in this enterprise as well as a recipient of the best available care.

The final chapters of *Lung Cancer* reflect important new initiatives. The first is prevention and early detection. The final chapter suggests the bases for future translations into clinical practice.

The interplay and coordination among all of the physicians and laboratory investigators contributing to this monograph cannot be overemphasized. There are few, if any, other types of cancer that call for such broad understanding and technological expertise among the many physicians involved as does lung cancer. The expertise and commitment the contributing physicians and scientists bring to this treatise reflect only a part of the commitment they bring to the care of their patients.

James D. Cox, MD
Waun Ki Hong, MD
Jack A. Roth, MD

PREFACE

It is estimated that 450,000 people in the United States will die of lung cancer and other tobacco-related disorders this year. The relationship between smoking and lung cancer is inarguable. It is strongly believed that changes in population behavior could in time almost eliminate this disease, and efforts to bring about such changes remain a challenge for those involved with public policy.

In contrast to efforts in breast cancer prevention, which have demonstrated that antiestrogens are effective in reducing the risk of disease development in high-risk women, attempts to identify pharmacologic interventions effective in secondary prevention of lung cancer have thus far met with little success. There remains, however, a strong interest in this area, and a number of novel agents are currently being tested in clinical trials.

The combined-modality treatment approach has resulted in modest gains in the survival of lung cancer patients. Specifically in locally advanced disease, neoadjuvant systemic therapy followed by local therapies, including surgery and radiation therapy, has had a favorable impact on disease-free and overall survival. The availability of novel cytotoxic agents and drugs with substantial antitumor activity as well as target-specific biologics has the potential to further favorably alter the prognosis of lung cancer patients.

This volume reflects M. D. Anderson Cancer Center's commitment to the multidisciplinary disease-oriented approach—an approach that has evolved here over a number of years and is contributing to the progress in patient outcomes. We would like to thank the volume editors—Dr. Frank V. Fossella, Dr. Ritsuko Komaki, and Dr. Joe B. Putnam, Jr.—for their significant efforts in putting this book together. This volume is a tribute to their continued dedication, as well as that of the faculty in their departments, to a resolution of the lung cancer problem. We would also like to thank the Department of Scientific Publications for their assistance with this volume, especially Walter Pagel for helping develop the series, Stephanie Deming for editing the manuscript, and Leigh Fink for editorial assistance, including help with permissions and illustrations.

Aman U. Buzdar, MD
Ralph S. Freedman, MD, PhD

Contents

CONTRIBUTORS

George R. Blumenschein, Jr., MD, Assistant Professor, Department of Thoracic/Head and Neck Medical Oncology

Yvette De Jesus, RN, CNS, AOCN®, Associate Director, Practice Outcomes

Jeremy J. Erasmus, MD, Associate Professor, Department of Diagnostic Radiology

Frank V. Fossella, MD, Professor, Department of Thoracic/Head and Neck Medical Oncology

Walter N. Hittelman, PhD, Professor, Department of Experimental Therapeutics

Jason F. Kelly, MD, Assistant Professor, Department of Radiation Oncology

Fadlo R. Khuri, MD, Associate Professor, Department of Thoracic/Head and Neck Medical Oncology

Edward S. Kim, MD, Assistant Professor, Department of Thoracic/Head and Neck Medical Oncology

Ritsuko Komaki, MD, Professor, Gloria Lupton Tennison Professorship in Lung Cancer Research, Department of Radiation Oncology

Jonathan M. Kurie, MD, Associate Professor, Department of Thoracic/Head and Neck Medical Oncology

Reginald F. Munden, MD, DMD, Associate Professor, Department of Diagnostic Radiology

Katherine M. W. Pisters, MD, Associate Professor, Department of Thoracic/Head and Neck Medical Oncology

Joe B. Putnam, Jr., MD, Professor, Department of Thoracic and Cardio-vascular Surgery

Jae Y. Ro, MD, PhD, Professor, Department of Pathology

W. Roy Smythe, MD, Assistant Professor, Department of Thoracic and Cardiovascular Surgery

Stephen G. Swisher, MD, Associate Professor, Department of Thoracic and Cardiovascular Surgery

Pheroze Tamboli, MD, Assistant Professor, Department of Pathology

Ara A. Vaporciyan, MD, Assistant Professor, Department of Thoracic and Cardiovascular Surgery

Garrett L. Walsh, MD, Professor, Department of Thoracic and Cardio-vascular Surgery

Ralph Zinner, MD, Assistant Professor, Department of Thoracic/Head and Neck Medical Oncology

1

IMPLEMENTATION OF MULTIDISCIPLINARY CARE IN THE TREATMENT OF PATIENTS WITH LUNG CANCER

Joe B. Putnam, Jr., Frank V. Fossella, and Ritsuko Komaki

CHAPTER OVERVIEW

The treatment of patients with lung cancer requires a committed multidisciplinary approach. A thorough pretreatment evaluation, including clinical staging based on chest radiography, computed tomography of the chest and upper abdomen, and other examinations plus evaluation of the patient's performance status, is essential for effective treatment planning. For patients with non–small cell lung cancer (NSCLC) with localized disease and clinically negative mediastinal lymph nodes, anatomic pulmonary resection and intrathoracic mediastinal lymph node dissection should be performed. In patients with NSCLC with histologically positive mediastinal lymph nodes or unresectable local disease, pulmonary resection is not performed as sole or initial treatment; rather, combined regimens of chemotherapy and radiation therapy or protocol-based therapy is recommended. Novel agents for treatment of metastatic NSCLC are being intensively evaluated; targeted receptor therapy, novel combination chemotherapy, and gene therapy with or without chemotherapy and radiation therapy are among the potential therapeutic modalities being investigated. Patients with small cell lung cancer (SCLC) are usually treated with combination chemotherapy. For both NSCLC and SCLC, clinical trials optimize therapy. The multidisciplinary program of the Thoracic Center at M. D. Anderson Cancer Center, involving specialists in thoracic surgery, medical oncology, and radiation oncology, is designed to provide each lung cancer patient with an optimal, individualized treatment plan. Our extensive use of clinical trials allows our patients to have constant access to the best treatment ideas for all stages of lung cancer. Our multidisciplinary planning conferences, clinical guidelines, patient care pathways, and programs for continuous quality improvement provide a scientifically sound, medically effective, and patient-centered program of care.

INTRODUCTION

Lung cancer is a significant public health problem in the United States and the world. In the United States, lung cancer is currently the most common cancer among both men and women and is the leading cause of cancer-related deaths. Despite improvements in treatment over the past few decades, survival in patients with lung cancer remains poor. One-year survival rates improved from 34% in 1975 to 41% in 1996; however, the 5-year survival rate for all stages combined is only about 14%. Five-year survival rates approach 50% for patients with localized disease, 20% for patients with regional disease, and 2% for patients with distant disease.

Only about 15% of lung cancers are discovered when they are still localized. Prevention and early detection of lung cancer have proven difficult. Population screening with chest radiography, cytologic examination of sputum (sputum cytology), and fiber-optic bronchoscopy have all shown only limited effectiveness. In the future, more sensitive radiographic imaging studies, such as low-dose helical computed tomography (CT), or examination of molecular markers in biopsy materials or sputum may be shown to be of value in lung cancer screening. Solving the problem of lung cancer will require the combined efforts of cancer prevention specialists, basic scientists, and clinicians in educating the public about lung cancer risk factors, elucidating the mechanisms of the disease process, and improving clinical care.

Local and systemic treatment interventions (surgery, radiation therapy, and chemotherapy) can improve survival in patients with lung cancer. However, successful treatment depends upon accurate pathologic staging prior to the initiation of definitive therapy. For patients with disease confined to the lung parenchyma, anatomic resection of the involved lobe and mediastinal lymph node dissection is the optimal approach for treatment and pathologic staging. In patients with more advanced disease, a structured multidisciplinary approach, including evaluations and recommendations by the surgeon, the medical oncologist, and the radiation oncologist *prior to treatment*, is the best way to ensure optimal treatment. Although resection alone is frequently performed for localized disease, long-term survival with this approach can be reduced in patients with larger tumors compared to those with smaller tumors. In time, multidisciplinary care may be shown to confer benefits to patients with larger localized disease similar to those experienced by patients with more advanced stage lung cancers.

In the future, knowledge of molecular changes that predispose to the development of lung cancer may lead to strategies for chemoprevention or treatments directed at genetic alterations in the cancer itself. Currently, numerous clinical trials, initiated through the efforts of oncologists throughout the world, are ongoing in an attempt to better understand and evaluate various combinations of multidisciplinary treatments.

The purpose of this monograph is to give practicing physicians an overview of our multidisciplinary approach to the care of lung cancer patients at M.D. Anderson Cancer Center. This introductory chapter will present an overview of the biological basis for multidisciplinary care, the outcomes of multidisciplinary interventions, and likely directions of future progress.

EPIDEMIOLOGY

In 2001, an estimated 169,500 new cases of lung cancer were diagnosed in the United States, and these accounted for 13% of all cancers diagnosed. In men, the incidence of lung cancer increased steadily between the mid-1960s and mid-1990s and did not begin to level off until 1997 (at 43.1 cases per 100,000). Although the incidence of lung cancer is now declining in men, the incidence in women continues to increase.

Lung cancer accounts for almost 154,900 deaths (28% of all cancer deaths) in the United States each year. The number of deaths from lung cancer exceeds the number of deaths from breast, prostate, and colorectal cancers combined (Figures 1–1 and 1–2). Although the death rate from lung cancer has recently begun to decline in men, the death rate from lung cancer in women continues to increase. In 1987, for the first time, the death rate from lung cancer in women exceeded the death rate from breast cancer.

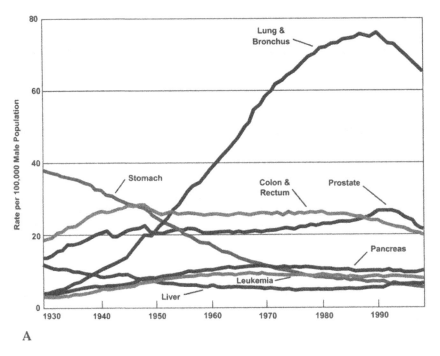

A

Figure 1–1. Age-adjusted cancer death rates, males (A) and females (B) by site, US, 1930–1998. (Per 100,000, age-adjusted to the 1970 US standard population.) † Uterus cancer death rates are for uterine cervix and uterine corpus combined. Note: Due to changes in ICD coding, numerator information has changed over time. Rates for cancers of the liver, lung & bronchus, and colon & rectum are affected by these coding changes. Data from: US Mortality Public Use Data Tapes 1960–1998, US Mortality Volumes 1930–1959, National Center for Health Statistics, Centers for Disease Control and Prevention, 2001. Source: American Cancer Society. *Cancer Facts and Figures—2002.* Reprinted by the permission of the American Cancer Society, Inc.

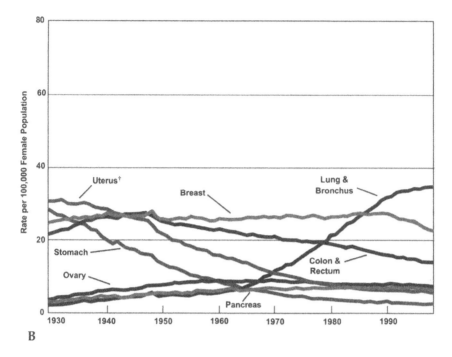

B

Figure 1–1. *(continued)*

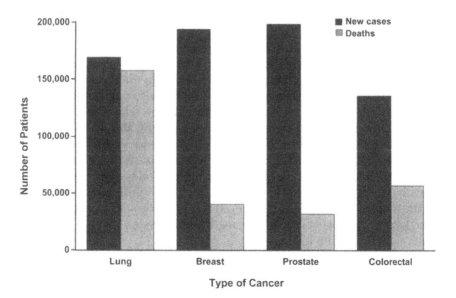

Figure 1–2. New cases of cancer and cancer deaths for the 4 leading cancers in the United States, 2001. Source: American Cancer Society. *Cancer Facts and Figures—2001.* Atlanta, Ga: American Cancer Society; 2001:5.

The decrease in lung cancer incidence and mortality in men probably reflects decreases in cigarette smoking over the past 30 years. Unfortunately, smoking cessation in women has lagged behind smoking cessation in men. Cigarette smoking among young people increased during the 1990s.

ETIOLOGY

Cigarette smoking is unequivocally the most important risk factor in the development of lung cancer. The American Cancer Society estimates that about 170,000 cancer deaths could be avoided each year if tobacco use were eliminated (American Cancer Society, 2002). Other environmental factors that may predispose individuals to lung cancer include iatrogenic radiation exposure and exposure to industrial substances such as asbestos, arsenic, chromium, and nickel; organic chemicals; radon; air pollution; and secondary smoke.

PATHOLOGY

In general, lung cancer is slightly more likely to develop in the right lung than in the left lung as the right lung has approximately 55% of the lung parenchyma. In addition, lung cancer occurs more frequently in the upper lobes than in the lower lobes. The blood supply to lung tumors, which arise from the bronchial epithelium, is from the bronchial arteries. A small percentage of patients with lung cancer have a second focus or metastasis of lung cancer at diagnosis.

Lung cancer can extend directly by local extension along the bronchus of origin, into the chest wall, across fissures, and into the great vessels, the pericardium, or the diaphragm. Lung cancer can also involve other thoracic structures, such as the superior vena cava, the recurrent or phrenic nerves, or the esophagus, by direct extension. Lung tumors commonly metastasize to the pulmonary (intraparenchymal) and mediastinal lymph nodes. Small cell lung cancer (SCLC) is more likely than non–small cell lung cancer (NSCLC) to metastasize to the lymph nodes and other organs. Typically, the pattern of spread is first to the hilar lymph nodes and then into the mediastinal (usually ipsilateral) lymph nodes. Tumors of the left lower lobe that metastasize to the mediastinal nodes involve the contralateral mediastinum in about 25% of patients.

Lung cancer can spread hematogenously to the liver, adrenals, lung, bones, kidneys, and brain. Bone metastases are usually osteolytic. Lung cancer is the second most common cause of bone metastases after breast cancer. Metastases rarely occur distal to the elbow or distal to the knee. Spread of lung cancer through the airways to another discontinuous area is extremely rare and frequently difficult to prove; second primary lung tumors are more common.

DETECTION AND DIAGNOSIS

Patients with lung cancer are usually 50 to 70 years of age; lung cancer is rarely seen in patients under the age of 30. As the lung parenchyma has no sensory nerve fibers, symptoms occur only with compression, invasion, or metastasis to other organs or structures. Many lung cancers grow to a large size before they cause local symptoms such as hemoptysis, a change in sputum production, dyspnea, obstruction, or pain. Few patients are asymptomatic at the time of diagnosis. Most patients have bronchopulmonary symptoms such as cough, dyspnea, chest pain, or hemoptysis. Fever, wheezing, or stridor may also be present. Some patients have asymptomatic pulmonary nodules identified on screening chest radiography performed as part of a routine physical examination or because of a related pulmonary problem. Other symptoms may include hoarseness, superior vena cava syndrome, chest wall pain, Horner's syndrome, dysphagia, pleural effusion, and phrenic nerve paralysis. Nonspecific symptoms such as anorexia, malaise, fatigue, and weight loss may also occur.

Obstruction of a main-stem bronchus or lobar bronchus may impair the passage of mucus. With this partial obstruction and bacterial overgrowth, pneumonia may develop. Frequently, patients with undiagnosed lung cancer present to their local physician with clinical evidence of pneumonia of several days' duration. The pneumonia may be treated intermittently with antibiotics for a period of several weeks. If the pneumonia does not clear, a chest radiograph is obtained, which frequently will identify the lung cancer.

Cytologic examination of sputum (sputum cytology), chest radiography, fiber-optic bronchoscopy, and fine-needle aspiration of the mass may assist clinicians in making the diagnosis of lung cancer and establishing more precisely the stage of disease.

Screening of patients at high risk for lung cancer has been proposed as a method of reducing mortality from this disease. However, sputum cytology and chest radiography, the screening methods most extensively examined to date, have proved to have low sensitivity in the detection of small, resectable lung tumors. More recently, the Early Lung Cancer Action Project showed that low-resolution CT of the chest revealed small nodules undetectable on routine chest radiography (Henschke et al, 1999). Some of these nodules have the potential to be lung cancer. The authors identified criteria that could be used to identify patients who have a high likelihood of early-stage lung cancer and thus are appropriate candidates for additional evaluation and possible resection.

It is hoped that a prospective randomized trial of lung cancer screening using low-resolution CT of the chest will be conducted to objectively measure the survival benefits of this approach compared to chest radiography alone.

STAGING

Lung cancer staging allows physicians to group patients on the basis of the extent of disease and the expected survival so that appropriate therapy can be applied in a systematic manner. Staging also assists physicians in counseling patients and family members regarding potential therapy and prognosis.

The staging system for lung cancer is the International System for Staging Lung Cancer, which was adopted in 1986 and is supported by the American Joint Committee on Cancer and the Union Internationale Contre Le Cancer. The system was revised in 1997 (Mountain, 1997; Mountain and Dresler, 1997) (Tables 1–1, 1–2, and 1–3). The stage categories were developed through a process in which patients with similar survival were grouped together and their clinical characteristics were examined (Mountain, 1997; Mountain and Dresler, 1997; Naruke et al, 2001). In the 1997 revision, stage I disease was divided into stages IA and IB. In addition, T3N0M0 disease was moved from stage IIIA to stage IIB since patients with this type of disease have survival outcomes closer to those of other patients with stage IIB disease.

NSCLC can be roughly grouped into 3 major categories on the basis of treatment options. The first category consists of disease that is completely contained within the lung and can be completely resected (stage I and II). The second category consists of primary tumors that are resectable but are associated with lymph node metastases or mediastinal involvement that cannot be controlled with surgery (stage IIIA with N2 involvement and stage IIIB). The third and final category consists of tumors associated with distant metastases (stage IV disease); these tumors are not treated with surgery except with palliative intent.

Despite our best surgical efforts, approximate 5-year survival rates by stage for patients with NSCLC are as follows: stage I, 65%; stage II, 40%; stage III, 15%; and stage IV, 5% (Nesbitt et al, 1995; Mountain, 1997; Naruke et al, 1998) (see Table 6–1, page 103).

The role of staging in SCLC is discussed in chapters 10 and 11.

PRETREATMENT EVALUATION

In patients with lung cancer, the goals of the pretreatment evaluation are to determine the clinical disease stage (the final clinical stage determined before the initiation of definitive therapy) and to determine the patient's

Table 1–1. TNM Definitions in the International System for Staging Lung Cancer

Primary Tumor (T)

TX   Primary tumor cannot be assessed, or tumor proven by the presence of malignant cells in sputum or bronchial washings but not visualized by imaging or bronchoscopy.

T0   No evidence of primary tumor.

Tis   Carcinoma in situ.

T1   Tumor ≤ 3 cm in greatest dimension, surrounded by lung or visceral pleura, without bronchoscopic evidence of invasion more proximal than the lobar bronchus* (i.e., not in the main bronchus).

T2   Tumor with any of the following features of size or extent:
       > 3 cm in greatest dimension
       Involves main bronchus, ≥ 2 cm distal to the carina
       Invades the visceral pleura
       Associated with atelectasis or obstructive pneumonitis that extends to the hilar region but does not involve the entire lung

T3   Tumor of any size that directly invades any of the following: chest wall (including superior sulcus tumors), diaphragm, mediastinal pleura, parietal pericardium; or tumor in the main bronchus < 2 cm distal to the carina, but without involvement of the carina; or associated atelectasis or obstructive pneumonitis of the entire lung.

T4   Tumor of any size that invades any of the following: mediastinum, heart, great vessels, trachea, esophagus, vertebral body, carina; or tumor with a malignant pleural or pericardial effusion,† or with satellite tumor nodule(s) within the ipsilateral primary tumor lobe of the lung.

Regional Lymph Nodes (N)

NX   Regional lymph nodes cannot be assessed.

N0   No regional lymph node metastasis.

N1   Metastasis to ipsilateral peribronchial and/or ipsilateral hilar lymph nodes, and intrapulmonary nodes involved by direct extension of the primary tumor.

N2   Metastasis to ipsilateral mediastinal and/or subcarinal lymph node(s).

N3   Metastasis to contralateral mediastinal, contralateral hilar, ipsilateral or contralateral scalene, or supraclavicular lymph node(s).

Distant Metastasis (M)

MX   Distant metastasis cannot be assessed.

M0   No distant metastasis.

M1   Distant metastasis present.‡ Specify site(s).

---

* The uncommon superficial tumor of any size with its invasive component limited to the bronchial wall, which may extend proximal to the main bronchus, is also classified T1.

† Most pleural effusions associated with lung cancer are due to tumor. However, there are a few patients in whom multiple cytopathologic examinations of pleural fluid show no tumor. In these cases, the fluid is nonbloody and is not an exudate. When these elements and clinical judgment dictate that the effusion is not related to the tumor, the effusion should be excluded as a staging element and the patient's disease should be staged T1, T2, or T3. Pericardial effusion is classified according to the same rules.

‡ Separate metastatic tumor nodules in the ipsilateral nonprimary-tumor lobe(s) of the lung also are classified M1.

Reprinted with permission from Mountain CF. Revisions in the International System for Staging Lung Cancer. *Chest* 1997;111:1710–1717.

Table 1–2.   Description of the Stage Groupings for Lung Cancer

The TNM subsets are combined to form 7 stage groups, in addition to stage 0, that reflect fairly precise levels of disease progression and their implications for treatment selection and prognosis. Staging is not relevant for occult carcinoma (TXN0M0).

Stage 0 is assigned to patients with carcinoma in situ, which is consistent with the staging of all other sites.

Stage IA includes only patients with tumors 3 cm or less in greatest dimension and no evidence of metastasis, the anatomic subset T1N0M0.

Stage IB includes only patients with a T2 primary tumor classification and no evidence of metastasis, the anatomic subset T2N0M0.

Stage IIA is reserved for patients with a T1 primary tumor classification and metastasis limited to the intrapulmonary, including hilar, lymph nodes, the anatomic subset T1N1M0.

Stage IIB includes 2 anatomic subsets: patients with a T2 primary tumor classification and metastasis limited to the ipsilateral intrapulmonary, including hilar, lymph nodes, the anatomic subset T2N1M0; and patients with primary tumor classification of T3 and no evidence of metastasis, the anatomic subset T3N0M0.

Stage IIIA includes 4 anatomic subsets that reflect the implications of ipsilateral, limited, extrapulmonary extension of lung cancer. Patients included are those with a T3 primary tumor classification and metastasis limited to the ipsilateral intrapulmonary, including hilar, lymph nodes, the anatomic subset T3N1M0; and patients with T1, T2, or T3 primary tumor classifications and metastasis limited to the ipsilateral mediastinal and subcarinal lymph nodes, the anatomic subsets T1N2M0, T2N2M0, and T3N2M0.

Stage IIIB designates patients with extensive primary tumor invasion of the mediastinum and metastases to the contralateral mediastinal, contralateral hilar, and ipsilateral and contralateral scalene/supraclavicular lymph nodes. Patients with a T4 primary tumor classification or N3 regional lymph node metastasis but no distant metastasis are included.

Stage IV is reserved for patients with evidence of distant metastatic disease, M1, such as metastases to brain, bone, liver, adrenal gland, contralateral lung, pancreas and other distant organs, and metastases to distant lymph node groups such as axillary, abdominal, and inguinal. Patients with metastasis in ipsilateral nonprimary tumor lobes of the lung are also designated as having M1 disease.

Source: Mountain CF. Revisions in the International System for Staging Lung Cancer. *Chest* 1997;111:1710–1717.

performance status. These 2 factors taken together will suggest the best treatment option.

History and Physical Examination

The pretreatment evaluation includes a history and a physical examination, with particular attention paid to extrathoracic symptoms suggestive of paraneoplastic syndromes (distant manifestations of lung cancer not re-

Table 1–3. Brief Description of the Stage Groupings for Lung Cancer

Stage 0	Carcinoma in situ		
Stage IA	T1	N0	M0
Stage IB	T2	N0	M0
Stage IIA	T1	N1	M0
Stage IIB	T2	N1	M0
	T3	N0	M0
Stage IIIA	T3	N1	M0
	T1	N2	M0
	T2	N2	M0
	T3	N2	M0
Stage IIIB	T4	N0	M0
	T4	N1	M0
	T4	N2	M0
	T1	N3	M0
	T2	N3	M0
	T3	N3	M0
	T4	N3	M0
Stage IV	Any T	Any N	M1

Reprinted with permission from Mountain CF. Revisions in the International System for Staging Lung Cancer. *Chest* 1997;111:1710–1717.

lated to metastases) and to the cervical and supraclavicular lymph nodes. Enlarged cervical or supraclavicular lymph nodes may be the first clues to extrathoracic nodal metastasis (N3 disease), the presence of which suggests treatment with nonsurgical means (chemotherapy, radiation therapy, or both).

The evaluation of performance status includes evaluation of cardiac function, pulmonary function, exercise tolerance, and associated comorbid conditions that will influence the patient's subsequent therapy.

Chest Radiography and Computed Tomography of the Chest and Upper Abdomen

Chest radiography and CT of the chest and upper abdomen (including the adrenal glands) are performed in all patients.

Chest radiography provides information on the size, shape, and density of the tumor and its location with respect to the mediastinal structures. Chest radiography also provides information about the presence of thoracic lymphadenopathy, pleural effusion, pericardial effusion, pulmonary infiltrates, pneumonia, and consolidation. Changes in the contour of the mediastinum secondary to lymphadenopathy and metastasis to ribs or other bone structures may be visualized. Chest radiography may also provide clues to the tumor's histologic subtype: squamous carcinomas tend to be large and centrally located, adenocarcinomas tend to be more peripherally located, and SCLCs tend to be large, located centrally or near the hilum, and associated with bulky mediastinal lymphadenopathy.

On chest radiography, the relationship of the mass to the thoracic structures and mediastinum and whether the mass appears limited or diffuse should be noted. In addition, attention should be paid to whether the following features are present: cavitation, segmental or lobar collapse or consolidation, hilar or mediastinal enlargement, evidence of intrathoracic metastasis, and evidence of extrapulmonary intrathoracic extension.

CT of the chest and upper abdomen provides more detail than chest radiography about the surface characteristics of the tumor, the location of the tumor in relation to the mediastinum and mediastinal structures, and metastasis to lung, bones, liver, and adrenals. CT will also reveal any enlargement of the mediastinal lymph nodes. Although CT cannot accurately or consistently predict invasion, it can reveal the size and the density of mediastinal nodes. CT of the chest and upper abdomen has a specificity of 65% and a sensitivity of 79% in the identification of mediastinal lymphadenopathy. When lymph nodes are larger than 1.5 cm in diameter, CT has a specificity of approximately 85% in the identification of metastasis to mediastinal lymph nodes.

Evaluation of Enlarged Mediastinal Lymph Nodes

If chest radiography or CT of the chest and upper abdomen indicates that mediastinal lymph nodes are enlarged (≥ 1 cm), biopsy is required to determine whether the nodes are involved with lung cancer metastases and to define the extent of such involvement. The probability of metastatic involvement in lymph nodes measuring 1 cm or larger is 30%. Other causes of mediastinal lymphadenopathy include mediastinal inflammation, peripheral pulmonary obstruction, atelectasis, consolidation, bronchitis, pneumonitis, and pneumonia; in addition, some patients may have normally enlarged mediastinal lymph nodes.

Methods available for mediastinal lymph node biopsy include transbronchial biopsy (for technical details, see the section Bronchoscopy later in this chapter), cervical mediastinoscopy, extended cervical mediastinoscopy, anterior mediastinotomy (Chamberlain procedure), video-assisted thoracoscopy, and fine-needle aspiration. The procedure of choice depends on the location of the enlarged nodes and the patient's performance status. Positron emission tomography (PET) is also being investigated as an alternative technique or more likely a technique complementary to mediastinoscopy for identifying potential metastatic involvement of mediastinal nodes. Pathologic review of the biopsy specimen is required before initiation of treatment.

Video-Assisted Thoracic Surgery

Video-assisted thoracic surgery techniques may be used to biopsy left hilar lymph nodes and to evaluate the intrathoracic manifestations of a lung tumor.

Bronchoscopy

Bronchoscopy is recommended in the case of planned pulmonary resection, positive findings on sputum cytology with negative findings on chest radiography, or persistence of atelectasis or an infiltrate despite medical management.

Surgeons always perform a bronchoscopy before resection to independently assess the endobronchial anatomy and exclude occult second primary tumors with an endobronchial component. The surgeon must ensure that all known tumor will be encompassed by the planned pulmonary resection. The precise location of an endobronchial tumor may modify the planned operation. For example, if the tumor is located in the right upper lobe orifice and involves a portion of the right primary bronchus or a portion of the right middle lobe bronchus, a sleeve lobectomy may be required to conserve the right middle and lower lobes and thereby avoid a pneumonectomy. Findings on bronchoscopy depend on the location of the lesion: more centrally located lung tumors are more likely to be associated with positive findings on bronchoscopy, whereas smaller and more peripheral lung tumors are more likely to be associated with negative findings on bronchoscopy.

Transbronchial biopsy may be performed by passing a special 21-gauge (Wang) needle through the flexible bronchoscope. This technique may be used to biopsy mediastinal nodes or other masses adjacent to the larger bronchi. Pulmonary parenchyma may be obtained with transbronchial biopsy by forcing the flexible biopsy forceps through the terminal bronchioles into the lung parenchyma. However, this technique must be performed with caution because of the potential for hemorrhage or pneumothorax.

Fluorescence bronchoscopy after intravenous injection of hematoporphyrin derivatives can be used to localize in situ and superficial tumors. These tumors will fluoresce when illuminated with light from a special laser.

Additional Diagnostic and Staging Studies

Various other preoperative studies are indicated selectively.

Transthoracic Needle Aspiration Biopsy

Fine-needle aspiration by a transthoracic route (transthoracic needle aspiration biopsy; TTNA biopsy) may be 95% accurate in confirming or ruling out lung cancer in patients who are unable to undergo surgery. TTNA biopsy is not recommended in patients with good physiologic reserve who are considered appropriate candidates for surgery (e.g., patients with clinical stage I or II disease).

In patients with hard palpable lymph nodes in the cervical or supra-clavicular area, fine-needle aspiration may provide an accurate diagnosis of metastatic (N3) involvement. Otherwise, a superficial lymph node biopsy or a scalene node biopsy can be performed to obtain tissue for further evaluation. If cervical or supraclavicular lymph nodes are positive, the disease is clinical stage IIIB, and surgery is not recommended.

Sputum Cytology

Sputum cytology may be an appropriate diagnostic procedure if the patient is unable to undergo surgery, has symptoms suggestive of cancer, and has severe emphysema and thus is not a candidate for TTNA biopsy because of the increased risk of pneumothorax.

Transesophageal Sonography

Transesophageal sonography may assist the clinician in evaluating lung cancer that may abut the esophagus, heart, or aorta. Directed trans-esophageal biopsies of subcarinal lymph nodes may also be performed.

Bone Scanning, Computed Tomography, and Magnetic Resonance Imaging

In patients with resectable lung cancer (stage I or II disease), bone scanning and CT of the brain are not recommended in the absence of related symptoms. A bone scan should be performed only if the patient complains of bone pain. Plain radiographic films of the affected area should be obtained to supplement the bone scan. If questions still exist after the studies are completed, magnetic resonance (MR) imaging of the painful area may also be performed. Finally, biopsy of the involved bony area may be required. Similarly, CT or MR imaging of the brain should be performed only if the patient has neurological symptoms or if the diagnosis of SCLC is suspected. It is not cost-effective to perform CT of the brain in an otherwise asymptomatic patient with lung cancer who has no neurological symptoms and is physiologically fit and stage-appropriate for surgery.

In patients with more advanced disease, bone scanning and CT or MR imaging of the brain may have a higher yield in revealing occult metastatic disease. MR imaging is frequently used to complement CT in evaluating the location of these tumors within the chest. Specifically, MR imaging is helpful for evaluating bony invasion of the chest wall or other mediastinal structures. In patients with superior sulcus tumors and patients with tumors involving the first and second or third ribs, MR imaging may provide additional information beyond that obtainable with CT regarding the extent of the tumor's involvement of the brachial plexus, thoracic inlet, great vessels, or other mediastinal structures (Komaki et al, 1990).

Positron Emission Tomography

Fluorodeoxyglucose PET (FDG-PET) is a method of determining the presence or absence of cancer on the basis of differences in glucose metabolism between cancer cells and normal cells. Cancer cells metabolize glucose more rapidly than normal cells. When FDG is injected intravenously as a substrate, cancer cells incorporate and metabolize the compound. With subsequent phosphorylation, FDG-phosphate with tracer is trapped within the cell and can be visualized with PET. Various nuclear scanning devices can be used to scan the patient for areas of increased uptake. Such areas are commonly associated with cancer metastases, and frequently these metastases are otherwise unsuspected.

PET coupled with CT may be more sensitive and specific than PET alone in the identification of nodal disease or distant metastases. The sensitivity and specificity of FDG-PET range from 94% to 97% for benign lesions and 80% to 100% for malignant lesions. Active inflammation may result in false-positive results. In patients previously treated with radiation therapy, FDG-PET may be helpful in distinguishing between recurrent or persistent lung cancer and radiation fibrosis.

PET is used most commonly to exclude occult metastases in patients with locally advanced NSCLC. Its use as a routine screening study in patients with early-stage disease (clinical stage I or II disease) may not be cost-effective.

Molecular Marker Assays

Various molecular markers may be associated with a worse prognosis in patients with lung cancer. DNA aneuploidy is associated with poor survival. Ki-67 status was a significant predictor of the distant metastatic control rate for adenocarcinoma.

Oncogenes, including k-*ras*, *myc*, and *neu*, serve to regulate, in a positive sense, the growth of tumors. Mutation in k-*ras* is the most frequent mutation found in lung cancer; it accounts for 90% of genetic mutations in adenocarcinoma. This oncogene codes for a protein associated with signal transduction. Mutations in k-*ras* are associated with poor survival. Overexpression of the HER-2/*neu* oncogene is associated with worse survival in patients with lung cancer.

Tumor suppressor genes, such as *p53*, normally provide a negative influence on cell growth. If a tumor suppressor gene is mutated, then this negative influence is removed and the tumor grows unchecked. Gene therapy trials to replace or modify *p53* mutation are under way and have shown that gene therapy is safe when used in a clinical environment (Roth et al, 1996; Swisher et al, 1999) (for more information, see chapter 15). Mutations in the retinoblastoma *(RB)* gene are also associated with poor survival. If both *p53* and *RB* mutations are present, survival is only 12 months, compared to 46 months in patients with normal expression of the corresponding proteins.

TREATMENT

Treatment options for lung cancer include surgery in patients with localized disease, chemotherapy in patients with metastatic disease, and radiation therapy for local control in patients with disease not amenable to surgery. Eligible patients should be offered enrollment in clinical trials. A multidisciplinary approach is the optimal treatment approach in patients with advanced-stage disease.

Multidisciplinary Therapy

A multidisciplinary team is critically important in the treatment of patients with lung cancer. A multidisciplinary approach improves treatment planning and survival time. In the treatment of locally advanced disease, chemotherapy, surgery, and radiation therapy may all be employed and must be coordinated and sequenced in an optimal manner. The use of ad hoc chemotherapy and radiation therapy strategies may do more harm than good. The use of carefully constructed clinical protocols, clinical guidelines, and multidisciplinary care creates an optimal environment in which to select the best treatment for the individual patient.

At M.D. Anderson, the multidisciplinary management of thoracic neoplasms is standard. At our institution, the thoracic surgical oncology service, the thoracic medical oncology service, and the thoracic radiation oncology service are all located within the same clinic area, the Thoracic Center. The proximity of these services facilitates the efficient care of patients with complex thoracic malignancies, such as lung cancer, esophageal cancer, mediastinal malignancies, and other, more rare, tumors, including sarcomas, chest wall neoplasms, and pulmonary metastases. The location of all related specialties in the same clinic, knowledge of the advantages and disadvantages of each modality of treatment, and a philosophical and moral commitment to optimizing each individual patient's care make for an ideal environment in which to provide the best care for patients with lung cancer.

Each week, we hold a major and enthusiastically supported combined conference with the thoracic surgical oncology service, the thoracic medical oncology service, the thoracic radiation oncology service, and the radiologists, pathologists, students, residents, and other allied health-care professionals involved in treating patients with lung cancer. The goals of these conferences are to discuss complex patient problems, discuss candidates for clinical trials, and facilitate transmission of new ideas in basic science, clinical research, translational research, and other aspects of patient care. These conferences are one way that we strive to accomplish our institutional mission: to eliminate cancer in Texas, the nation and the world through outstanding integrated programs in patient care, research, education and prevention.

Non–Small Cell Lung Cancer

NSCLC is treated on the basis of the best clinical staging information available prior to the initiation of definitive therapy. Survival depends on the cumulative mechanical and biological effects of treatment on the primary tumor and micro- and macrometastases. Despite our best efforts, survival in patients with advanced-stage NSCLC remains dismal. Even in patients with earlier-stage disease, survival rates are poor; 5-year survival rates are about 55%, 50%, and 40%, respectively, for patients with stage IB, IIA, and IIB disease. In selected patients, combinations of surgery, chemotherapy, and radiation therapy may provide better survival results than treatment with a single modality alone. The choice of initial therapy (whether single-modality or multimodality therapy) depends on the patient's clinical stage at presentation and the availability of relevant clinical trials. However, treatment options may vary even among different subsets of patients with the same clinical disease stage.

Early-Stage Disease

In patients with early-stage NSCLC (stage I, II, or early IIIA [T3N1]), treatment with surgery alone can result in long-term survival. Lobectomy is the procedure of choice for lung cancer confined to a single lobe. In certain patients with lung cancer and chest wall involvement (T3N0M0), surgery alone as a local control modality may be an effective treatment. En bloc resection of the lung and involved chest wall with mediastinal lymphadenectomy results in a 5-year survival rate of approximately 50%. In addition, patients with T3N0M0 disease with tumors less than 2 cm from the carina have a 5-year survival rate of 36% with surgical resection alone.

Anatomic resection of lung cancer is the gold standard for treatment of early-stage NSCLC. Lobectomy has been shown to be superior to lesser resection even in patients with stage IA disease (T1N0) (Ginsberg and Rubinstein, 1995). Lesser resection, such as wedge resection or segmentectomy, is reserved for patients in whom anatomic resection would carry a prohibitive risk of complications. In patients unable to tolerate surgery, radiation therapy can also be used as primary treatment. Potential complications of radiation therapy include esophagitis and fatigue. Radiation-induced myelitis of the spinal cord is devastating; the risk of this complication can be minimized by careful administration of treatment. Three-dimensional radiation therapy may further focus the dose on the target area while minimizing radiation injury to surrounding tissues.

Preoperative radiation therapy has been investigated in clinical trials and has been shown not to improve survival compared to surgery alone (Komaki, 1985; Komaki et al, 1985).

The favorable results of trials of chemotherapy in patients with advanced-stage disease suggest that chemotherapy may also improve survival in patients with earlier stages of lung cancer. Pisters and colleagues conducted a phase II trial of perioperative paclitaxel and carboplatin in patients with stage IB, IIA, IIB, or T3N1 NSCLC (Pisters et al, 2000). The end points assessed were response, side effects, resectability, and morbidity. All patients underwent invasive staging with mediastinoscopy, and all were free of metastases to ipsilateral mediastinal or subcarinal lymph nodes. Chemotherapy consisted of paclitaxel 225 mg/m^2 given as a 3-hour infusion and carboplatin AUC = 6 every 21 days for 2 cycles before surgery. After resection, patients with R0 resections (complete resection with negative margins) received an additional 3 cycles. Patients with R1 and R2 resections (R1, complete resection with microscopic residual disease or positive margins; R2, incomplete resection with macroscopic residual disease) were treated with "best therapy" off study. A total of 94 patients were entered. Ninety patients (96%) completed both cycles of preoperative chemotherapy. A major (complete or partial) response to chemotherapy occurred in 50 patients (54%). Four patients had a complete pathologic response. Eighty-three patients (90%) underwent surgery, and 75 patients (82%) had a complete resection. Two postoperative deaths occurred. The authors concluded that induction chemotherapy in this population is feasible and is associated with a high response rate. A randomized Intergroup trial comparing surgery alone with induction chemotherapy and surgery is ongoing.

Pathologic examination of the resected specimen is critical to ensure optimal pathologic staging, which may influence subsequent therapy. The bronchial, parenchymal, and pleural margins and the pulmonary, hilar, and mediastinal lymph nodes are evaluated. If all the margins and lymph nodes are negative, no postoperative radiation therapy is required. Postoperative radiation therapy has no significant survival benefit in patients without evidence of lymphatic metastasis (Weisenburger, 1994). If a patient has microscopic disease at any margin or within any mediastinal lymph nodes, postoperative radiation therapy is recommended as it may improve local control.

Advanced-Stage Disease

Most patients with NSCLC with histologically confirmed N2 or more advanced disease have a biologically aggressive tumor with probable occult metastatic disease. While pulmonary resection and mediastinal lymphadenectomy can provide some patients with improved survival and enhanced local control, most patients with pathologically confirmed N2 or more advanced disease will not benefit from surgery as the sole treatment modality. Neoadjuvant platinum-based chemotherapy before surgery improves survival over surgery alone in these patients (Rosell et al, 1994; Roth et al, 1994; Roth et al, 1998) (Table 1–4). Currently a prospective clinical trial (Radiation Therapy Oncology Group trial 93–09) is comparing neoadjuvant chemoradiation therapy and surgical resection with definitive chemotherapy and radiation therapy in patients with N2 stage IIIA

Table 1–4. Results of Randomized Trials of Surgery versus
            Neoadjuvant Chemotherapy plus Surgery
            for Advanced-Stage NSCLC

Investigators and Treatment	No. of Patients	Resection Rate (%)	Median Survival (mo)	3-Year Survival Rate (%)
Rosell et al, 1994				
Surgery [+ XRT]	30	90	8.0	0
Chemo + surgery [+XRT]	29	85	26.0	29
Roth et al, 1994				
Surgery	32	66	11.0	15
Chemo + surgery	28	61	64.0	56
Pass et al, 1992				
Surgery	14	86	15.6	23
Chemo + surgery	13	85	28.7	50

Chemo indicates chemotherapy; XRT, radiation therapy.

NSCLC. Advanced-stage NSCLC (stages IIIA with N2 involvement, IIIB, and IV) cannot typically be treated effectively with a single modality (i.e., chemotherapy or radiation therapy).

Surgery. Most patients with advanced-stage NSCLC are treated nonsurgically. However, some patients with advanced-stage disease may benefit from surgical resection. In deciding whether surgery is appropriate, the surgeon must balance the value of mechanical extirpation of the local disease (e.g., local disease control, pain relief, and the potential for improved survival) with the risks associated with a surgical procedure. Typically, the risks exceed the potential benefits and surgery is not considered; however, in some patients, surgery for advanced-stage lung cancer may provide benefit in the form of local tumor control, palliation of symptoms, improved quality of life, and the potential for improved survival.

Surgery is warranted in patients with an isolated brain metastasis because surgery in this situation can improve quality of life and survival. The primary lung tumor can then be treated according to the T and N stage.

Multispecialty surgical care may be beneficial for resection of complex tumors that extend into the spinal column. In such cases, neurosurgical or orthopedic reconstruction and stabilization of the spine are performed concurrently with resection of the primary tumor. A multispecialty surgical approach can render previously "unresectable" disease resectable with negative margins. Tumors that involve contiguous structures such as the great vessels or portions of the heart, diaphragm, or chest wall can be resected using cardiovascular reconstruction and surgical techniques.

Such multispecialty surgical treatments may also be used to treat more aggressive variants of superior sulcus tumors and other thoracic malignancies.

Surgery may also be used for palliation of the symptoms of advanced disease. Surgery along with laser ablative techniques and stent placement can be used to manage or relieve obstruction of the trachea or main-stem bronchi. We have shown that treatment of recurrent symptomatic pleural effusions with surgical placement of a chronic indwelling pleural catheter (Pleurx; Denver Biomedical Inc., Golden, Colorado) provides excellent relief of dyspnea and allows patients to function independently outside the hospital (Putnam et al, 1999).

Combination Chemotherapy. Combination chemotherapy in patients with advanced-stage NSCLC is well tolerated and is associated with modest but significant improvement in survival compared to single-agent chemotherapy or to supportive care alone. Quality-of-life analyses in patients treated with chemotherapy have demonstrated maintenance of or improvement in quality of life.

Radiation Therapy. Radiation therapy can be used as primary therapy in patients with unresectable NSCLC. As mentioned earlier, in the section Early-Stage Disease, care must be taken to minimize radiation-related complications.

Radiation therapy can also be used to stop hemoptysis if the bleeding site is identified on bronchoscopy and relieve airway obstruction, superior vena cava obstruction, and pain caused by tumor invasion, bone destruction, cord compression, or other metastasis-related problems.

Chemotherapy with Radiation Therapy. Prospective randomized studies have shown that induction cisplatin-based chemotherapy followed by radiation therapy appears to improve survival compared with radiation therapy alone in patients with locally advanced lung cancer (Dillman et al, 1990; Le Chevalier et al, 1991; Sause et al, 1995; Dillman et al, 1996; Fong et al, 1999). Dillman and colleagues (1990) showed that patients treated with cisplatin 100 mg/m^2 and vinblastine 5 mg/m^2 prior to radiation therapy (60 Gy over 6 weeks) had better survival than patients who received the same radiation therapy regimen immediately with no prior chemotherapy. In a second published analysis of the study, when the median follow-up time for the induction chemotherapy arm was 7 years, the radiographic response rate was 56% for the chemotherapy group and only 43% for the radiation-therapy-alone group ($P = .092$). Median survival was 13.7 months in the chemotherapy group, compared with 9.6 months in the radiation-therapy-alone group ($P = .012$). The authors concluded that sequential chemotherapy and radiation therapy increased survival compared to radiation therapy alone.

Le Chevalier and colleagues reported the results of a large prospective study comparing radiation therapy (65 Gy) with radiation therapy and chemotherapy consisting of cisplatin, vindesine, cyclophosphamide, and lomustine. The 2-year survival rate was 14% for radiation therapy alone and 21% for chemotherapy and radiation therapy ($P = .08$). Distant metastasis was significantly less common in the combined treatment group. The local control rate at 1 year was poor in both groups (17% in patients treated with radiation therapy alone and 15% in patients treated with combined therapy) (Le Chevalier et al, 1991; Fong et al, 1999).

Sause and colleagues (1995) examined 3 treatments in patients with locally advanced, surgically unresectable lung cancer: standard radiation therapy, induction chemotherapy followed by standard radiation therapy, and twice-daily radiation therapy. They observed that chemotherapy plus radiation therapy was superior to the other treatments (log-rank $P = .03$). One-year survival rates and median survival times (months) were 46% and 11.4 months for standard radiation therapy; 60% and 13.8 months for chemotherapy plus radiation therapy; and 51% and 12.3 months for hyperfractionated radiation therapy.

Concurrent chemotherapy and radiation therapy may be better tolerated and result in improved survival compared to sequential chemotherapy and radiation therapy. Patients with inoperable clinical stage IIIA or IIIB disease and good pulmonary status and performance status should be treated with chemotherapy and radiation therapy. Trials of these modalities for patients with clinical stage IIIA NSCLC showed a modest but significant improvement in survival compared to survival after radiation therapy alone. An ongoing prospective multi-institutional trial is comparing chemotherapy, radiation therapy, and surgery versus chemotherapy and radiation therapy to define the role of surgery in improving local control beyond that obtained with radiation therapy alone. Although concurrent therapy may improve survival, this approach is associated with greater toxicity. The role of protective agents such as amifostine and WR21–27 (ethyol) in protecting patients from the side effects of radiation therapy and chemotherapy and the use of 3-dimensional conformal radiation therapy to reduce radiation-induced damage to the esophagus and lungs are currently being investigated.

Novel Modalities. Novel agents for treatment of metastatic NSCLC are being intensively evaluated. Targeted receptor therapy, novel combination chemotherapy, and gene therapy with or without chemotherapy and radiation therapy are all potential therapeutic modalities.

Small Cell Lung Cancer

SCLCs have a tendency to metastasize aggressively, and the majority of SCLCs are extensive-stage at presentation. For these reasons, SCLCs are typically not treated with surgery. Chemotherapy is the preferred method

KEY PRACTICE POINTS

- Chest radiography, sputum cytology, and fiber-optic bronchoscopy have shown only limited effectiveness in lung cancer screening.
- Most patients with advanced lung cancer have symptoms at the time of diagnosis; common symptoms include cough, dyspnea, chest pain, and hemoptysis.
- In patients with lung cancer, a thorough pretreatment evaluation, including clinical staging based on chest radiography, CT of the chest and upper abdomen, and other examinations plus evaluation of the patient's performance status, is essential for effective treatment planning.
- SCLC is more aggressive than NSCLC and is often extensive-stage at diagnosis.
- Clinical trials offer access to the best available treatment ideas, and enrollment of eligible patients in such trials is encouraged.
- In patients with localized NSCLC, lobectomy with intrathoracic mediastinal lymph node dissection should be performed.
- In patients with NSCLC with histologically positive mediastinal lymph nodes or unresectable local disease, various combinations of surgery, chemotherapy, and radiation therapy are recommended.
- Patients with SCLC are usually treated with combination chemotherapy.

of treatment. Radiation therapy may be used for palliation of symptoms or treatment of metastasis.

In rare situations in which SCLC is suspected but not confirmed after fine-needle aspiration and radiographic staging, surgical techniques (e.g., bronchoscopy) may be helpful for staging or diagnosis (Lassen and Hansen, 1999). In patients who present with a solitary pulmonary nodule characterized as early stage ($\leq$ 3 cm), pulmonary resection (e.g., wedge resection or lobectomy and mediastinal lymph node dissection) may be viewed as "treatment" after the fact in those cases in which SCLC is confirmed. Postoperative chemotherapy may be considered in these cases.

Suggested Readings

American Cancer Society. *Cancer Facts and Figures—2002.* Atlanta, Ga: American Cancer Society; 2002;3.

Dillman RO, Herndon J, Seagren SL, et al. Improved survival in stage III non-small-cell lung cancer: seven-year follow-up of Cancer and Leukemia Group B (CALGB) 8433 trial. *J Natl Cancer Inst* 1996;88:1210–1215.

Dillman RO, Seagren SL, Propert KJ, et al. A randomized trial of induction chemotherapy plus high-dose radiation versus radiation alone in stage III non-small-cell lung cancer. *N Engl J Med* 1990;323:940–945.

Fong KM, Sekido Y, Minna JD. Molecular pathogenesis of lung cancer. *J Thorac Cardiovasc Surg* 1999;118:1136–1152.

Ginsberg RJ, Rubinstein LV. Randomized trial of lobectomy versus limited resection for T1 N0 non-small cell lung cancer. Lung Cancer Study Group. *Ann Thorac Surg* 1995;60:615–622.

Henschke CI, McCauley DI, Yankelevitz DF, et al. Early Lung Cancer Action Project: overall design and findings from baseline screening. *Lancet* 1999;354 (9173):99–105.

Komaki R. Preoperative and postoperative irradiation for cancer of the lung. *J Belge Radiol* 1985;68:195–198.

Komaki R, Cox JD, Hartz AJ, et al. Characteristics of long-term survivors after treatment for inoperable carcinoma of the lung. *Am J Clin Oncol* 1985; 8:362–370.

Komaki R, Milas L, Ro JY, et al. Prognostic biomarker study in pathologically staged N1 non-small cell lung cancer. *Int J Radiat Oncol Biol Phys* 1998;40:787–796.

Komaki R, Mountain CF, Holbert JM, et al. Superior sulcus tumors: treatment selection and results for 85 patients without metastasis (M0) at presentation. *Int J Radiat Oncol Biol Phys* 1990;19:31–36.

Lassen U, Hansen HH. Surgery in limited stage small cell lung cancer. *Cancer Treat Rev* 1999;25:67–72.

Le Chevalier T, Arriagada R, Quoix E, et al. Radiotherapy alone versus combined chemotherapy and radiotherapy in nonresectable non-small-cell lung cancer: first analysis of a randomized trial in 353 patients. *J Natl Cancer Inst* 1991;83:417–423.

Mountain CF. Revisions in the International System for Staging Lung Cancer. *Chest* 1997;111:1710–1717.

Mountain CF, Dresler CM. Regional lymph node classification for lung cancer staging. *Chest* 1997;111:1718–1723.

Naruke T, Goya T, Tsuchiya R, et al. Prognosis and survival in resected lung carcinoma based on the new international staging system. *J Thorac Cardiovasc Surg* 1988;96:440–447.

Naruke T, Tsuchiya R, Kondo H, et al. Prognosis and survival after resection for bronchogenic carcinoma based on the 1997 TNM-staging classification: the Japanese experience. *Ann Thorac Surg* 2001;71:1759–1764.

Nesbitt JC, Putnam JB Jr, Walsh GL, et al. Survival in early-stage non-small cell lung cancer. *Ann Thorac Surg* 1995;60:466–472.

Pass HI, Pogrebniak HW, Steinberg SM, et al. Randomized trial of neoadjuvant therapy for lung cancer: interim analysis. *Ann Thorac Surg* 1992;53:992–998.

Pisters KM, Ginsberg RJ, Giroux DJ, et al. Induction chemotherapy before surgery for early-stage lung cancer: a novel approach. Bimodality Lung Oncology Team. *J Thorac Cardiovasc Surg* 2000;119:429–439.

Putnam JB Jr, Light RW, Rodriguez RM, et al. A randomized comparison of indwelling pleural catheter and doxycycline pleurodesis in the management of malignant pleural effusions. *Cancer* 1999;86:1992–1999.

Rosell R, Gomez-Codina J, Camps C, et al. A randomized trial comparing preoperative chemotherapy plus surgery with surgery alone in patients with non-small-cell lung cancer. *N Engl J Med* 1994;330:153–158.

Roth JA, Atkinson EN, Fossella F, et al. Long-term follow-up of patients enrolled in a randomized trial comparing perioperative chemotherapy and surgery with surgery alone in resectable stage IIIA non-small-cell lung cancer. *Lung Cancer* 1998;21:1–6.

Roth JA, Fossella F, Komaki R, et al. A randomized trial comparing perioperative chemotherapy and surgery with surgery alone in resectable stage IIIA non-small-cell lung cancer. *J Natl Cancer Inst* 1994;86:673–680.

Roth JA, Nguyen D, Lawrence DD, et al. Retrovirus-mediated wild-type p53 gene transfer to tumors of patients with lung cancer. *Nat Med* 1996;2:985–991.

Sause WT, Scott C, Taylor S, et al. Radiation Therapy Oncology Group (RTOG) 88–08 and Eastern Cooperative Oncology Group (ECOG) 4588: preliminary results of a phase III trial in regionally advanced, unresectable non-small-cell lung cancer. *J Natl Cancer Inst* 1995;87:198–205.

Swisher SG, Roth JA, Nemunaitis J, et al. Adenovirus-mediated p53 gene transfer in advanced non-small-cell lung cancer. *J Natl Cancer Inst* 1999;91:763–771.

Weisenburger TH. Effects of postoperative mediastinal radiation on completely resected stage II and III epidermoid cancer of the lung. LCSG 773. *Chest* 1994;106(6 suppl):297S–301S.

2   CLINICAL EXAMINATION OF PATIENTS WITH SUSPECTED LUNG CANCER

Frank V. Fossella

CHAPTER OVERVIEW

In patients with suspected lung cancer, the goals of the clinical examination are to confirm the histologic diagnosis, establish the extent of disease for the purpose of treatment planning, and identify any associated symptoms or complications of the disease that might warrant immediate attention. The basic components of the clinical examination are a history and physical examination, routine blood work, chest radiography, computed tomography of the chest, additional imaging studies as needed, diagnostic biopsy, and, in patients with operable disease, preoperative testing to ensure a reasonably low risk of postsurgical complications. The most common sites of lung cancer metastases are the adrenal glands, liver, central nervous system, and bone. Blood work in patients with lung cancer can suggest possible sites of metastastic disease, suggest underlying metabolic disorders related to the cancer, and reveal comorbid conditions (e.g., diabetes mellitus) that need to be addressed in planning further therapy. Chest radiography can reveal the size and location of the primary tumor, the presence of adenopathy or pleural effusion, and possible associated pneumonia. Computed tomography of the chest is more precise than chest radiography in the detection of enlarged hilar and mediastinal lymph nodes, pleural and pericardial effusion, invasion into the chest wall and mediastinal structures, lymphangitic carcinomatosis, and smaller lung parenchymal metastases. Methods available for obtaining tissue for histologic diagnosis include sputum cytology, fine-needle aspiration, flexible fiber-optic bronchoscopy, and transthoracic needle aspiration biopsy.

INTRODUCTION

The goals of the clinical examination of patients with suspected lung cancer are to confirm the histologic diagnosis, establish the extent of disease for the purpose of treatment planning, and identify any associated symptoms or complications of the disease that might warrant immediate attention. The basic components of the clinical examination include the history and physical examination, routine blood work, chest radiography, computed tomography (CT) of the chest, other radiographic imaging as dictated by the findings on these preliminary studies and the patient's symptoms, appropriate diagnostic biopsy, and preoperative testing of patients whose disease is deemed potentially operable.

HISTORY AND PHYSICAL EXAMINATION

The history and physical examination is an important initial step in evaluating patients with suspected lung cancer as it usually will uncover important information regarding a patient's stage of disease and prognosis and associated medical complications of the underlying cancer. The symptoms and signs of lung cancer may be caused by local effects of the primary tumor or regional lymph node metastases; distant metastases; or paraneoplastic disorders.

Symptoms and Signs Due to Local Effects

Symptoms and signs of disease due to local effects of the primary tumor or regional lymph node metastases include cough, hemoptysis, dyspnea, fever, chest pain, hoarseness, and swelling and venous distension of the face, neck, and chest wall. Cough may result from endobronchial tumor, pneumonia, or pleural effusion. Hemoptysis is commonly seen in patients with endobronchial lesions and may also result from associated complications of lung cancer, such as pulmonary embolus or pneumonia. Dyspnea may be due to a variety of factors, including endobronchial disease, atelectasis, postobstructive pneumonia, pleural effusion, pulmonary embolus, and lymphangitic spread. Dyspnea may also be due to arrhythmia or tamponade resulting from pericardial effusion.

Fever may result from pneumonia, or it may occur in the absence of frank infection in patients with postobstructive atelectasis. Chest pain commonly occurs in patients whose disease involves the pleura or chest wall. Hoarseness may result from vocal cord paralysis in patients with mediastinal disease affecting the recurrent laryngeal nerve; occasionally, patients with massive mediastinal disease may develop bilateral vocal cord paralysis, resulting in stridor due to upper airway obstruction. Patients with large right-sided central tumors may develop obstruction of the superior vena cava, resulting in a typical syndrome of swelling and venous distension of the face, neck, and chest wall, sometimes associated with shortness of breath, headache, and, in extreme cases, altered mental status.

Symptoms and Signs Due to Distant Metastases

Distant metastatic disease may also cause symptoms and findings on physical examination that are pertinent to treatment planning and prognosis. The most common sites of metastasis of lung cancer are the adrenal glands, liver, central nervous system (CNS), and bone.

Adrenal metastases are quite common in patients with non–small cell lung cancer (NSCLC) but rather uncommon in patients with small cell lung cancer (SCLC). Adrenal metastases are rarely symptomatic, are not typically associated with any findings on physical examination, and are usually only discovered on routine radiographic studies (chest radiography and CT of the chest). Occasionally, however, massive adrenal metastases can cause flank pain. In addition, patients with advanced bilateral adrenal metastases may develop symptoms of adrenal insufficiency.

Liver metastases occur frequently in patients with lung cancer, more commonly with SCLC than with NSCLC. The symptoms of hepatic metastases may include jaundice and right upper quadrant pain associated with the findings of hepatomegaly and liver tenderness on examination. However, these findings usually occur only in patients with very advanced liver disease. More commonly, hepatic metastases present with less specific symptoms, such as anorexia, malaise, and weight loss.

Metastases to the CNS are commonly seen in both SCLC and NSCLC (particularly adenocarcinoma). While CNS metastases are often asymptomatic and discovered only incidentally during radiographic evaluation, there are certainly many symptoms and physical findings related to CNS involvement that the clinician should be attuned to when doing the baseline history and physical examination. Symptoms of brain metastases may include headache, altered mental status, seizure, nausea and vomiting, focal motor or sensory deficits, cranial nerve palsies, and cerebellar symptoms, such as ataxia.

Another form of CNS metastasis from lung cancer is involvement of the spinal cord. This may occur in the form of spinal cord compression (usually due to direct extension of vertebral body metastases into the spinal canal), intramedullary metastases (relatively uncommon), or leptomeningeal seeding of the spinal canal. Spinal cord compression and intramedullary metastases are rarely asymptomatic and should be identified rapidly as they constitute neurological emergencies necessitating immediate treatment. About 90% of patients complain of back pain—either localized or radicular—as their first symptom. At diagnosis, about 75% of patients will note muscle weakness, and 50% will have associated sensory loss below the level of the metastasis. Bowel or bladder incontinence is another less common symptom of cord compression. On physical examination, patients with spinal cord compression typically have back tenderness at the site of metastasis. Other associated findings on physical examination may include sensory loss or paresis below the level of the metastasis, decrease in anal sphincter tone, muscle spasticity, and abnormal deep tendon reflexes.

Leptomeningeal metastases are most commonly seen with adenocarcinoma of the lung. Symptoms and physical findings associated with this relatively uncommon complication may include headache, seizure, altered mental status, cranial nerve deficits (typically involving multiple nerves bilaterally), radicular pain, and incontinence.

Skeletal metastases occur in about one third of patients with lung cancer. Patients with bone metastases often complain of pain and are found to have bone tenderness on physical examination. Many patients, however, may be asymptomatic, with this finding discovered incidentally on a routine bone scan or because of elevated alkaline phosphatase levels or hypercalcemia. Bone marrow involvement, which may occur with SCLC but is uncommon with NSCLC, may result in nonspecific symptoms of fatigue.

Symptoms and Signs Due to Paraneoplastic Disorders

In addition to symptoms related to local disease or metastatic disease, lung cancer may cause symptoms mediated by ectopic production of various peptides, cytokines, and other biologically active substances. These paraneoplastic symptoms include nonspecific constitutional complaints of fatigue, anorexia, weight loss, cachexia, fever, and malaise. Eliciting such nonspecific constitutional symptoms in the history is important because their existence may direct the remainder of the workup and, just as important, may offer useful prognostic information and help the physician determine which palliative care measures would be most appropriate.

Paraneoplastic symptoms may also be the result of discrete syndromes associated with bronchogenic carcinoma. For example, SCLC may cause the syndrome of inappropriate production of antidiuretic hormone (SIADH) and ectopic adrenocorticotropic hormone production, and squamous carcinoma of the lung may result in hypercalcemia due to production of an ectopic parathyroid hormone–like substance. (Hypercalcemia may also be seen with any histologic subtype of lung cancer in the presence of bone metastases.) It is important to elicit symptoms referable to these metabolic aberrations (e.g., altered mental status, constipation, or weakness) that might indicate the presence of one of these underlying syndromes.

Laboratory Studies

The clinical evaluation of patients with suspected lung cancer generally includes routine laboratory work, consisting of a complete blood count (including a differential blood count and a platelet count) and a full set of serum chemistry studies. These laboratory tests may be useful indicators of possible sites of metastatic disease (e.g., elevated results on liver function tests or an elevated alkaline phosphatase level might direct the clinician to look for liver or bone metastases, respectively). The laboratory tests may also uncover important underlying metabolic aberrations due to paraneoplastic syndromes (e.g., hyponatremia due to SIADH, hypokalemia and hyperglycemia due to ectopic adrenocorticotropic hormone production, or hypercalcemia). They may provide important prognostic information; for example, a low albumin level and an elevated serum lactate dehydrogenase level both portend a worse prognosis in lung cancer patients. Finally, laboratory tests may reveal other significant comorbid conditions that need to be addressed in planning further therapy (e.g., diabetes mellitus, anemia, renal insufficiency, or leukocytosis due to concurrent infection).

The use of serum marker assays, such as assays for carcinoembryonic antigen, is not routine in the evaluation of lung cancer patients.

Radiographic Imaging

Chest Radiography

Routine posteroanterior and lateral chest radiography is usually the first test to suggest an underlying bronchogenic carcinoma. Chest radiography is typically done by the patient's primary physician because of symptoms such as dyspnea, hemoptysis, suspected pneumonia, or chest pain. The findings on chest radiography that might help guide further evaluation and treatment include the size and location of the primary tumor, the presence of adenopathy or pleural effusion, and possible associated pneumonia. However, because chest radiography is relatively imprecise with regard to detecting enlarged mediastinal lymph nodes and small parenchymal metastases, CT of the chest invariably follows.

Computed Tomography of the Chest

CT of the chest is much more precise than chest radiography in detecting enlarged hilar and mediastinal lymph nodes, pleural and pericardial effusion, invasion into the chest wall and mediastinal structures, lymphangitic carcinomatosis, and smaller lung parenchymal metastases. All of these findings would have an important bearing on subsequent diagnostic or therapeutic measures and also on the patient's prognosis.

When chest CT is used to evaluate mediastinal node metastases, one must recognize the limitations of this imaging modality. Generally, mediastinal lymph nodes larger than 1 cm are considered abnormal. However, the incidence of false-positive findings on chest CT (i.e., detection of an enlarged node that is not malignant) is about 30%. One reason for this relatively high incidence of false-positives is the frequent occurrence of benign causes of mediastinal lymphadenopathy in the lung cancer patient. These include, for example, reactive hyperplasia from postobstructive pneumonia, granulomatous inflammation, and anthracosis. The rate of false-negative findings on chest CT (i.e., failure of CT to show any enlargement of mediastinal nodes followed by subsequent documentation of nodal metastasis at mediastinoscopy or thoracotomy) is about 10%.

Computed Tomography of the Abdomen

A dedicated CT scan of the abdomen is generally not required in the routine evaluation of lung cancer patients because the chest CT typically includes enough of the upper abdomen to permit evaluation for metastasis to the liver and adrenals. However, if the clinician's index of suspicion of liver metastasis is high (e.g., if the chest CT suggests hepatic involvement or if the patient has unexplained elevation of the results of liver function tests), then a dedicated CT scan of the abdomen with a contrast agent is warranted to conclusively rule out liver metastases if this finding would affect the patient's treatment (e.g., if the patient otherwise has potentially operable NSCLC or if the patient otherwise has limited-stage SCLC).

Because the incidence of benign adrenal adenoma in the general population is significant, ranging from 2% to 10%, patients in whom adrenal enlargement of uncertain etiology noted on a CT scan of the chest or abdomen is the sole indication of possible metastasis should have further evaluation to exclude a benign tumor. CT-guided adrenal biopsy would provide a conclusive diagnosis in this setting. Magnetic resonance (MR) imaging of the abdomen has also proven useful in this setting, offering a sensitivity of 96% and a specificity of 100%.

Additional Radiographic Studies

In the "routine" staging of lung cancer, additional radiographic studies, including CT and MR imaging of the brain and bone scans, should be dictated by the circumstances of the case. Certainly, in patients experiencing neurological symptoms for which palliative radiation therapy or resection would be considered, CT or MR imaging of the brain is indicated. Similarly, patients experiencing bone pain for which palliative radiation therapy would be offered should have a bone scan with or without plain films.

However, in the absence of neurological symptoms and bone pain, routine imaging of the brain and bones is not necessary unless the finding of occult metastases in these sites would significantly alter treatment. For example, in patients who otherwise have limited-stage SCLC and patients who have stage III NSCLC, we typically do brain and bone scans even in the absence of symptoms because finding occult brain or bone metastases in these patients would drastically alter therapy—from multimodality treatment with "curative" intent to, generally, chemotherapy only. In contrast, in patients who already have documented extensive-stage SCLC or stage IV NSCLC, these scans need not be done as the discovery of additional occult metastases will generally not alter treatment. In the staging of patients with potentially operable stage I or II NSCLC, brain and bone scans are generally not recommended in the absence of other findings that would indicate metastasis to these sites unless the clinician's index of suspicion remains high. For example, brain and bone scans might be considered in an asymptomatic patient with stage I or II poorly differentiated adenocarcinoma but would probably not be necessary in a patient with operable bronchioloalveolar carcinoma, a tumor with a much lower likelihood of occult metastasis.

In addition to the roles of MR imaging in screening for brain metastasis and evaluation of suspicious adrenal enlargement, MR imaging also has a role in the preoperative evaluation of patients with superior sulcus tumors and patients with other potentially operable T4 lesions. The presence of chest wall or vertebral body invasion is often difficult to distinguish with chest CT alone. MR imaging of the chest is generally superior in this regard and is helpful to the thoracic surgeon in planning resection.

Positron emission tomography (PET) is able to characterize lung lesions reliably in most cases, failing to detect only very small lesions and tumors of a very indolent nature. PET may therefore play a role in the evaluation of patients with solitary pulmonary nodules. PET scanning is also a useful tool in documenting the presence of mediastinal lymph node metastases, with reported sensitivity and specificity of more than 90%. In this regard, PET is more accurate than CT scanning, although PET images lack the anatomic precision seen with CT scans. PET scans also have potential utility in detecting otherwise undetected widespread metastases in patients for whom curative resection is being considered. At this time, our recommendations regarding the optimal use of PET scans in the staging of lung cancer are still evolving. The controversy surrounding PET is discussed in more detail in chapter 3.

Pulmonary Function Tests

All patients who are being considered for surgical treatment of their lung cancer should undergo complete pulmonary function testing, including analysis of the diffusing capacity of the lung for carbon monoxide and arterial blood gas analysis, to identify patients at increased risk of postoperative pulmonary complications of lung resection. Generally, patients with a forced expiratory volume in 1 second (FEV_1) of greater than 2 L and a maximum voluntary ventilation of greater than 55% of predicted can tolerate a pneumonectomy. A lobectomy is considered feasible in patients with FEV_1 of more than 1 L and a maximum voluntary ventilation of at least 40% of predicted. If results on routine pulmonary function tests are borderline, then a xenon ventilation perfusion scan and oxygen consumption studies may be done to further evaluate a patient's suitability to undergo potentially curative resection of lung cancer.

The preoperative evaluation of patients with lung cancer is covered in more detail in chapters 6 and 7.

Histologic Confirmation
of Diagnosis

Ultimately, of course, the final diagnosis of lung cancer rests upon the histologic confirmation of malignancy. The diagnosis of malignancy in patients with suspected lung cancer should be obtained with the least invasive procedure needed to obtain tissue.

Sputum Cytology

Sputum cytology is a simple, noninvasive way to confirm cancer, but this approach is often nondiagnostic and is highly dependent on factors such as the location and size of the tumor with respect to the major airways and the patient's ability to produce adequate sputum specimens. Thus, the yield with sputum cytology is less than 20% for patients with small peripheral lesions. The usefulness of sputum cytology is further limited by the necessity of a thorough head and neck examination to rule out head and neck primary lesions in patients in whom findings on sputum cytology are positive for squamous cancer.

Fine-Needle Aspiration

In patients with easily accessible superficial lymph nodes or dermal metastases, fine-needle aspiration will generally yield a positive diagnosis with little risk or discomfort to the patient. In patients with suspected pleural effusion, diagnostic thoracentesis is a low-risk procedure with a relatively high yield.

KEY PRACTICE POINTS

- In patients with suspected lung cancer, the clinical examination should include a history and physical examination, routine blood work, chest radiography, CT of the chest, other radiographic imaging as dictated by the findings on these preliminary studies and the patient's symptoms, appropriate diagnostic biopsy, and preoperative testing of patients whose disease is deemed potentially operable.

- Eliciting nonspecific constitutional symptoms (e.g., fatigue and weight loss) in the history is important because their existence may direct the remainder of the workup, offer useful prognostic information, and help the physician determine which palliative care measures would be most appropriate.

- CT of the chest is more precise than chest radiography in the detection of enlarged hilar and mediastinal lymph nodes, pleural and pericardial effusion, invasion into the chest wall and mediastinal structures, lymphangitic carcinomatosis, and smaller lung parenchymal metastases.

- When chest CT is used to determine whether mediastinal lymph node metastases are present, the rate of false-positive findings is 30%, and the rate of false-negative findings is 10%.

- CT of the abdomen with a contrast agent is warranted if the index of suspicion of liver metastasis is high and the finding of liver metastases would affect the patient's treatment.

- Owing to the 2% to 10% incidence of benign adrenal adenoma in the general population, patients in whom the sole indication of possible metastases is adrenal enlargement of uncertain etiology noted on a CT scan of the chest or abdomen should have further evaluation to exclude a benign tumor.

- MR imaging of the chest is generally superior to chest CT in determining the presence of chest wall or vertebral body invasion.

- The diagnosis of malignancy in patients with suspected lung cancer should be obtained with the least invasive procedure needed to obtain tissue.

Flexible Fiber-Optic Bronchoscopy

Flexible fiber-optic bronchoscopy is a useful tool for diagnosing suspected lung cancer, although this method is somewhat dependent on the size, location, and accessibility of the primary tumor. Endobronchial lesions that can be directly visualized are sampled with the use of biopsy forceps, washings, and brushings; the yield of bronchoscopy for such lesions is greater than 80%. More peripheral lesions may be sampled with transbronchial biopsy, washings, and brushings, with the diagnostic yield highly dependent on the size of the lesion. For example, the yield is about 25% for lesions smaller than 2 cm but may be as high as 80% for lesions larger than 4 cm. Submucosal tumors (e.g., small cell carcinoma) may be sampled with transbronchial biopsy as well.

The use of flexible fiber-optic bronchoscopy to document the histologic subtype has the added advantage of providing important staging information in patients whose disease is potentially operable. For example, bronchoscopy will document the proximity of the primary lesion to the carina and may also occasionally reveal a synchronous lesion within the airways, both important factors for the surgeon to consider in deciding whether surgery is feasible. In addition, in selected patients, mediastinal lymph nodes may also be sampled at bronchoscopy with transbronchial needle aspiration.

Transthoracic Needle Aspiration Biopsy

Peripheral lesions that are inaccessible on flexible fiber-optic bronchoscopy and mediastinal lymph nodes may be biopsied with transthoracic needle aspiration (TTNA) under CT or fluoroscopic guidance. TTNA biopsy is a relatively safe procedure; a severe pneumothorax (i.e., one requiring chest tube placement) occurs in about 10% to 15% of procedures, and patients with severe bullous disease are at higher risk. The yield of TTNA biopsy is more than 90%, but the false-negative rate may be as high as 20% to 30%. Therefore, if findings on TTNA biopsy are negative in a patient in whom suspicion of cancer remains high, additional diagnostic measures should be considered. These might include repeat TTNA biopsy, fine-needle aspiration of another site of suspected disease (e.g., a liver mass), open lung biopsy, or, in selected patients with small peripheral nodules, video-assisted thoracoscopic surgery.

Suggested Readings

American Thoracic Society and European Respiratory Society. Pretreatment evaluation of non-small-cell lung cancer. *Am J Respir Crit Care Med* 1997;156:320–332.

Arcasoy SM, Jett JR. Superior pulmonary sulcus tumors and Pancoast's syndrome. *N Engl J Med* 1997;337:1370–1376.

Broderick LS, Tarver RD, Conces DJ Jr. Imaging of lung cancer: old and new. *Semin Oncol* 1997;24:411–418.

Midthun DE, Jett JR. Early detection of lung cancer: today's approach. *J Respir Dis* 1998;19:56–69.

Patel AM, Peters SG. Clinical manifestations of lung cancer. *Mayo Clin Proc* 1993;68:273–277.

3   THORACIC IMAGING TECHNIQUES FOR NON–SMALL CELL AND SMALL CELL LUNG CANCER

Reginald F. Munden and Jeremy J. Erasmus

CHAPTER OVERVIEW

Lung cancer is the most common malignancy and the leading cause of cancer-related deaths in the United States. Thoracic imaging has an important role in the evaluation of lung cancer: it is used in the detection, diagnosis, and staging of the disease and in assessing response to therapy and monitoring for recurrence after treatment.

Screening for lung cancer—efforts to detect lung cancer before symptoms develop—has been advocated as a means for improving outcomes in patients with this disease. However, while lung cancer screening trials have shown a reduction in the stage at diagnosis and improvement in long-term survival rates, these trials have not shown an effect of screening on disease-specific mortality. Thus screening for lung cancer remains controversial. Large randomized controlled studies are currently being established to evaluate the impact of screening on mortality in patients with lung cancer. Until these trials are completed, routine screening for lung cancer is not recommended.

Twenty to 30% of patients with lung cancer present with a solitary lung opacity on thoracic imaging. Assessment of morphologic features and growth rate can be useful in differentiating malignant from benign solitary lesions. However, often the nature of a solitary lung opacity cannot be determined with conventional anatomic imaging (radiographs and/or routine nonenhanced and contrast-enhanced computed tomography [CT] and magnetic resonance [MR] images). In such cases, the opacity can be further evaluated with dynamic contrast-enhanced CT or with positron emission tomography (PET) using a radioactive glucose analog, fluorodeoxyglucose F 18 (FDG), the metabolism of which is typically increased in malignant cells compared to benign cells. Lesions with indeterminate etiology after comprehensive radiologic assessment are observed, biopsied, or resected.

Once a diagnosis of non–small cell lung cancer (NSCLC) has been established, the disease is staged according to the International System for Staging Lung Cancer. This system describes the extent of NSCLC in terms of the primary tumor (T descriptor), lymph nodes (N descriptor), and metastases (M descriptor). The T descriptor defines the size, location, and extent of the primary tumor. Because the extent of the primary tumor determines whether the disease will be treated with surgical resection or with palliative radiation therapy or chemotherapy, CT is usually used to assess the degree of pleural, chest wall, and mediastinal invasion. MR imaging has superior soft-tissue contrast resolution and multiplanar capability and is thus particularly useful in the evaluation of superior sulcus tumors.

The presence of nodal metastases and their location are of major importance in determining the most appropriate management. However, the accuracy of CT and MR imaging in the detection of mediastinal nodal metastases (N2 and N3 disease) is not optimal. FDG-PET is a more accurate modality for assessing nodal metabolism (disease) and is particularly useful in detecting metastases in normal-sized nodes. Although the role of imaging in the evaluation of distant metastasis is not clearly defined, imaging can be used to evaluate patients at initial presentation for the presence of metastases to the adrenal glands, kidneys, liver, brain, bones, and lymph nodes.

Imaging also has an important role in the assessment of patients after surgical resection and in the determination of response to therapy after the initiation of chemotherapy or radiation therapy.

Introduction

Lung cancer, an uncommon disease before 1900, became a major health problem in the 20th century. In the United States, lung cancer is the most common malignancy and the leading cause of cancer-related deaths in both men and women. This chapter will review the current applications of thoracic imaging techniques in lung cancer patients at M. D. Anderson Cancer Center, including screening for lung cancer, evaluation of focal pulmonary abnormalities, staging of lung cancer, assessment of response to treatment, and monitoring for tumor recurrence after treatment.

Screening

Screening for lung cancer—efforts to detect lung cancer before symptoms develop—has been advocated as a means for improving the prognosis of patients with this disease. The concept is supported by 2 main observations: most patients with lung cancer have advanced disease at the time of clinical presentation, and the diagnosis of lung cancer at an early stage is usually associated with improved prognosis. However, the role of imaging in screening is not clearly defined.

Currently, the American Cancer Society does not recommend screening but rather advocates primary prevention. This recommendation is based on the results of 4 large randomized trials undertaken in the 1970s that evaluated the utility of chest radiography and sputum cytology in lung cancer screening (Kubik et al, 1990; Strauss, 1997). These trials showed that screening improved long-term survival rates but did not reduce disease-specific mortality, which is considered the best indicator of screening effectiveness because mortality is not affected by lead-time bias, length-time bias, or overdiagnosis bias.

Recently, there has been renewed interest in evaluating lung cancer screening, in part because of a belief that the older trials were flawed in design and methodology and also because of advances in radiologic imaging that have occurred in the interim (Kaneko et al, 1996; Strauss, 1997; Henschke et al, 1999). In particular, the advent of computed tomography (CT) has allowed detection of small lung cancers not apparent on conventional chest radiographs. Two recent small studies have confirmed that there is increased detection of small lung cancers when CT is used to screen patients considered to be at high risk for developing lung cancer (Kaneko et al, 1996; Henschke et al, 1999). In one of these studies, the Early Lung Cancer Action Project, low-dose helical CT was used to screen for lung cancer in 1,000 patients (Henschke et al, 1999). Lung cancer was detected in 2.7% of these patients with CT but in only 0.7% with chest radiography. Furthermore, 23 (85%) of the 27 lung cancers detected with CT were stage I, compared to only 4 (67%) of the 7 lung cancers detected with chest radiography. However, neither of these 2 small studies has shown an effect of screening on disease-specific mortality. Routine screening for lung cancer should not be instituted until screening has been demonstrated to produce a reduction in mortality. We believe that a large, randomized controlled study is needed to address this issue. In this regard, M.D. Anderson will participate in the American College of Radiology Imaging Network Trial, a multi-institutional randomized controlled study that is designed to evaluate screening for lung cancer.

DIAGNOSIS

Most patients with lung cancer have advanced disease at presentation, and thus diagnosis is usually not difficult. However, 20% to 30% of patients present with a solitary lung opacity, and it is often challenging, both clinically and radiologically, to differentiate these malignancies from benign abnormalities. A number of management strategies are available to M.D. Anderson radiologists for determining whether a focal lung opacity revealed by chest radiography or CT represents lung cancer.

Initially, radiographs or CT scans are reviewed to determine the calcification pattern and the growth rate. If the opacity is diffusely calcified or if comparison studies show that the size of the opacity has been stable for more than 2 years, the abnormality is most likely benign, and usually no further evaluation is done. However, pre-existing radiographs or CT scans are often not available for review, and it can be difficult to determine whether a small opacity is calcified or stable in size on radiographs. Thus, many focal lung opacities require further radiologic evaluation. This additional evaluation is described in the following paragraphs.

Evaluation of Morphology and Growth

Evaluation of the morphologic features of a lung opacity, including size, margins, contour, and presence of calcification and/or fat, can be useful in determining whether an opacity is benign or malignant.

The likelihood of malignancy increases with increasing opacity size, but small size alone is not sufficient to exclude malignancy. The widespread use of CT and the recent introduction of CT to screen patients for lung cancer have resulted in the frequent detection of small opacities (1–5 mm) not visible on chest radiographs. While the majority of these opacities are most likely benign, recent studies of resected small nodules have shown that a considerable number are either primary or secondary pulmonary malignancies (Munden et al, 1997; Ginsberg et al, 1999). Consequently, the use of small size to exclude malignancy is unreliable and is not advocated.

Typically, benign opacities have well-defined margins and a smooth contour while malignant opacities have poorly defined or spiculated margins and a lobular or irregular contour. There is, however, considerable overlap in the typical appearances.

Two aspects of the internal morphology of an opacity—fat (x-ray attenuation -40 to -120 Hounsfield units [HU]) and calcification—are reliable in distinguishing malignant from benign opacities. Fat within a nodule is a characteristic finding of hamartomas and obviates further evaluation. Calcification of an opacity can be useful in determining benignity, although the majority of benign opacities are not calcified. Calcification that has a diffuse solid, central punctate, laminated, or "popcorn-like" appearance is diagnostic of a benign opacity except in patients with primary extrathoracic osteoid-forming tumors, such as osteosarcomas. Metastases in these patients can occasionally manifest as nodules with benign-appearing calcification. Calcification can be detected histologically in up to 14% of lung cancers and is occasionally visible on CT (Mahoney et al, 1990). This calcification is typically amorphous and correlates with a high probability of malignancy.

CT is considerably more sensitive than radiographic evaluation in the detection of calcification. In most small, calcified opacities, calcification is detected visually when thinly collimated slices (1–3 mm) are obtained through the lesion. With the partial volume averaging that occurs when more thickly collimated slices (7–10 mm) are obtained, calcification within a small opacity may not be visible. Measurement of CT attenuation values (CT densitometry) can be used to infer the presence of calcium within an opacity. The use of this technique is, however, inappropriate if the opacity is spiculated or is greater than 3 cm in diameter (Swensen et al, 1991). A CT attenuation value of 200 HU is usually used to distinguish between calcified and noncalcified opacities. If the density of the opacity is in the benign range (> 200 HU), serial radiologic studies (radiographs or CT scans) are obtained at 3, 6, 12, 18, and 24 months to confirm the absence of growth. The sensitivity and specificity of this technique in the detection of benign disease are, however, not optimal, and consequently CT densitometry is not routinely used at M. D. Anderson.

Nodule growth is evaluated by reviewing pre-existing chest radiographs or CT scans. The majority of malignant opacities double in volume within 30 to 400 days. Nodular opacities that double in volume more rapidly or more slowly are usually infectious or inflammatory. Absence of growth over a 2-year period is generally a reliable indicator of benignity. Recently, however, the appropriateness of this standard—particularly in the setting of small nodules—has been questioned (Yankelevitz and Henschke, 1997). For growth to be detectable on successive radiographs, an opacity must increase in diameter by 3 to 5 mm. In the case of a small opacity, doubling in volume may produce a change in diameter of less than 3 to 5 mm. For example, the diameter of an 8-mm opacity will increase by only 2 mm with a doubling in volume, and consequently, the opacity will appear stable on chest radiographs. Although this change in diameter could theoretically be detected with CT, slight differences between one CT study and the next in the level at which an image is obtained are common and make the confident detection of a small change in size difficult. In most cases, however, the use of CT does allow an accurate assessment of growth, and recently it has been reported that growth can be detected in lung cancers as small as 5 mm when CT is repeated within 30 days (Yankelevitz et al, 1999). Furthermore, the measurement of serial volumes (using CT), which increase proportionally faster than diameter, has been suggested to be an accurate and potentially useful method for assessing growth rate in small opacities (Yankelevitz et al, 2000). Presently, however, there is no consensus as to which parameters should be measured to determine growth or what growth-free interval is required to ascertain that a small nodule is benign.

Evaluation of Nodule Enhancement and Metabolism

Perfusion and metabolism differ qualitatively and quantitatively between malignant and benign lesions, and thus dynamic contrast-enhanced CT can be used to differentiate between benign and malignant opacities. This technique has recently been shown in a multi-institutional prospective trial to be useful in the evaluation of opacities with indeterminate etiology after standard radiologic evaluation (Swensen et al, 2000). High-resolution CT images of the lesion with 3-mm collimation are obtained before and after intravenous administration of contrast material (2 mL/sec; 300 mg iodine/mm; 420 mg iodine/kg). After administration of contrast, serial 5-second spiral acquisitions are performed at 1, 2, 3, and 4 minutes. Enhancement is determined by subtracting the precontrast nodule density from the maximal nodule density after contrast administration. Typically, malignant opacities enhance more than 20 HU, while benign opacities enhance less than 15 HU.

While the use of contrast-enhanced CT reduces the number of benign opacities resected, a significant proportion of benign opacities will enhance more than 15 HU and require additional radiologic evaluation, biopsy, or resection. At M.D. Anderson, an alternative to dynamic contrast-enhanced CT that we have found useful in assessing lesions is the determination of glucose metabolism. Metabolism of glucose is typically increased in malignant cells, and this metabolism can be imaged using positron emission tomography (PET) and a radioactive glucose analog, fluorodeoxyglucose F 18 (FDG) (Figure 3–1). FDG-PET often allows diagnosis of malignant and benign nodules with indeterminate etiology after conventional imaging. Increased FDG uptake has been reported to have a sensitivity of 96.8% and a specificity of 77.8% in the diagnosis of malignancy when used in the evaluation of opacities measuring 10 mm or larger

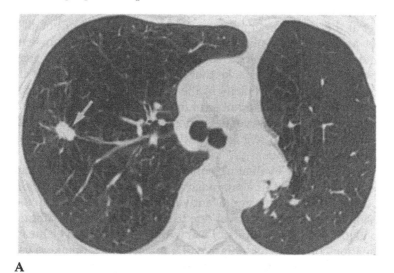

A

B

Figure 3–1. Non–small cell lung cancer manifesting as a hypermetabolic nodule on FDG-PET. CT scan (A) shows a small nodule in the right upper lobe (arrow). Note the emphysematous lung disease. Axial PET image (B) shows increased FDG uptake within the nodule (arrow) compared with the uptake in the mediastinum. These findings are suggestive of malignancy. M = mediastinum, V = vertebral body.

(Gupta et al, 1992; Dewan et al, 1993; Patz et al, 1993; Knight et al, 1996; Gould et al, 2001). False-negative results are uncommon; however, at M.D. Anderson, serial radiologic assessment is performed for 2 years on all opacities with low FDG uptake that are not biopsied or resected. Low FDG uptake has a high specificity in the diagnosis of benign lesions and can substantially reduce the number of unnecessary biopsies and surgical resections performed. However, false-positive results can occur with infection and inflammation (e.g., lesions due to tuberculosis, histoplasmosis, or rheumatoid arthritis).

Preliminary studies evaluating solitary lung opacities also suggest a possible role of FDG-PET as a prognostic indicator (Ahuja et al, 1998; Dhital et al, 2000). Patients with significantly increased FDG uptake in the primary lesion have a worse survival rate than that of patients with modest FDG uptake. The concentration of FDG within a nodule can be measured on attenuation-corrected, quantitative PET images. FDG uptake is usually expressed as the standardized uptake value, also referred to as the differential uptake ratio. This semiquantitative measure is calculated by dividing the mean activity of the nodule by the injected dose and multiplying the result by the body weight—i.e.,

$$\text{Standardized Uptake Value} = \frac{\text{Mean Activity of Nodule (mCi/mL)} \times \text{Body Weight (kg)}}{\text{Injected Dose (mCi)}}$$

Image-Guided Transthoracic Needle Aspiration Biopsy

Many lesions have indeterminate etiology even after comprehensive radiologic assessment. These lesions can be observed, biopsied, or resected. The choice of approach is usually subjective and based on the perceived probability that the opacity is malignant (according to clinical parameters such as the patient's age and cigarette-smoking history as well as the radiologic features of the nodule).

Advances in CT and cytopathology have led to an expanded role for image-guided transthoracic needle aspiration (TTNA) biopsy in the diagnostic evaluation of thoracic lesions. TTNA biopsy is now widely accepted as a safe, accurate procedure with a high yield in establishing the diagnosis of pulmonary and mediastinal masses. TTNA biopsy has been shown to frequently alter management in patients with lung cancer and, if the likelihood of malignancy is low, is the best initial diagnostic procedure (Klein and Zarka, 1997). In the case of peripheral opacities, TTNA should be used instead of bronchoscopy because TTNA is more likely to yield a diagnosis. Most radiographically visible lesions can be biopsied with a TTNA approach if biopsy is clinically indicated.

TTNA biopsy has a high sensitivity for the diagnosis of malignancy, and even in the case of small lesions (10–15 mm in diameter) the yield is

95% to 100% (Li et al, 1996; Klein and Zarka, 1997; Westcott et al, 1997). Specific benign diagnoses are more difficult but have been made in up to 91% of patients with a benign lesion undergoing TTNA biopsy (Klein et al, 1996). Complications, most notably pneumothorax and hemorrhage, occur in approximately 5% to 30% of patients. Hemorrhage is almost always self-limiting, and only about 15% of patients with pneumothoraces eventually require chest tube placement (Klein and Zarka, 1997).

TTNA biopsy of enlarged hilar and mediastinal nodes is useful in determining the stage of lung cancer. CT-guided TTNA biopsy has been proven to be more cost-effective and less invasive than mediastinoscopy and can be used to sample nodes that are inaccessible at mediastinoscopy (e.g., nodes in the aortopulmonary window or in the subcarinal/azygoesophageal region).

STAGING OF LUNG CANCER

Non–Small Cell Lung Cancer

In patients with non–small cell lung cancer (NSCLC), treatment and prognosis are usually determined on the basis of the disease stage. Patients with NSCLC are staged according to the International System for Staging Lung Cancer (Mountain, 1997). This system describes the extent of NSCLC in terms of the primary tumor (T descriptor), lymph nodes (N descriptor), and metastases (M descriptor). The TNM descriptors can be determined clinically with a history, a physical examination, and radiologic imaging or by pathologic analysis of samples obtained with biopsy or surgery.

Primary Tumor

The T descriptor defines the size, location, and extent of the primary tumor. Because the extent of the primary tumor determines whether the disease will be treated with surgical resection or palliative radiation therapy or chemotherapy, imaging is used to assess the degree of pleural, chest wall, and mediastinal invasion. CT and magnetic resonance (MR) imaging are useful in confirming gross chest wall or mediastinal invasion but are inaccurate in differentiating between anatomic contiguity and subtle invasion. MR imaging has superior soft-tissue contrast resolution and multiplanar ability and is thus particularly useful in the evaluation of superior sulcus tumors—i.e., assessment of invasion of the brachial plexus, subclavian vessels, and vertebral bodies (Figure 3–2).

Up to 33% of patients with NSCLC have a malignant pleural effusion or pleural metastases at presentation. Such tumors are classified as T4 lesions and are not resectable. The diagnosis of pleural metastases or malignant pleural effusion can be difficult: CT often fails to show pleural thickening

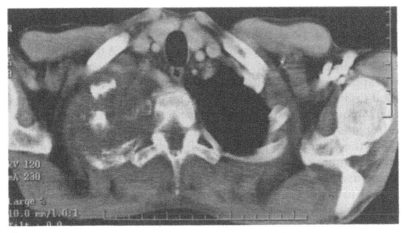

A

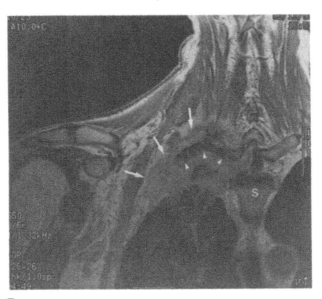

B

Figure 3–2. Pancoast tumor with mediastinal and chest wall invasion. Chest CT scan (A) shows a mass in the apex of the right hemithorax with destruction of the adjacent ribs. Coronal T1-weighted MR image (B) shows a mass (arrows) in the apex of the right hemithorax with loss of the adjacent soft-tissue plane consistent with local invasion of the mediastinum and chest wall. Note the tumor extension along the brachiocephalic vein (arrowheads). S = sternum.

and nodularity, findings suggestive of pleural metastases, and cytologic evaluation is positive for malignancy in only approximately 66% of patients who have a malignant pleural effusion at presentation (American Thoracic Society/European Respiratory Society, 1997; Mountain 1997). In the most recent version of the International System for Staging Lung Cancer, primary tumors associated with satellite nodules in the same lobe are also classified as T4 disease (Mountain, 1997). This new classification may, however, imply a worse prognosis than is warranted, and it has been advocated that patients with satellite nodules undergo definitive resection if there are no other contraindications to surgery.

Regional Lymph Nodes

The presence of nodal metastases and their location are of major importance in determining management and prognosis in patients with NSCLC. Size is the only criterion used to diagnose nodal metastases, with nodes greater than 10 mm in short-axis diameter considered abnormal (Figure 3–3). Because enlarged nodes can be hyperplastic or reactive and small nodes can contain metastases, the accuracy of CT in the detection of metastases to hilar and mediastinal nodes is only 62% to 88%, and the accuracy of MR imaging is only 50% to 82% (Martini et al, 1985; Musset et al, 1986; Klein and Webb, 1991; Webb et al, 1991; Quint et al, 1995).

FDG-PET is more accurate (accuracy, 81%–96%) than CT and MR imaging in the detection of nodal disease (Valk et al, 1995; Dwamena et al, 1999; Dietlein et al, 2000; Kalff et al, 2001). FDG-PET is particularly useful

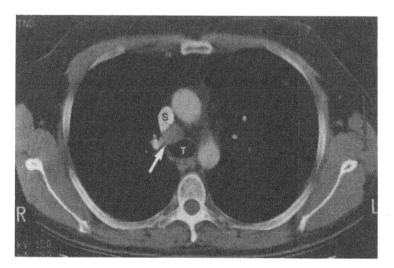

Figure 3–3. NSCLC with intrathoracic nodal metastasis. CT scan shows a 15-mm right paratracheal node (arrow). Mediastinoscopy confirmed metastatic disease. S = superior vena cava, T = trachea.

in detecting metastatic disease in normal-sized nodes and in differentiating hyperplastic nodes from nodes enlarged because of metastases. Recently, it has been advocated that mediastinoscopy be avoided in patients with normal uptake of FDG-PET in mediastinal nodes and potentially resectable lung cancer.

Metastatic Disease

Patients with NSCLC commonly have metastases to the adrenal glands, kidneys, liver, brain, bones, and lymph nodes at presentation. The role of imaging in the detection of these metastases is, however, not clearly defined. Because the combination of normal findings on clinical examination and normal findings on routine laboratory tests (hematocrit and measurement of alkaline phosphatase, gamma-glutamyltranspeptidase, and aspartate aminotransferase) has a negative predictive value of greater than 95% with respect to the presence of metastatic disease, routine radiologic evaluation for occult extrathoracic metastases may not be required. In fact, considering the low incidence (0.5%–0.9%) of metastases in patients with limited intrathoracic disease (T1–2N0) and no clinical findings of metastases and the high cost of detecting these metastases, it has been suggested that extrathoracic imaging may not be required in the staging evaluation of these patients. At M. D. Anderson, however, routine imaging of the upper abdomen is still performed in these patients because of the poor reliability of clinical and laboratory findings in the detection of intra-abdominal metastases.

Metastases to the adrenal glands are common and are detected in up to 20% of patients at presentation. A small (< 3 cm) adrenal mass is more likely to be benign if it occurs in the absence of other extrathoracic metastases. CT and MR imaging can be useful in the evaluation of adrenal masses. A confident diagnosis of benignity can be made if an adrenal mass has an attenuation value of less than 10 HU on a noncontrast CT scan. MR imaging using chemical shift analysis and dynamic gadolinium enhancement can also be used to determine whether an adrenal mass is benign (Figure 3–4). Unfortunately, with some adrenal lesions, the etiology remains indeterminate after radiologic evaluation, and biopsy is required.

Central nervous system metastases are present at presentation in 18% of patients with NSCLC, and 10% of patients with central nervous system metastases have no associated symptoms (Hooper et al, 1984; Mintz et al, 1984; Colice et al, 1995). Consequently, it has been suggested that routine CT of the brain should be performed in the initial staging evaluation of all patients with NSCLC. However, because central nervous system metastases are usually associated with neurological signs and symptoms, imaging for central nervous system metastases in asymptomatic patients with NSCLC is not generally performed at M. D. Anderson.

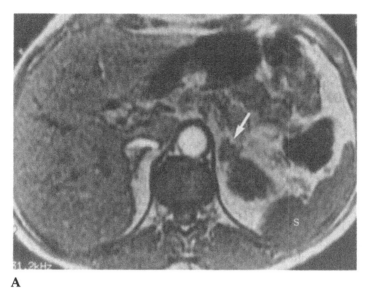

A

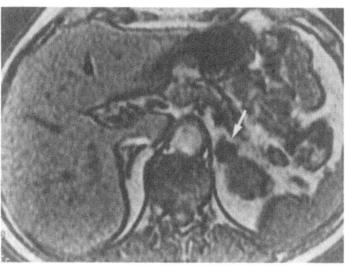

B

Figure 3–4. NSCLC with an indeterminate adrenal mass revealed on CT. Chemical-shift MR imaging was performed to further evaluate the adrenal mass. In-phase (TR 110, TE 4.2) spoiled gradient-recalled echo MR image (A) shows a left adrenal mass (arrow) with signal intensity similar to that of the spleen (S). Opposed-phase (TR 110, TE 1.8) spoiled gradient-recalled echo MR image (B) shows that the left adrenal mass (arrow) is now markedly hypointense. These findings are typical of adenoma. The patient underwent resection of the primary lung malignancy.

Patients with skeletal metastases usually have related symptoms or have laboratory abnormalities suggestive of bone metastases. Because imaging rarely reveals occult skeletal metastases in asymptomatic patients, it is recommended that bone radiographs, technetium Tc 99m-labeled methylene diphosphonate bone scintigraphy, and MR imaging be performed only to evaluate a history of focal bone pain or an elevated alkaline phosphatase level.

Because staging of NSCLC performed on the basis of symptoms, abnormal laboratory findings, and abnormal findings on conventional radiologic imaging is sometimes inaccurate, physicians are using FDG-PET to improve the accuracy of staging. FDG-PET has a higher sensitivity and specificity than CT in detecting metastases to the adrenal glands, bones, and extrathoracic lymph nodes. Whole-body PET permits staging of intra- and extrathoracic disease with a single study, reveals occult extrathoracic metastases in 11% to 14% of patients initially selected for curative resection, and alters management in up to 40% of patients (Valk et al, 1995; Weder et al, 1998; Dwamena et al, 1999; Dietlein et al, 2000) (Figure 3–5).

Small Cell Lung Cancer

Small cell lung cancer (SCLC) is generally staged according to the Veteran's Administration Lung Cancer Study Group recommendations as limited disease or extensive disease (Darling, 1997). Limited disease is defined as tumor confined to a hemithorax and the regional lymph nodes. In the staging system for SCLC, unlike in the TNM classification for NSCLC, metastases to the ipsilateral supraclavicular, contralateral supraclavicular, and mediastinal lymph nodes are considered local disease. Extensive disease is defined as tumor with noncontiguous metastases to the contralateral lung or distant metastases.

The majority of patients with SCLC have extensive disease at presentation, and common sites of metastatic disease include the liver, bones, bone marrow, brain, and retroperitoneal lymph nodes. There is no consensus regarding the imaging studies and invasive procedures that should be performed in the staging evaluation of SCLC, but at M. D. Anderson, our usual workup for extrathoracic metastatic disease is as described in the following paragraphs.

Figure 3–5. NSCLC in a 63-year-old woman. The patient complained of chronic cough but otherwise had no symptoms. Contrast CT scan (A) shows a mass (large arrows) surrounding the bronchus intermedius (asterisk) and atelectasis of the right lower lobe due to occlusion of the lower lobe bronchus. Note the adenopathy in the left hilum (small arrow). Technetium Tc 99m-labeled methylene diphosphonate bone scintigram (B) shows minimal uptake in the right shoulder, which was interpreted as a sign of degenerative disease. Note the increased uptake in the right antecubital fossa at the injection site. (*Figure continues on page 50*)

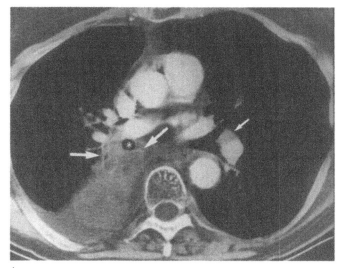

A

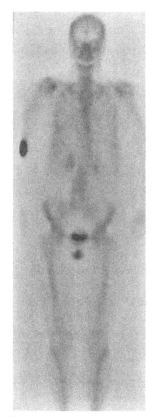

B

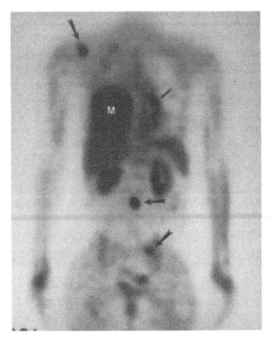

C

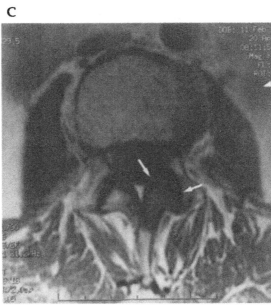

D

Patients with SCLC with bone and bone marrow metastases are often asymptomatic and frequently have normal blood alkaline phosphatase levels. However, because isolated bone and bone marrow metastases are uncommon, bone marrow aspiration and technetium Tc 99m-labeled methylene diphosphonate bone scintigraphy and MR imaging are usually performed only if the patient has other findings of extensive disease.

Central nervous system metastases are common at presentation in patients with SCLC, and approximately 10% of patients will have no associated symptoms. Because therapeutic central nervous system irradiation and chemotherapy can decrease morbidity and improve prognosis, MR imaging of the brain is routinely performed in patients with SCLC.

Routine CT or MR imaging of the abdomen is performed because metastases to the liver and abdominal nodes are common at presentation and patients with such metastases often have no associated symptoms and can have normal findings on liver function tests.

EVALUATION OF PATIENTS AFTER TREATMENT

After surgical resection or the initiation of chemotherapy or radiation therapy, radiologic imaging has an important role in the assessment of response to therapy. At M. D. Anderson, patients are closely monitored clinically to assess response to treatment. Patients also usually undergo routine chest radiography and CT to determine if a change in therapy is required. Furthermore, because relying on patient symptoms to determine local recurrence can delay diagnosis and compromise further treatment after successful first-line therapy, evaluation with chest radiography or CT or both is usually performed at yearly intervals. However, chest radiography, CT, and MR imaging often do not permit persistent or recurrent tumor to be distinguished from necrotic tumor, posttreatment scarring, or fibrosis. PET may have an important role in guiding patient care after surgery or radiation therapy as it is more accurate than conventional studies in detecting recurrent tumor (accuracy of 78%–98%, sensitivity of 97%–100%, and specificity of 62%–100%) (Figure 3–6). False-positive findings on PET can be caused by postirradiation inflammatory changes, and therefore it is recommended that PET studies not be obtained until 4 to 6 months after irradiation. The usefulness of PET in the posttreatment evaluation of lung cancer patients is currently under investigation at M. D. Anderson.

Figure 3–5. *(continued)* Coronal whole-body PET (C) shows markedly increased FDG uptake in the mass and atelectatic lobe (M) and reveals focal areas of increased FDG uptake in the clavicle, pelvis, and lumbar spine (large arrows). Note the increased uptake in the left hilum (small arrow), which is indicative of metastasis. Axial fast spin-echo T2-weighted MR image (D) of the lumbar spine shows decreased signal intensity in the lamina of the vertebral body (arrows), consistent with metastasis.

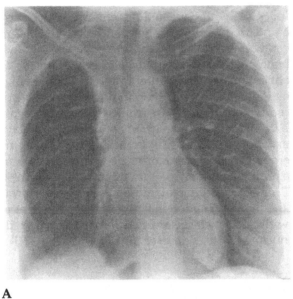

A

B

Figure 3–6. Recurrence of NSCLC 3 years after treatment of a nonresectable malignancy with chemotherapy and radiation therapy. Posteroanterior chest radiograph (A) shows radiation fibrosis in the right upper lobe. The radiographic appearance had been stable for 2 years. Coronal PET image (B) reveals marked uptake of FDG in the region of postirradiation change in the right lung that was suspicious for tumor (arrows). Radiographic assessment 3 months later showed destruction of the first right rib consistent with recurrent disease. M = mediastinum, L = liver.

KEY PRACTICE POINTS

- Lung cancer is the most common malignancy and the leading cause of cancer-related deaths in the United States.

- Lung cancer screening with CT is under investigation, and prospective randomized trials may prove this practice to be beneficial in reducing patient mortality.

- Assessment of the morphologic features (size, margins, contour, and density) and growth rate can be useful in differentiating malignant from benign lung lesions.

- Assessment of perfusion with dynamic contrast-enhanced CT and assessment of glucose metabolism with FDG-PET can be used to further evaluate lung lesions for which conventional radiologic imaging fails to establish the etiology.

- TTNA is a safe, accurate procedure with a high diagnostic yield in establishing the diagnosis of lung cancer and evaluating enlarged mediastinal nodes.

- Patients with NSCLC are staged according to the International System for Staging Lung Cancer. This system describes the extent of NSCLC in terms of the primary tumor (T descriptor), lymph nodes (N descriptor), and metastases (M descriptor).

- MR imaging is particularly useful in the evaluation of superior sulcus tumors.

- The accuracy of CT and MR imaging in the detection of mediastinal nodal metastases (N2 and N3 disease), a major determinant of treatment, is not optimal.

- FDG-PET is more accurate than CT and MR imaging in the assessment of nodal metastases and is particularly useful in detecting metastatic disease in normal-sized nodes.

- Imaging has an important role in the detection of metastases to the adrenal glands, kidneys, liver, brain, bones, and lymph nodes.

- Whole-body PET imaging permits staging of intra- and extrathoracic disease with a single study and alters management in up to 40% of patients with NSCLC.

- SCLC is usually staged as limited disease or extensive disease.

SUGGESTED READINGS

Abrams J, Doyle LA, Aisner J. Staging, prognostic factors, and special considerations in small cell lung cancer. *Semin Oncol* 1988;15:261–277.

Ahuja V, Coleman RE, Herndon J, et al. The prognostic significance of fluorodeoxyglucose positron emission tomography imaging for patients with non-small cell lung carcinoma. *Cancer* 1998;83:918–924.

American Thoracic Society and European Respiratory Society. Pretreatment evaluation of non-small-cell lung cancer. *Am J Respir Crit Care Med* 1997; 156:320–332.

Boland GW, Lee MJ. Magnetic resonance imaging of the adrenal gland. *Crit Rev Diagn Imaging* 1995;36:115–174.

Boland GW, Lee MJ, Gazelle GS, et al. Characterization of adrenal masses using unenhanced CT: an analysis of the CT literature. *AJR Am J Roentgenol* 1998;171:201–204.

Bury T, Corhay JL, Duysinx B, et al. Value of FDG-PET in detecting residual or recurrent nonsmall cell lung cancer. *Eur Respir J* 1999;14:1376–1380.

Colice GL, Birkmeyer JD, Black WC, et al. Cost-effectiveness of head CT in patients with lung cancer without clinical evidence of metastases. *Chest* 1995; 108:1264–1271.

Darling GE. Staging of the patient with small cell lung cancer. *Chest Surg Clin N Am* 1997;7:81–94.

Dewan NA, Gupta NC, Redepenning LS, et al. Diagnostic efficacy of PET-FDG imaging in solitary pulmonary nodules. Potential role in evaluation and management. *Chest* 1993;104:997–1002.

Dhital K, Saunders CA, Seed PT, et al. [(18)F]Fluorodeoxyglucose positron emission tomography and its prognostic value in lung cancer. *Eur J Cardiothorac Surg* 2000;18:425–428.

Dietlein M, Weber K, Gandjour A, et al. Cost-effectiveness of FDG-PET for the management of potentially operable non-small cell lung cancer: priority for a PET-based strategy after nodal-negative CT results. *Eur J Nucl Med* 2000;27:1598–1609.

Dwamena BA, Sonnad SS, Angobaldo JO, et al. Metastases from non-small cell lung cancer: mediastinal staging in the 1990s—meta-analytic comparison of PET and CT. *Radiology* 1999;213:530–536.

Ginsberg MS, Griff SK, Go BD, et al. Pulmonary nodules resected at video-assisted thoracoscopic surgery: etiology in 426 patients. *Radiology* 1999;213:277–282.

Gould MK, Maclean CC, Kuschner WG, et al. Accuracy of positron emission tomography for diagnosis of pulmonary nodules and mass lesions: a meta-analysis. *JAMA* 2001;285:936–937.

Gupta NC, Frank AR, Dewan NA, et al. Solitary pulmonary nodules: detection of malignancy with PET with 2-[F-18]-fluoro-2-deoxy-D-glucose. *Radiology* 1992; 184:441–444.

Henschke CI, McCauley DI, Yankelevitz DF, et al. Early Lung Cancer Action Project: overall design and findings from baseline screening. *Lancet* 1999; 354:99–105.

Hooper RG, Tenholder MF, Underwood GH, et al. Computed tomographic scanning of the brain in initial staging of bronchogenic carcinoma. *Chest* 1984;85:774–776.

Kalff V, Hicks RJ, MacManus M, et al. Clinical impact of (18)F fluorodeoxyglucose positron emission tomography in patients with non-small-cell lung cancer: a prospective study. *J Clin Oncol* 2001;19:111–118.

Kaneko N, Eguchi K, Ohmatsu H, et al. Peripheral lung cancer: screening and detection with low-dose spiral CT vs. radiography. *Radiology* 1996;201:798–802.

Klein JS, Salomon G, Stewart EA. Transthoracic needle biopsy with a coaxially placed 20-gauge automated cutting needle: results in 122 patients. *Radiology* 1996;198:715–720.

Klein JS, Webb WR. The radiologic staging of lung cancer. *J Thorac Imaging* 1991;7:29–47.

Klein JS, Zarka MA. Transthoracic needle biopsy: an overview. *J Thorac Imaging* 1997;12:232–249.

Knight SB, Delbeke D, Stewart JR, et al. Evaluation of pulmonary lesions with FDG-PET. Comparison of findings in patients with and without a history of prior malignancy. *Chest* 1996;109:982–988.

Kubik A, Parkin DM, Khlat M, et al. Lack of benefit from semi-annual screening of the lung: follow-up report of a randomized controlled trial on a population of high-risk males in Czechoslovakia. *Int J Cancer* 1990;45:26–33.

Li H, Boiselle PM, Shepard JO, et al. Diagnostic accuracy and safety of CT-guided percutaneous needle aspiration biopsy of the lung: comparison of small and large pulmonary nodules. *AJR Am J Roentgenol* 1996;167:105–109.

Mahoney MC, Shipley RT, Corcoran HL, et al. CT demonstration of calcification in carcinoma of the lung. *AJR Am J Roentgenol* 1990;154:255–258.

Martini N, Heelan R, Westcott J, et al. Comparative merits of conventional, computed tomographic, and magnetic resonance imaging in assessing mediastinal involvement in surgically confirmed lung carcinoma. *J Thorac Cardiovasc Surg* 1985;90:639–648.

McLoud TC, Bourgouin PM, Greenberg RW, et al. Bronchogenic carcinoma: analysis of staging in the mediastinum with CT by correlative lymph node mapping and sampling. *Radiology* 1992;182:319–323.

Mintz BJ, Tuhrim S, Alexander S, et al. Intracranial metastases in the initial staging of bronchogenic carcinoma. *Chest* 1984;86:850–853.

Moore EH. Needle-aspiration lung biopsy: a comprehensive approach to complication reduction. *J Thorac Imaging* 1997;12:259–271.

Mori K, Tominaga K, Hirose T, et al. Utility of low-dose helical CT as a second step after plain chest radiography for mass screening for lung cancer. *J Thorac Imaging* 1997;12:173–180.

Mountain CF. Revisions in the International System for Staging Lung Cancer. *Chest* 1997;111:1710–1717.

Munden RF, Pugatch RD, Liptay MJ, et al. Small pulmonary lesions detected at CT: clinical importance. *Radiology* 1997;202:105–110.

Musset D, Grenier P, Carette MF, et al. Primary lung cancer staging: prospective comparative study of MR imaging with CT. *Radiology* 1986;160:607–611.

Patz EF Jr, Lowe VJ, Hoffman JM, et al. Focal pulmonary abnormalities: evaluation with F-18 fluorodeoxyglucose PET scanning. *Radiology* 1993;188:487–490.

Protopapas Z, Westcott JL. Transthoracic hilar and mediastinal biopsy. *J Thorac Imaging* 1997;12:250–258.

Quint LE, Francis IR, Wahl RL, et al. Preoperative staging of non-small-cell carcinoma of the lung: imaging methods. *AJR Am J Roentgenol* 1995;164:1349–1359.

Richert-Boe K, Humphrey LL. Screening for cancers of the lung and colon. *Arch Intern Med* 1992;152:2398–2404.

Seemann MD, Staebler A, Beinert T, et al. Usefulness of morphological characteristics for the differentiation of benign from malignant solitary pulmonary lesions using HRCT. *Eur Radiol* 1999;9:409–417.

Strauss GM. Measuring effectiveness of lung cancer screening: from consensus to controversy and back. *Chest* 1997;112:216S–228S.

Swensen SJ, Harms GF, Morin RL, et al. CT evaluation of solitary pulmonary nodules: value of 185-H reference phantom. *AJR Am J Roentgenol* 1991;156:925–929.

Swensen SJ, Viggiano RW, Midthun DE, et al. Lung nodule enhancement at CT: multicenter study. *Radiology* 2000;214:73–80.

Valk PE, Pounds TR, Hopkins DM, et al. Staging non-small cell lung cancer by whole-body positron emission tomographic imaging. *Ann Thorac Surg* 1995; 60:1573–1581.

Webb WR, Gatsonis C, Zerhouni EA, et al. CT and MR imaging in staging non-small cell bronchogenic carcinoma: report of the Radiologic Diagnostic Oncology Group. *Radiology* 1991;178:705–713.

Weder W, Schmid RA, Bruchhaus H, et al. Detection of extrathoracic metastases by positron emission tomography in lung cancer. *Ann Thorac Surg* 1998;66:886–892.

Westcott JL, Rao N, Colley DP. Transthoracic needle biopsy of small pulmonary nodules. *Radiology* 1997;202:97–103.

Yankelevitz DF, Gupta R, Zhao B, et al. Small pulmonary nodules: evaluation with repeat CT—preliminary experience. *Radiology* 1999;212:561–566.

Yankelevitz DF, Henschke CI. Does 2-year stability imply that pulmonary nodules are benign? *AJR Am J Roentgenol* 1997;168:325–328.

Yankelevitz DF, Reeves AP, Kostis WJ, et al. Determination of malignancy in small pulmonary nodules based on volumetrically determined growth rates. *Radiology* 2000;209(suppl): 375.

4 PATHOLOGIC EVALUATION OF LUNG CANCER

Pheroze Tamboli and Jae Y. Ro

CHAPTER OVERVIEW

The goals of pathologic evaluation of lung cancer are to accurately classify the tumor and to determine the extent of invasion (pleural, vascular-lymphatic, and chest-wall soft tissue) and the status of the surgical margins. The pathologic classification of lung tumors set out by the World Health Organization has been changed significantly in recent years. The most important changes are the revisions in the definitions of the neuroendocrine tumors (typical carcinoid, atypical carcinoid, small cell carcinoma, and large cell neuroendocrine carcinoma) and bronchioloalveolar adenocarcinoma. Because adenocarcinoma of the lung is becoming one of the most common malignant tumors of the lung, recognition of atypical adenomatous hyperplasia, the putative precursor lesion for adenocarcinoma, is becoming more important. The use of immunohistochemical stains, such as stains for thyroid transcription factor 1 and cytokeratin subsets, is recommended for distinguishing between primary adenocarcinoma of the lung and metastatic adenocarcinoma. Electron microscopy has a limited role in the diagnosis of lung cancer; it is useful for recognizing neuroendocrine granules in tumors and for differentiating adenocarcinoma from mesothelioma. At present, molecular biology techniques have a very limited role in the diagnosis and classification of lung cancer; however, with further advances in knowledge, it is likely that these techniques will come to have clinical applications.

INTRODUCTION

Lung cancer will be diagnosed in approximately 169,400 new patients in the United States in the year 2002. Many lung tumors are detected in asymptomatic individuals during routine examination or during follow-up for other diseases. Solitary pulmonary nodules are detected in 0.1% to 0.2% of routine chest radiographs. Of these nodules, 60% are benign, while the remaining 40% turn out to be malignant. The pathologist's main role in the management of lung tumors is to promptly evaluate lung nodules to confirm or rule out malignancy. Prompt and accurate pathologic evaluation minimizes the number of invasive procedures performed for benign processes and expedites resection of malignant nodules, thereby affording the best chance for cure.

DIAGNOSIS OF LUNG CANCER

Diagnostic Algorithm

The diagnostic algorithm shown in Figure 4–1 is useful in the pathologic evaluation of a lung nodule. Because infectious and other nonneoplastic

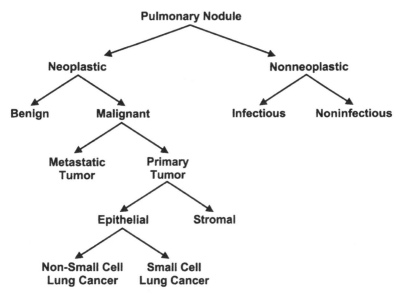

Figure 4–1.   Algorithm for pathologic diagnosis of lung nodules.

processes may result in pulmonary nodules that mimic neoplasia, the first step in the algorithm is to decide whether the nodule is neoplastic or non-neoplastic.

If the lesion is neoplastic, the next step is to decide whether it is benign or malignant. Benign tumors are usually expansile or encapsulated, are well-differentiated, resemble the tissue of origin, have a slow rate of growth, have no mitoses or rare normal mitoses, and—most important—do not metastasize. Malignant tumors show an infiltrative growth pattern, are usually not encapsulated, have an atypical structure with anaplasia, grow rapidly, have high mitotic counts and abnormal mitoses, and have the ability to metastasize.

Because metastases in the lung are more common than primary lung tumors, the next step once a malignant lung tumor has been identified is to decide whether it is a primary lung tumor or a metastasis. Primary lung tumors are usually single; usually have an ill-defined margin, with dysplasia in the adjacent epithelium; and occasionally show vascular-lymphatic invasion. Metastases, in contrast, may be single or multiple, usually are small, possess a well-defined margin, are not associated with dysplasia in the adjacent epithelium, and frequently show vascular-lymphatic invasion.

Primary malignant tumors of the lung may be epithelial or mesenchymal. Epithelial tumors are generally arranged in nests or cords and have oval, round, or polygonal cells set within a desmoplastic stroma with blood

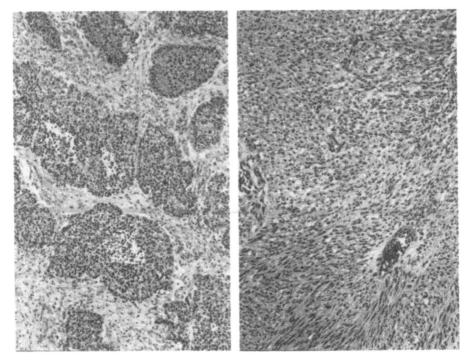

Figure 4–2. Comparison of epithelial and mesenchymal tumors. The epithelial tumor (left panel) is arranged in nests, while the mesenchymal tumor (right panel) grows as a sheet of cells.

vessels within the stroma (Figure 4–2). Mesenchymal tumors usually grow in a diffuse pattern with spindled or ovoid cells, lack a desmoplastic stroma, and have blood vessels between tumor cells (Figure 4–2). The epithelial tumors are broadly divided into small cell lung cancer and non–small cell lung cancer (NSCLC). NSCLC is further divided into squamous cell carcinoma, adenocarcinoma, and large cell carcinoma.

Preoperative Evaluation

The pathologist plays a pivotal role in the preoperative evaluation of radiographically detected lung nodules. The pathologist is responsible for establishing the definitive tissue diagnosis of benignity or malignancy—often on the basis of a limited tissue sample. Methods for obtaining preoperative specimens include bronchial brushing, bronchial washing, fine-needle aspiration biopsy, core needle biopsy, endobronchial biopsy, and transbronchial biopsy. Bronchial brushing, bronchial washing, and endobronchial biopsy are used for sampling endobronchial tumors, while the other techniques are generally utilized for more peripherally located lesions. Open lung biopsy is generally utilized for diagnosis of lesions that do not yield sufficient tissue with use of the above-mentioned less invasive procedures and for nonneoplastic lung disease.

Bronchial brushing, bronchial washing, and fine-needle aspiration biopsy yield single cells or small groups of cells that are evaluated by a cytopathologist. Bronchial brushing and bronchial washing are performed endoscopically, while fine-needle aspiration biopsy is done under direct imaging guidance. During the acquisition of these specimens, a cytopathologist is usually on hand to comment on whether the specimen is adequate for establishing the diagnosis and to divide the specimen for different diagnostic and research tests. At M. D. Anderson Cancer Center, the cytopathology laboratory is located adjacent to the interventional radiology suite to facilitate the expeditious analysis of fine-needle aspirates obtained under imaging guidance. This close working relationship between the cytopathologists and radiologists benefits patients by reducing the number of procedures they must undergo to have the diagnosis of lung cancer established and by reducing the time needed to establish the diagnosis.

Endobronchial biopsy and transbronchial biopsy yield small pieces of tissue, usually measuring less than 5.0 mm in maximal dimension. Core needle biopsy yields a tissue fragment that measures approximately 1.0 mm in diameter, with a length of 5.0 mm to 20.0 mm depending on the type of needle and the technique employed.

Occasionally the mediastinal lymph nodes are examined as part of the preoperative evaluation to confirm the diagnosis of metastatic disease in clinically suspicious lymph nodes to help plan treatment. The lymph nodes are either sampled using fine-needle aspiration biopsy or removed in their entirety during mediastinoscopy.

Especially in the case of a limited tissue sample, it may not be possible to accurately classify a lung cancer before surgery except with regard to its being small cell carcinoma or NSCLC (Edwards et al, 2000). The difficulty of subclassifying NSCLC on the basis of small tissue samples is due to the well-known morphologic heterogeneity of lung cancer. However, as the recommended treatment for patients with NSCLC does not differ on the basis of histologic subtype, rendering the diagnosis of NSCLC in a biopsy specimen is usually adequate.

Intraoperative Evaluation

At M. D. Anderson, intraoperative pathologic evaluation is an important component of the surgical management of lung cancer. Frozen section examination is routinely performed to evaluate the bronchial margin of lobectomy and pneumonectomy specimens, to establish the diagnosis of nodules detected incidentally at the time of surgery, and to evaluate regional lymph nodes. Sometimes, the soft tissue margins of a chest wall resection specimen may also be examined using the frozen section technique.

Postoperative Evaluation

Postoperative evaluation of lung cancer specimens is important for accurate classification of tumor type, tumor staging, and determination of prognostic factors. The most common types of lung cancer specimens seen are lobectomy specimens, pneumonectomy specimens, chest wall resection specimens, and mediastinal lymph node dissection specimens. The important factors to be evaluated and reported include the tumor size; the tumor type; the degree of differentiation; the extent of the tumor, including the distance from the bronchial margin and the presence or absence of pleural invasion; the presence or absence of vascular invasion; the status of the surgical margins; and the number of lymph nodes involved by metastatic tumor. In addition, any associated atelectasis or obstructive pneumonitis should be evaluated and reported.

CLASSIFICATION OF LUNG TUMORS

The classification of lung tumors has recently undergone numerous changes because of progress in the understanding of the biology of these tumors. The latest World Health Organization (WHO) classification of lung tumors, published in 1999, is shown in Tables 4–1 and 4–2 (Travis et al, 1999). This classification schema is based on the light-microscopic morphologic appearance of the most well differentiated component of the tumors. As of yet, ancillary evaluation techniques, such as immunohistochemical analysis, electron microscopy, and molecular biology techniques, have only a limited role in tumor classification. In this section, we will limit our description of pathologic features to the more important aspects of the preinvasive lesions and some of the more common malignant tumors. More detailed information about pathologic classification of lung tumors is available elsewhere (Colby et al, 1995; Travis et al, 1999).

Preinvasive Lesions

The concept of preinvasive or precancerous lesions of the lung is not as evolved as the concept of preinvasive lesions in some other organs, including the cervix, colon, and urinary bladder. However, in the past 2 decades, there has been considerable work on the concept of incipient neoplasia of the lung (Colby et al, 1998). Three possible precancerous lesions are now listed in the WHO classification: squamous dysplasia and carcinoma in situ, atypical adenomatous hyperplasia (AAH), and diffuse idiopathic pulmonary neuroendocrine cell hyperplasia (DIPNECH). That these 3 lesions are considered preinvasive does not mean that they will naturally evolve into invasive carcinoma in all patients. In some patients, these lesions may serve as a marker of the possibility of developing lung cancer at a later time.

**Table 4–1. World Health Organization Classification
of Epithelial Tumors of the Lung**

Benign Tumors

Papilloma
   Squamous cell papilloma
      Exophytic
      Inverted
   Glandular papilloma
   Mixed squamous cell and glandular papilloma
Adenoma
   Alveolar adenoma
   Papillary adenoma
   Adenoma of salivary-gland type
   Mucous gland adenoma
   Pleomorphic adenoma
   Mucinous cystadenoma

Preinvasive Lesions

Squamous dysplasia and carcinoma in situ
Atypical adenomatous hyperplasia
Diffuse idiopathic pulmonary neuroendocrine cell hyperplasia

Malignant Tumors

Squamous cell carcinoma
   Papillary squamous cell carcinoma
   Clear cell squamous cell carcinoma
   Small cell squamous cell carcinoma
   Basaloid squamous cell carcinoma
Small cell carcinoma
   Small cell carcinoma
   Combined small cell carcinoma
Adenocarcinoma
   Acinar adenocarcinoma
   Papillary adenocarcinoma
   Bronchioloalveolar adenocarcinoma
      Nonmucinous
      Mucinous
      Mixed mucinous and nonmucinous or indeterminate cell type
   Solid adenocarcinoma with mucin
   Adenocarcinoma with mixed subtypes
   Well-differentiated fetal adenocarcinoma
   Mucinous (colloid) adenocarcinoma
   Mucinous cystadenocarcinoma
   Signet-ring adenocarcinoma
   Clear cell adenocarcinoma *(continued)*

Table 4–1. *(continued)* **World Health Organization Classification of Epithelial Tumors of the Lung**

Malignant Tumors (continued)

Large cell carcinoma
    Large cell neuroendocrine carcinoma
    Combined large cell neuroendocrine carcinoma
    Basaloid carcinoma
    Lymphoepithelioma-like carcinoma
    Clear cell carcinoma
    Large cell carcinoma with rhabdoid phenotype
Adenosquamous carcinoma
Carcinoma with pleomorphic, sarcomatoid, or sarcomatous elements
    Carcinoma with spindle and/or giant cells
        Pleomorphic carcinoma
        Spindle cell carcinoma
        Giant cell carcinoma
    Carcinosarcoma
    Pulmonary blastoma
Carcinoid tumor
    Typical carcinoid
    Atypical carcinoid
Carcinoma of salivary-gland type
    Mucoepidermoid carcinoma
    Adenoid cystic carcinoma
    Acinic cell carcinoma
    Epimyoepithelial carcinoma
    Malignant mixed tumor
Unclassified carcinoma

Source: Travis et al, 1999.

Squamous Dysplasia and Carcinoma in Situ

Squamous mucosa is not a normal component of the tracheobronchial tree but rather develops as a metaplastic response to certain stimuli, most notably cigarette smoke. The presence of squamous metaplasia in the bronchial epithelium does not necessarily mean that squamous dysplasia and carcinoma in situ will follow. Rather, squamous metaplasia is part of the normal physiologic response to injurious stimuli affecting the bronchial mucosa.

Squamous dysplasia is the development of abnormalities in the squamous mucosa, including an increase in the number of cell layers, an increase in cell size, variation in cell size, an increased nucleus-to-cytoplasm

Table 4–2. World Health Organization Classification of Nonepithelial Tumors of the Lung

Soft Tissue Tumors	Lymphoproliferative Diseases	Miscellaneous Tumors	Tumor-Like Lesions
Localized fibrous tumor	Lymphoid interstitial pneumonia (LIP)	Hamartoma	Tumorlet
Epithelioid hemangioendothelioma	Nodular lymphoid hyperplasia	Sclerosing hemangioma	Minute meningothelioid nodules
Pleuropulmonary blastoma	Low-grade marginal zone B-cell lymphoma of the mucosa-associated lymphoid tissue (MALT)	Clear cell tumor	Langerhans cell histiocytosis
Chondroma		Germ cell tumors: teratoma, mature; teratoma, immature	Inflammatory pseudotumor (inflammatory myofibroblastic tumor)
Calcifying fibrous pseudotumor of the pleura		Thymoma	
Congenital peribronchial myofibroblastic tumor	Lymphomatoid granulomatosis	Malignant melanoma	Localized organizing pneumonia
Diffuse pulmonary lymphangiomatosis			Amyloid tumor (nodular amyloid)
Desmoplastic round cell tumor			Hyalinizing granuloma
			Lymphangioleiomyomatosis
			Micronodular pneumocyte hyperplasia
			Endometriosis
			Bronchial inflammatory polyp

Source: Travis et al, 1999.

ratio, abnormalities in nuclear contour and nuclear chromatin, increased numbers of nucleoli and mitoses, and loss of normal maturation with alteration of polarity. Squamous dysplasia is graded as mild, moderate, or severe depending on the thickness of the involved epithelium and the severity of the changes.

Carcinoma in situ is full-thickness involvement of the squamous mucosa by neoplastic cells that show all the morphologic features of squamous cell carcinoma but are confined by the basement membrane. These cells have the potential to invade into the underlying stroma, at which point they would be classified as squamous cell carcinoma. Carcinoma in situ cells may extend into submucosal glands, but such extension is not considered invasion as long as the basement membrane is not breached.

Atypical Adenomatous Hyperplasia

AAH is defined as a lesion measuring 5.0 mm or less that is composed of atypical epithelial cells lining the alveoli and respiratory bronchioles (Travis et al, 1999). The morphologic appearance of this lesion is similar to that of nonmucinous bronchioloalveolar adenocarcinoma (BAC). In AAH, the alveolar septae are thickened and lined by a monotonous layer of cuboidal or low columnar cells with scant cytoplasm, enlarged hyperchromatic nuclei, and inconspicuous nucleoli (Figure 4–3). When examined with an electron microscope, these cells show the features of either type II pneumocytes or Clara cells.

AAH has been referred to in the past by various names, including atypical bronchioloalveolar cell hyperplasia, bronchioloalveolar adenoma, atypical alveolar hyperplasia, alveolar epithelial hyperplasia, and atypical alveolar cuboidal cell hyperplasia. AAH is thought to be the most likely precursor for pulmonary adenocarcinoma, especially nonmucinous BAC. There is no conclusive evidence of this association, but there is much circumstantial evidence, including the frequent association of AAH with adenocarcinoma, the presence of multifocal AAH in lungs removed for adenocarcinoma, and the observation of a morphologic transformation from AAH to adenocarcinoma (Kitamura et al, 1999). A study using analysis of the human androgen receptor gene has shown AAH to be a monoclonal proliferation (Niho et al, 1999). Additional corroborating evidence of the malignant potential of AAH and its similarity to adenocarcinoma includes reports indicating that AAH has the following features: *p53* mutations (Kitamura et al, 1999), expression of carcinoembryonic antigen (Kitamura et al, 1999), expression of blood group antigens, increased proliferative activity as measured by Ki-67 antibody, higher mean nuclear area as measured by nuclear morphometry (Kitamura et al, 1999), loss of heterozygosity of loci on chromosomes 3p, 9p, and 17p, telomerase activity, and the presence of mutations of codon 12 of the K-*ras* gene.

The lesions included in the differential diagnosis of AAH are reactive alveolar epithelial hyperplasia, nodular type II pneumocyte hyperplasia, bronchiolization of the alveolar septae, and small BAC. Of these, small BAC is the most important differential diagnostic consideration because in the 1997 TNM staging system for lung cancer, multiple tumor nodules within the same lobe are considered pT4 disease but the presence of a tumor nodule in a different lobe is classified as M1 disease (Sobin and Wittekind, 1997). Thus, in the case of a separate nodule in another lobe (i.e., not the lobe containing the main tumor), confusing AAH for a small BAC or vice versa could potentially affect management decisions for the patient. Morphologic features that favor BAC are loss of alveolar architecture with prominent papillary growth, marked cell

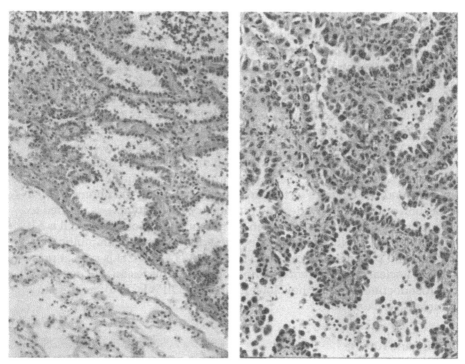

Figure 4–3. Composite photomicrograph showing AAH (left panel) and BAC (right panel).

crowding, overlapping of nuclei, and cytologic atypia, including enlarged hyperchromatic nuclei with prominent nucleoli (Figure 4–3).

Grading of AAH remains controversial, but most authorities now divide AAH into low grade and high grade. However, as interobserver reproducibility is suspect, the WHO does not recommend grading these lesions.

While all the evidence points to a link between AAH and adenocarcinoma, much work needs to be done to establish the clinical significance of AAH lesions detected radiographically and in biopsy specimens obtained for nonneoplastic diseases as most of the information we have available is based on resection specimens and some autopsy specimens. As yet we do not have conclusive proof that AAH lesions progress to adenocarcinoma. Therefore, the diagnosis of AAH in biopsy specimens needs to be made with caution and should take into account the radiographic picture and clinical findings, especially in the absence of a mass lesion.

Diffuse Idiopathic Pulmonary Neuroendocrine Cell Hyperplasia

DIPNECH is a very rare phenomenon that is defined as a diffuse proliferation of neuroendocrine cells confined to the bronchiolar epithelium without extension beyond the bronchiolar basement membrane. These lesions are typically associated with obliterative bronchiolar fibrosis but without interstitial lung disease. The neuroendocrine cells in DIPNECH may be present as an increased number of scattered single cells, small nodules of cells (referred to as neuroendocrine bodies), or linear proliferations. The sine qua non for DIPNECH is the presence of increased numbers of neuroendocrine cells within the bronchiolar mucosa without breach of the basement membrane. The presence of a proliferation of neuroendocrine cells beyond the confines of the bronchiolar basement membrane—i.e., a collection of cells that invades into pulmonary parenchyma—is referred to as a tumorlet if it measures less than 5.0 mm or a carcinoid tumor if it is 5.0 mm or larger. DIPNECH may also be present in patients with multiple tumorlets and patients with carcinoid tumors. As DIPNECH is rare, at present it is unclear what percentage of patients with this lesion will develop a neuroendocrine tumor or how long it takes for DIPNECH to progress to a neuroendocrine tumor.

Malignant Tumors

A variety of malignant tumors arise in the lung, but the vast majority are bronchogenic carcinomas. Other lung tumors include neuroendocrine tumors (carcinoids, small cell carcinoma, large cell neuroendocrine carcinoma), mesenchymal tumors, and other miscellaneous neoplasms. The term bronchogenic carcinoma is used for the epithelial tumors and refers to the origin of most of these tumors in the bronchial (and sometimes bronchiolar) epithelium. Bronchogenic carcinoma arises most often in and about the hilus of the lung. Most bronchogenic carcinomas arise from first-order, second-order, and third-order bronchi. A small number of lung tumors arise in the periphery of the lung. These are predominantly adenocarcinoma, including the bronchioloalveolar type.

The malignant epithelial tumors may be heterogeneous, having different mixtures of histologic patterns within the same tumor. Tumors containing both squamous cell carcinoma and adenocarcinoma or both small cell and squamous cell carcinoma are not infrequent. In the latest WHO classification system, a minimum of 10% of the tumor must show a specific morphologic subtype for the tumor to be classified as belonging to that subtype—e.g., at least 10% of a tumor must show squamous differentiation and another 10% must show adenocarcinoma differentiation if the tumor is to be classified as adenosquamous carcinoma (Travis et al, 1999). The 10% cut-off is arbitrary and is obviously dependent on adequate sampling of the tumor. This is one of the reasons for assigning a histologic subtype only on the basis of resection specimens and using the terms small cell carcinoma and NSCLC for classification of epithelial tumors diagnosed on the basis of small tissue samples.

Squamous Cell Carcinoma

Squamous cell carcinoma is the classic smoking-related lung carcinoma. It usually arises from the bronchi, but rarely tumors originate in the peripheral lung parenchyma. Squamous cell carcinoma used to be the most common type of lung cancer, accounting for 25% to 40% of all lung tumors, but has now been overtaken by adenocarcinoma, which is the most common lung cancer in many countries around the world.

Squamous cell carcinoma by definition shows polygonal tumor cells with intercellular bridges with or without keratinization. There are 4 histologic variants of this cancer: papillary, clear cell, small cell, and basaloid. It is important to recognize these variants as squamous cell carcinoma and to avoid confusion between these variants and the other subtypes of lung cancer. The small cell and basaloid variants may be misdiagnosed as small cell carcinoma in small biopsy samples. These histologic variants have no prognostic significance, except possibly for basaloid squamous carcinoma, which has been reported to behave more aggressively than the other variants.

Neuroendocrine Tumors of the Lung

There are 4 well-recognized neuroendocrine tumors of the lung: typical carcinoid, atypical carcinoid, small cell carcinoma, and large cell neuroendocrine carcinoma (Travis et al, 1998a,b). Until recently, a slew of names had been used for these tumors, including neuroendocrine carcinoma, malignant carcinoid, intermediate cell neuroendocrine carcinoma, and peripheral small cell carcinoma resembling carcinoid. With the publication of the latest WHO classification system, it is hoped that the confusing older terminology will become a thing of the past.

Neuroendocrine tumors of the lung form a morphologic spectrum, with typical carcinoid at one end and small cell carcinoma and large cell neuroendocrine carcinoma at the other end. The 4 types of neuroendocrine carcinoma have in common certain characteristic features that are apparent on light microscopy, electron microscopy, and immunohistochemical staining and with molecular biology techniques. However, the 4 tumor types differ in terms of incidence, epidemiology, clinical features, response to therapy, and survival. Of course it needs to be stressed that all these tumors, including typical carcinoid, are malignant tumors, albeit with differing biological potential.

Small cell carcinoma is the most common neuroendocrine tumor, comprising 20% to 25% of all lung cancers; the other 3 tumor types are relatively uncommon, together comprising only 2% to 3% of all malignant lung tumors. Typical and atypical carcinoids usually affect younger patients than do small cell carcinoma and large cell neuroendocrine carcinoma. Cigarette smoking is an important risk factor for all neuroendocrine tumors. However, while almost all small cell carcinomas and large cell neuroendocrine carcinomas affect smokers, 20% to 40% of carcinoid tumors occur in nonsmokers. Both types of carcinoid tumor may be found in patients with type I multiple endocrine neoplasia syndrome, but there is no association between this syndrome and the other 2 neuroendocrine tumor types (small cell carcinoma and large cell neuroendocrine carcinoma).

Typical Carcinoid. Typical carcinoid of the lung is morphologically similar to carcinoid tumors seen in other sites. Tumor cells are arranged in nests, trabeculae, or cords or form rosettes. The tumor cells are uniform, small, have a small amount of eosinophilic cytoplasm, and have round or oval nuclei with finely granular chromatin and rare small nucleoli. These tumors may show increased cellularity, nuclear atypia, and rare mitoses. By definition, typical carcinoids measure 5.0 mm or more, have fewer than 2 mitoses per 10 high-power fields, and lack necrosis. Up to 15% of typical carcinoids metastasize to the regional lymph nodes, but these tumors rarely metastasize to distant sites or cause death.

Atypical Carcinoid. Atypical carcinoids have morphologic features similar to those of typical carcinoids except that atypical carcinoids are characterized by necrosis or 2 to 10 mitoses per 10 high-power fields (Figure 4–4), are more cellular, and have a greater degree of nuclear atypia. Neuroendocrine tumors with similar morphologic features but with more than 10 mitoses per 10 high-power fields are classified as large cell neuroendocrine

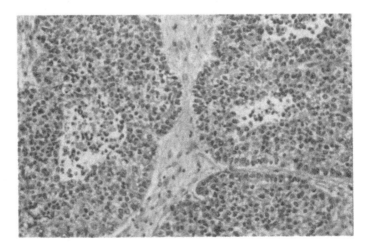

Figure 4–4. Atypical carcinoid. The tumor is arranged in nests and shows mitoses and necrosis.

carcinomas. Atypical carcinoid is distinguished from typical carcinoid by the number of mitoses and the presence of necrosis. For this reason, this distinction may be difficult in small biopsy samples. Atypical carcinoids may metastasize and cause death (Beasley et al, 2000).

Small Cell Carcinoma. In the past, small cell carcinoma was divided into oat cell carcinoma; small cell carcinoma, intermediate cell type; mixed small cell/large cell carcinoma; and combined oat cell carcinoma. However, these categories lacked prognostic significance, and there was poor interobserver reproducibility in the assignment of tumors to these categories. Therefore, in 1998, it was recommended that the terms "oat cell carcinoma" and "small cell carcinoma, intermediate cell type" be discarded and that all tumors with pure small cell carcinoma histologic features be referred to as "small cell carcinoma" (Travis et al, 1998a). The category "mixed small cell/large cell carcinoma" persisted and was defined as a tumor with both small cell and large cell carcinoma components, but subsequent studies failed to confirm the clinical significance of this categorization and there was poor interobserver reproducibility.

In the recent WHO classification, small cell carcinoma is divided into small cell carcinoma and combined small cell carcinoma. The term "small cell carcinoma" is used for tumors with pure small cell carcinoma histologic features without a NSCLC component. Combined small cell carcinoma is a mixture of small cell carcinoma and any NSCLC component, including squamous cell carcinoma, adenocarcinoma, sarcomatoid carcinoma, or large cell carcinoma—even large cell neuroendocrine carcinoma.

Small cell carcinoma is defined as a malignant tumor composed of small round to oval cells with scant cytoplasm, ill-defined cell boundaries, prominent nuclear molding, and nuclei with finely granular chromatin that either lack nucleoli or have small inconspicuous nucleoli (Figure 4–5). These tumors have a very high mitotic rate (by definition 11 or more mitoses per 10 high-power fields), and necrosis tends to be extensive.

Small cell carcinoma is distinguished from atypical carcinoid on the basis of the mitotic rate and the amount of necrosis. Atypical carcinoids have only up to 10 mitoses per 10 high-power fields, and necrosis tends to be focal. As small cell carcinomas undergo extensive necrosis, they show the Azzopardi effect within necrotic areas—i.e., a hematoxyphilic deposit of DNA from necrotic cells that is encrusted on blood vessel walls. This effect is uncommon in atypical carcinoids. Neuroendocrine differentiation is less pronounced in small cell carcinoma as assessed by both immunohistochemical staining and electron microscopy. Small cell carcinomas show focal or weak staining for chromogranin and synaptophysin, while atypical carcinoids show diffuse and strong immunoreactivity for these markers. On electron microscopy, cytoplasmic dense core neuroendocrine granules can be seen but are usually sparse in small cell carcinoma; in contrast, these granules are usually numerous and dif-

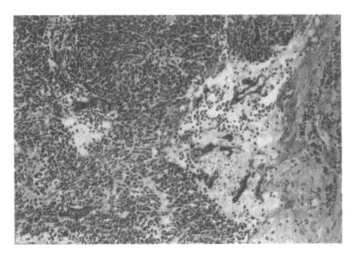

Figure 4–5. Small cell carcinoma of the lung. The tumor cells have a small amount of cytoplasm, the nuclei exhibit molding, and nucleoli are not visible. Foci of necrosis and multiple mitoses are present.

fusely distributed in the cytoplasm in atypical carcinoid. In a small crushed specimen, it may be difficult to identify mitosis and extensive tumor necrosis. However, the cells in small cell carcinoma have less cytoplasm than do the cells in carcinoids, and thus small cell carcinomas appear more hyperchromatic.

In our experience, immunohistochemical staining with chromogranin and synaptophysin is useful for differentiating small cell carcinoma from atypical carcinoid, particularly in small crushed specimens, as atypical carcinoids usually show diffuse and strong immunoreactivity for neuroendocrine markers while small cell carcinomas reveal weak and focal or no reactivity for neuroendocrine markers.

Large Cell Neuroendocrine Carcinoma. According to the WHO classification, a large cell neuroendocrine carcinoma is one that shows histologic features of large cell carcinoma with neuroendocrine differentiation and expression of neuroendocrine markers detected by either immunohistochemistry or electron microscopy. Large cell neuroendocrine carcinoma cells are more polygonal than small cell carcinoma cells, have more abundant cytoplasm, have larger nuclei with prominent nucleoli, and lack nuclear molding. Large cell neuroendocrine carcinomas resemble small cell carcinoma in 2 aspects: large areas of necrosis and high mitotic activity (large cell neuroendocrine carcinomas usually have more than 50 mitoses per 10 high-power fields) (Figure 4–6).

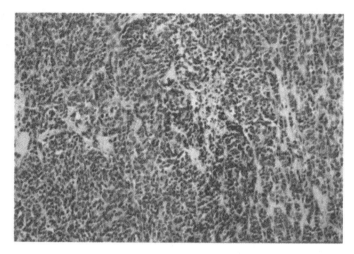

Figure 4–6. Large cell neuroendocrine carcinoma. The tumor cells are large, with hyperchromatic nuclei and prominent nucleoli.

Adenocarcinoma

Adenocarcinoma is a malignant epithelial tumor that forms glands with or without mucin production. The incidence of adenocarcinoma has significantly increased in the last 2 decades; 25% to 40% of lung cancers are now classified as adenocarcinoma, and this tumor is now the most common form of lung cancer in women and, in many studies, in men as well. Adenocarcinomas are subdivided into acinar, papillary, bronchioloalveolar, solid adenocarcinoma with mucin, adenocarcinoma with mixed subtypes, and other uncommon types. Adenocarcinoma with mixed subtypes is the most frequent adenocarcinoma encountered in routine practice. These tumors usually contain a mixture of acinar, papillary, and solid components with mucin formation and bronchioloalveolar patterns. Any of the above-mentioned subtypes may also be seen in pure form. Rare variants of adenocarcinoma include well-differentiated fetal adenocarcinoma (WDFA), mucinous (colloid) adenocarcinoma, mucinous cystadenocarcinoma, signet-ring adenocarcinoma, and clear cell adenocarcinoma.

One of the most important changes in the current WHO classification system has been in the definition of BAC. These tumors are defined as adenocarcinomas with a pure bronchioloalveolar pattern with no evidence of stromal, vascular, or pleural invasion. If invasion is present, tumors are best classified as adenocarcinoma mixed type with bronchioloalveolar features. To be sure that invasion is not overlooked, BAC should be diagnosed only after examination of resection specimens to ensure adequate sampling, and not after examination of biopsy samples alone. BAC, when defined using these strict criteria, is associated with a much better patient outcome than the other subtypes of adenocarcinoma.

In the acinar subtype of adenocarcinoma, tumor cells form acini or tubules. The papillary subtype has an abundance of papillary structures. In the solid adenocarcinoma with mucin subtype, tumor cells by definition have 5 or more mucin-positive cells in at least 2 high-power fields and lack acini, tubules, and papillae. WDFA is a very distinctive subtype that resembles fetal lung; this subtype should be distinguished from pulmonary blastoma, a biphasic tumor with a much worse prognosis. In the past, WDFA was classified as a variant of pulmonary blastoma; however, the recent WHO classification classifies WDFA as a variant of adenocarcinoma.

Histologic grading of adenocarcinomas is based on a relatively simple 3-grade system: tumors are classified as well differentiated, moderately differentiated, or poorly differentiated. Most tumors (70%) are moderately differentiated; about 25% are poorly differentiated, and only about 5% are well differentiated. The grading is based on the morphologic features of the predominant histologic pattern. Well-differentiated tumors show architectural regularity, relatively mild cytologic atypia, focal solid growth, and minimal necrosis. Most BACs are well differentiated, and most cases of solid adenocarcinoma with mucin production are poorly differentiated. Most reports confirm that well-differentiated adenocarcinomas behave better than poorly differentiated adenocarcinomas. In general, BAC and papillary adenocarcinoma behave better than the other types of adenocarcinoma. However, the degree of differentiation is not an independent prognostic factor, and prognosis is associated more with clinical stage.

Large Cell Carcinoma

Large cell carcinomas are NSCLCs that lack the morphologic features of squamous cell carcinoma, adenocarcinoma, and small cell carcinoma; in essence, large cell carcinoma is a diagnosis of exclusion. In the past, large cell carcinoma was referred to as large cell undifferentiated carcinoma. Large cell carcinoma is the least common of the major types of lung cancer, accounting for 10% to 15% of all lung cancer cases. These tumors are composed of cells with a moderate amount of cytoplasm, large nuclei, and prominent nucleoli.

Large cell carcinomas that show the morphologic features of large cell neuroendocrine carcinoma but lack expression of neuroendocrine markers as assessed with immunohistochemical staining and electron microscopy are termed large cell carcinoma with neuroendocrine morphology. In contrast, large cell carcinomas that show expression of neuroendocrine markers but lack the morphologic features of neuroendocrine carcinoma are called large cell carcinoma with neuroendocrine differentiation. It should be noted that these 2 tumor types are not considered to be distinct variants of large cell carcinoma, and their clinical significance remains to be determined.

The variants of large cell carcinoma are distinct tumors. These include large cell neuroendocrine carcinoma (described earlier, in the section Neuroendocrine Tumors of the Lung); combined large cell neuroendocrine carcinoma, which shows a mixture of NSCLC and large cell neuroendocrine carcinoma; basaloid carcinoma; lymphoepithelioma-like carcinoma; clear cell carcinoma; and large cell carcinoma with rhabdoid phenotype. The last 4 variants are very unusual and rare tumors.

Adenosquamous Carcinoma

Adenosquamous carcinoma is defined as a lung cancer showing both squamous cell carcinoma and adenocarcinoma. As mentioned earlier, near the beginning of the Malignant Tumors section, each component must comprise a minimum of 10% of the tumor. Strict criteria must be used in making this diagnosis as squamous cell carcinoma may exhibit rare foci of mucin on histochemical staining and solid adenocarcinoma may show squamoid areas, i.e., foci that resemble squamous cell carcinoma. The diagnosis of adenosquamous carcinoma should be used for tumors in which both the components show unequivocal morphologic features of squamous cell carcinoma and adenocarcinoma and per definition comprise at least 10% of the tumor.

Carcinomas with Pleomorphic, Sarcomatoid,
or Sarcomatous Elements

Carcinomas with pleomorphic, sarcomatoid, or sarcomatous elements comprise a set of NSCLC that is divided into 3 categories: carcinoma with spindle and/or giant cells; carcinosarcoma; and pulmonary blastoma.

The "carcinoma with spindle and/or giant cells" category is divided into pleomorphic carcinomas, tumors with a recognizable NSCLC component in addition to pleomorphic or spindle cells; spindle cell carcinomas, tumors composed predominantly of spindle cells without a recognizable NSCLC component; and giant cell carcinomas, tumors composed predominantly of giant cells without a recognizable NSCLC component.

Carcinosarcoma is the term used by the WHO classification for NSCLC with heterologous sarcomatous elements, such as rhabdomyosarcoma, osteosarcoma, or chondrosarcoma. At M.D. Anderson, we prefer the term "sarcomatoid carcinoma" for tumors showing a malignant spindle cell component regardless of the presence or absence of heterologous elements. The WHO definition of carcinosarcoma seems somewhat arbitrary and may be dependent on adequate sampling. As carcinosarcomas are rare, it may take some time to sort out their proper classification.

Pulmonary blastoma is a distinct biphasic tumor composed of an epithelial component that resembles well-differentiated fetal adenocarcinoma and primitive mesenchymal stroma. Pulmonary blastoma affects adults and should not be confused with pleuropulmonary blastoma, which is a tumor occurring in children.

Other Malignant Epithelial Lung Tumors

In addition to the above-mentioned malignant epithelial tumors, carcinomas of the salivary-gland type may arise from the bronchial glands. These include mucoepidermoid carcinoma, adenoid cystic carcinoma, acinic cell carcinoma, epimyoepithelial carcinoma, and malignant mixed tumor. All these tumors have morphologic features similar to their namesakes that originate in the salivary glands. Finally, malignant epithelial tumors may occur that cannot be classified in any of the above-mentioned categories; these tumors are termed "unclassified carcinoma."

ANCILLARY EVALUATION TECHNIQUES

Immunohistochemical Staining

Immunohistochemical stains are used regularly in our laboratory for the routine diagnosis of lung tumors and also for research purposes. These stains are routinely used to differentiate primary pulmonary adenocarcinoma from adenocarcinoma that has metastasized to the lung, to determine the neuroendocrine status of tumors, and to distinguish lung adenocarcinoma from epithelioid mesothelioma.

Distinguishing Primary Tumors from Metastases

Morphologically, primary adenocarcinoma of the lung may be remarkably similar to metastatic adenocarcinoma. The presence of multiple nodules in the lung in a patient with a history of a primary adenocarcinoma at another site often leads to the presumptive diagnosis of metastases. However, multifocal adenocarcinoma of the lung is not rare and needs to be distinguished from metastases. Also, some patients may develop a second primary tumor in the lung. Hence, during the evaluation of a solitary nodule of adenocarcinoma in a patient with a known history of an extrapulmonary tumor, primary adenocarcinoma of the lung needs to be ruled out.

Pulmonary adenocarcinomas stain positive for thyroid transcription factor 1 (TTF-1), cytokeratin 7, and surfactant apoprotein A but do not stain for cytokeratin 20. TTF-1 is a relatively new marker that is very useful for distinguishing between adenocarcinomas of pulmonary origin and adenocarcinomas from other sites (Ordonez, 2000a,b). TTF-1 is a transcription factor expressed by type II pneumocytes and Clara cells in the lung and also expressed in the thyroid gland, parathyroid gland, anterior pituitary, and tumors of thyroid gland and lung origin. Most carcinomas of the lung express TTF-1; however, the percentage of cases showing expression varies according to the subtype. Most adenocarcinomas of the lung and most small cell carcinomas express TTF-1; a smaller percentage of squamous cell carcinomas and large cell carcinomas express TTF-1. TTF-1 is useful for differentiating primary adenocarcinoma of the lung from adenocarcinomas that have metastasized to the lung from other sites (except in the case of metastatic thyroid carcinomas, which also express this factor).

Determining the Neuroendocrine Status of Tumors

The neuroendocrine markers used on a routine basis in our laboratory include chromogranin and synaptophysin. These 2 antibodies react with different cellular proteins—chromogranin reacts with cytoplasmic neuroendocrine granules, and synaptophysin reacts with a cell membrane glycoprotein. Thus it is important to use both markers and not use them interchangeably. The neuron-specific enolase antibody has fallen out of favor because of its lack of specificity. All typical and atypical carcinoids stain positive for chromogranin and synaptophysin. Small cell carcinomas also stain for these 2 markers, but the staining intensity is less than that seen in carcinoids because small cell carcinoma has fewer neuroendocrine granules. In up to one quarter of cases of small cell carcinoma, neuroendocrine granules are absent and thus the tumor does not stain for neuroendocrine markers. NSCLC may stain with chromogranin and synaptophysin to a variable degree.

Distinguishing Mesothelioma from Adenocarcinoma

Distinguishing mesothelioma from adenocarcinoma is one of the most important uses for immunohistochemical stains in the field of lung tumors (Ordonez, 1999a,b). In the past, only "negative" markers were available, meaning that diagnosis of mesothelioma was established with a lack of staining. The stains that are positive in adenocarcinoma but not in mesothelioma include carcinoembryonic antigen, B72.3, Ber-EP4, and MOC-31. At present, there are 2 valuable stains that are sensitive and specific for mesotheliomas: calretinin (Ordonez, 1999a,b) and cytokeratin 5/6 (Ordonez, 1999a,b). Both of these stains are usually negative in pulmonary adenocarcinoma. A note of caution is in order regarding the cytokeratin 5/6 stain, as it will stain squamous cell carcinoma of the lung. This entity, however, does not usually enter into the differential diagnosis of epithelioid mesothelioma.

Staining for Her-2/Neu and Epidermal Growth Factor Receptor

At M.D. Anderson, immunohistochemical staining for Her-2/Neu is performed using the HercepTest, developed by the Dako Corporation (Carpinteria, CA). This test is used as part of an ongoing study on the utility of the Her-2/Neu antibody for treating NSCLC. The stain for epithelial growth factor receptor antibody is another research-related immunohistochemical stain; it is used as part of a protocol using the epidermal growth factor receptor antibody for treatment of NSCLC. At present, these 2 immunohistochemical stains are used only for patients enrolled in these treatment protocols and are not part of the routine diagnostic workup.

Electron Microscopy

Electron microscopy is useful for studying the ultrastructural features of tumors. In its heyday, electron microscopy was used extensively for studying all types of tumors. At present, however, the only indicated use for electron microscopy in routine diagnostic pathology of lung tumors is to distinguish adenocarcinoma from mesothelioma in cases in which the results of immunohistochemical staining are equivocal. On electron microscopy, epithelioid mesothelioma shows characteristic abundant long and slender microvilli that are not seen in adenocarcinoma of the lung.

Molecular Biology Techniques

Molecular biology techniques have led to significant improvements in our understanding of human neoplasia, including lung cancer. At present, molecular biology techniques in lung cancer are used for research purposes only. However, in the future, these techniques will have clinical applications—for example, they may be used to stratify patients with respect to tumor characteristics and thus to indicate which patients are or are not appropriate candidates for a given therapeutic modality. In this section, we will briefly describe some of the more common abnormalities that have been reported in lung cancer.

In the past decade, the *p53* gene has been identified as one of the most common genes to be affected in human cancer. Mutations in *p53* have been reported in the preinvasive lung lesions—squamous dysplasia and carcinoma in situ and AAH. In squamous dysplasia, *p53* abnormalities have been reported in 10% to 50% of cases, with a higher incidence in the high-grade dysplasia category. In squamous carcinoma in situ, *p53* mutations have been detected by immunohistochemical staining in 60% to 90% of cases. In AAH, *p53* mutations have been reported in up to 70% of lesions. Among the malignant lung tumors, squamous cell carcinomas have the highest frequency of *p53* mutations—50% to 75% by immunohistochemical staining. Mutations in *p53* have also been reported in adenocarcinoma, atypical carcinoid, small cell carcinoma, large cell neuroendocrine carcinoma, and sarcomatoid carcinoma, although the incidence in these lesions is less than in squamous cell carcinoma.

Other genes mutated in lung cancer include the retinoblastoma gene (*Rb*), bcl-2, and K-*ras*. The *Rb* gene is mutated in almost all types of lung cancer. Mutations in *Rb* are seen most frequently in small cell carcinoma and large cell neuroendocrine carcinoma, in which the incidence of *Rb* mutations is 80% to 100%. The bcl-2 gene is strongly expressed in up to 90% of small cell carcinomas but in only 10% to 20% of atypical carcinoids; typical carcinoids do not express bcl-2. The K-*ras* gene, specifically codon 12, is mutated in AAH and adenocarcinoma. Mutations of this gene are rare in squamous cell carcinoma and in the neuroendocrine tumors. Other allelic losses reported in lung cancer include those related to chromosomes 1q, 2q, 3p, 5q, 8q, 9p, 13q, and 17p.

KEY PRACTICE POINTS

- The pathologic evaluation of a lung nodule should follow a diagnostic algorithm as up to 60% of nodules are due to nonneoplastic disease.

- The accurate classification of a lung tumor is dependent on the sampling technique. When only a limited sample is available, the pathologist may only be able to determine whether an epithelial tumor is a small cell carcinoma or a non–small cell carcinoma.

- The latest WHO classification of lung tumors includes significant changes in the definition of neuroendocrine tumors of the lung and in BAC.

- Three preinvasive lesions need to be recognized and reported: squamous dysplasia and carcinoma in situ, AAH, and DIPNECH.

- Strict criteria, as defined by the WHO classification scheme, should be used to categorize the neuroendocrine tumors of the lung as typical carcinoid, atypical carcinoid, small cell carcinoma, or large cell neuroendocrine carcinoma.

- BAC is a noninvasive carcinoma, the diagnosis of which should be rendered only after examination of a resection specimen and only after the presence of invasion has been carefully excluded.

- The TTF-1 immunohistochemical stain, used in conjunction with stains for cytokeratins 7 and 20, is useful for differentiating primary adenocarcinoma of the lung from metastatic adenocarcinoma.

- Calretinin and cytokeratin 5/6 immunohistochemical stains are useful for differentiating epithelioid mesothelioma from adenocarcinoma.

SUGGESTED READINGS

Beasley MB, Thunnissen FB, Brambilla E, et al. Pulmonary atypical carcinoid: predictors of survival in 106 cases. *Hum Pathol* 2000;31:1255–1265.

Colby TV, Koss MN, Travis WD. *Tumors of the Lower Respiratory Tract.* Washington, DC: Armed Forces Institute of Pathology and Universities Associated for Research and Education in Pathology; 1995. Atlas of Tumor Pathology, 3rd Series, fasc. 13.

Colby TV, Wistuba II, Gazdar A. Precursors to pulmonary neoplasia. *Adv Anat Pathol* 1998;5:205–215.

Edwards SL, Roberts C, McKean ME, et al. Preoperative histological classification of primary lung cancer: accuracy of diagnosis and use of the non–small cell category. *J Clin Pathol* 2000;53:537–540.

Kitamura H, Kameda Y, Ito T, et al. Atypical adenomatous hyperplasia of the lung. Implications for the pathogenesis of peripheral lung adenocarcinoma. *Am J Clin Pathol* 1999;111:610–622.

Kitamura H, Kameda Y, Nakamura N, et al. Atypical adenomatous hyperplasia and bronchoalveolar lung carcinoma. Analysis by morphometry and the expressions of p53 and carcinoembryonic antigen. *Am J Surg Pathol* 1996; 20:553–562.

Niho S, Yokose T, Suzuki K, et al. Monoclonality of atypical adenomatous hyperplasia of the lung. *Am J Pathol* 1999;154:249–254.

Ordonez NG. The immunohistochemical diagnosis of epithelial mesothelioma. *Hum Pathol* 1999a;30:313–323.

Ordonez NG. Role of immunohistochemistry in differentiating epithelial mesothelioma from adenocarcinoma. Review and update. *Am J Clin Pathol* 1999b; 112:75–89.

Ordonez NG. Thyroid transcription factor-1 is a marker of lung and thyroid carcinomas. *Adv Anat Pathol* 2000a;7:123–127.

Ordonez NG. Value of thyroid transcription factor-1 immunostaining in distinguishing small cell lung carcinomas from other small cell carcinomas. *Am J Surg Pathol* 2000b;24:1217–1223.

Sobin LH, Wittekind CH, eds. *TNM Classification of Malignant Tumors.* 5th ed. New York, NY: J. Wiley; 1997:93–100.

Travis WD, Colby TV, Corrin B, et al. *Histological Typing of Lung and Pleural Tumors.* 3rd ed. New York, NY: Springer-Verlag; 1999.

Travis WD, Gal AA, Colby TV, et al. Reproducibility of neuroendocrine lung tumor classification. *Hum Pathol* 1998a;29:272–279.

Travis WD, Rush W, Flieder DB, et al. Survival analysis of 200 pulmonary neuroendocrine tumors with clarification of criteria for atypical carcinoid and its separation from typical carcinoid. *Am J Surg Pathol* 1998b;22:934–944.

5 ROLE OF CLINICAL PRACTICE GUIDELINES AND CLINICAL PATHWAYS IN THE TREATMENT OF PATIENTS WITH LUNG CANCER

Yvette De Jesus and Garrett L. Walsh

CHAPTER OVERVIEW

Over the past decade, many health care institutions have developed and implemented clinical practice guidelines and clinical pathways as a means of standardizing patient care and managing costs while preserving the quality of services delivered. A clinical practice guideline is a framework for treating a specific disease entity and includes all treatment modalities supported by the medical literature, current practice standards, and expert opinion. Guidelines are often presented in the form of flowcharts. Clinical pathways are detailed, step-by-step descriptions of how to deliver the various treatments that form a practice guideline.

At M. D. Anderson Cancer Center, guidelines and pathways are used to guide care for patients with non–small cell lung cancer and small cell lung cancer. Use of these tools has enabled us to standardize our approach to patient care, analyze differences in patient outcomes between physicians, and discover where current practice patterns need to be changed. Guidelines and pathways also serve as valuable educational tools for residents and fellows training at our institution and help to optimize trainees' clinical practice behavior, leading to optimal patient care with minimal unnecessary laboratory and radiographic testing.

INTRODUCTION

More than 180,000 patients will be diagnosed with lung cancer in 2002, and nearly 85% of these patients will ultimately die of their disease. The initial evaluation, clinical staging, and treatment of these patients must be conducted in a structured and cost-effective manner to ensure that optimum care is delivered with the most efficacious use of health care resources. Over the past decade, the expansion in managed care coverage has put health care institutions increasingly under pressure to monitor costs while preserving the quality of their services. Many facilities have accomplished this by developing and implementing evidence-based tools such as clinical practice guidelines and clinical pathways. The purpose of using these evidence-based tools is to enhance, manage, and evaluate patient care while maintaining appropriate outcomes using a cost-effective approach. Clinical practice guidelines and clinical pathways have proven to be highly effective for managing patient populations with varying medical and oncologic diagnoses and different stages of disease.

This chapter will describe our collective efforts at M. D. Anderson Cancer Center in the development and implementation of guidelines for evaluating and treating patients with lung cancer. We will describe our pathway for pulmonary resection to illustrate how pathways can streamline the daily care of patients who undergo thoracic surgery.

CLINICAL PRACTICE GUIDELINES AND
CLINICAL PATHWAYS—DEFINITIONS

Clinical Practice Guidelines

A clinical practice guideline is a framework for treating a specific disease entity. Guidelines, which are often presented as flowcharts, include all possible treatment modalities supported by the medical literature, current practice standards, and expert opinion. Guidelines, therefore, are relatively broad brush stroke treatment strategies. Guidelines are developed after an extensive review of the medical literature, including consensus statements.

Clinical Pathways

Clinical pathways are detailed descriptions of the specific treatment options that form a practice guideline. A clinical pathway is a standardized, detailed sequence of events that occurs during an episode of care. Like guidelines, pathways are multidisciplinary, requiring the collaboration of all health care providers at the design, implementation, and evaluation phases. Categories of care covered in clinical pathways might include consultations, diagnostic tests, treatments, medications, diet, teaching and psychosocial counseling, and discharge planning. Pathways are the "to do" lists for episodes of care and are developed for "ideal" patients. Pathways are, however, merely guides and cannot take the place of clinicians' independent clinical judgment.

The documents prepared for clinical pathways include procedure-specific informed consent forms, preprinted physician order sheets (Figure 5–1), patient education materials, and patient outcomes documentation. Physicians and other appropriate health care providers review the completed draft documents, and a consensus is sought. The approved and implemented pathway documents require revisions as the health care team members identify new clinical issues that can be addressed in the plan of care.

In academic centers, with frequent rotations of residents and fellows, pathways serve as valuable educational guides for these trainees by quickly outlining "how we do it on our service." The use of structured pathways can significantly guide residents' and fellows' practice behavior and optimize quality patient care while minimizing unnecessary laboratory and radiographic testing.

DEVELOPMENT AND USE OF
GUIDELINES AT M. D. ANDERSON

At M.D. Anderson, institutional clinical practice guidelines are used to better understand and evaluate our own practices and serve as tools to

THE UNIVERSITY OF TEXAS
MD ANDERSON
CANCER CENTER

Inpatient
Physician Orders

Pulmonary Resection Post-Op Orders

Attending Physician: _____
Height: _____ cm   Weight: _____ kg   Start Date: _____
Allergies: _____

MD's signature indicates all orders are activated. To delete an order, draw one line through the item, write "delete," and initial your entry.

Primary Diagnosis _____
Admitting Diagnosis _____

Admit To
☐ PACU, then monitored bed   ☐ PACU, then non-monitored room
☐ PACU overnight   ☐ SICU

Diagnostic Tests
☐ PCXR stat   ☐ PCXR in arm   ☐ PA & Lat CXR in arm
☐ CBC stat   ☐ CBC in arm   ☐ ABG stat

Vital Signs
Routine per PACU/SICR/Telemetry Unit, then q4h x 48 hours, then every shift. Call HO if:
HR > 110 or < 50   Temp > 38.5°C   SBP > 180 or < 90
DBP ≥ 110   Urine output < 30 mL over 2 h or < 200 mL per shift
For pain score ≥ 5, call team managing pain.

Activity
☐   Bed rest.
☐   Ambulate on ward > TID with assistance.
☐   Out of bed to chair > TID for 1 hour and/or for each meal.

Treatment
1.   If in SICU, call Thoracic on call. Pager 404-3147 for ALL calls after 6:00 p.m.
2.   Head of bed at 30°.
3.   Foley to dependent drainage.
4.   DVT prophylaxis:
     a. TED stockings (thigh high).
     b. Compression stockings until fully ambulatory.
5.   Document input and output.
6.   Chest tubes:
     ☐ Water seal OR   ☐ Pleurevac suction 20 cm OR   ☐ Emerson suction 40 cm

Respiratory Care
1.   Ventilator settings as indicated below:
     ☐ SIMV _____   ☐ AC _____   ☐ TV _____   ☐ Other: _____
     ☐ PEEP _____   ☐ FiO₂ _____   ☐ PS _____
2.   Administer medication(s) indicated below:
     ☐ Albuterol 0.3 mL ☐ with 3 mL NS q4h
     ☐ Albuterol 0.5 mL ☐ with 2 mL 10% Mucomyst q4h
     ☐ Ipratropium bromide 0.5 mg in 2.5 mL NS q6h
3.   Chest physiotherapy q4h.
                    See Next Page—Respiratory Care and other orders continued

Physician's Signature: _____   Physician's Number: _____
Pager: _____   Date: _____   Time: _____
Orders transcribed by: ____ Date/time: _____ Orders verified by: _____ Date/time: ____

FAX COMPLETED ORDERS TO PHARMACY .
File under: Physician Orders   Page 1 of 2

Figure 5–1. Preprinted physician order form for postoperative care after pulmonary resection. Reprinted with permission from The University of Texas M.D. Anderson Cancer Center.

THE UNIVERSITY OF TEXAS
MD ANDERSON
CANCER CENTER

**Inpatient
Physician Orders**

Pulmonary Resection Post-Op Orders
See Previous Page

Respiratory Care, continued

4. If cough ineffective, NT suction q4h with soft coude tip catheter.
5. O_2 therapy via nasal cannula or face shield: titrate O_2 to maintain O_2 saturation to $\geq$ 92%.
6. Incentive spirometry (x10) and cough and deep breathe exercise by nurse every hour while awake, q2h at night.
7. O_2 tank for ambulation.

Diet

1. POD 1 NPO except for ice chips.
2. POD 2 clear liquids if not nauseated, then diet as tolerated.

IV Fluids

1. D5 _ NS with 20 mEq KCl @ 75 mL/h. Decrease IVFs to 15 mL/h on POD 1
   (Date:_____) if patient tolerating PO fluids.

Medications

    Antibiotics

    Administer as indicated below:

    ☐   Unasyn 1.5 gm IV q8h x 3 doses (no PCN allergy).
    ☐   Ciprofloxacin 400 mg IVPB q12h x 3 doses (PCN allergy).
    ☐   Other _____

    DVT Prophylaxis

    Heparin 5,000 units SC q12h.

    Pain Medications

    1. PCA:
       Med: _____

	Loading Dose (optional)	Basal (optional)	PRN Dose	Lockout Time	Hourly Max (optional)
_____	____ mg	____ mg/h	____ mg	____ min	____ mg/h

    2. When epidural or PCA discontinued, begin:
       a. Hydrocodone 7.5 mg/acetaminophen 500 mg 1-2 tablets PO q4h PRN or
       b. Hydrocodone 2.5 mg/acetaminophen 167 mg per 5 mL elixir 15-30 mL PO/per J-tube q3-4 h PRN.
    3. May wean PCA to PO analgesics after 4 days per patient tolerance.

    Scheduled Medications

    Surfak 1 PO daily.

    Medications as Needed (PRN)

    1. Ondansetron 4-8 mg IVPB q6h PRN nausea.
    2. Acetaminophen 650 mg PO/PT q4h PRN temp > 38°C.
       (Note: maximum dose of acetaminophen = 4 gm/24 hours.)
    3. Laxative of choice.
    4. Dulcolax suppository 1 PR qd as needed for constipation. May repeat 1 x if needed.
    5. Diphenhydramine 12.5 mg IVPB q4h PRN itching.

    Consults

    Anesthesia consult for management of epidural.

Physician's Signature: _____ Physician's Number: _____
Orders transcribed by: _____ Date/time: _____ Orders verified by: _____ Date/time: _____

FAX COMPLETED ORDERS TO PHARMACY
File under: Physician Orders   **Page 2 of 2**

Figure 5–1. *(continued)*

guide quality oncologic care on our campus as well as at institutions with whom we are affiliated. Guidelines are frequently referred to during multidisciplinary planning conferences during review of the specific oncology practice standards and treatment options. Our institutional guidelines not only outline options for initial treatment of the primary lesion but also address the indications for and timing of neoadjuvant and adjuvant therapies; outline how follow-up and surveillance testing should be performed after a given therapy is completed; and describe when salvage treatment and supportive care measures should be considered. Because M. D. Anderson is a research institution, our guidelines also mention the possibility of patients' eligibility for institutional or cooperative-group protocols whenever appropriate.

Many M. D. Anderson faculty members have participated in the development of the National Comprehensive Cancer Network guidelines (available at www.nccn.org), and many of these guidelines have been expanded to meet our specific institutional practice and protocol research strategies. The M. D. Anderson guidelines are available on our Web site: www.mdanderson.org.

Guidelines for Treatment of Lung Cancer Patients

When lung cancer patients are referred to M. D. Anderson with a lesion that has already been biopsied, their diagnosis places them in one of 2 categories, each with a corresponding clinical practice guideline: non–small cell lung carcinoma (large cell, adenocarcinoma, squamous cell, or bronchoalveolar histologic subtypes) or small cell lung carcinoma. Following are some of the salient features of these guidelines.

Clinical Guideline for Non–Small Cell Lung Cancer

All patients with non–small cell lung cancer have a history and physical examination, along with basic complete blood cell counts and liver function tests. In addition, all patients, regardless of the histologic subtype of their disease, undergo chest radiography and computed tomography (CT) of the chest, including the upper cross-sections of the abdomen and the adrenals. The CT scan of the chest is one of the most important imaging studies obtained as it allows initial clinical staging of the disease. A formal CT scan of the abdomen or pelvis is not requested as this has low yield in the detection of metastases. Brain scans and bone scans are performed if they are indicated on the basis of a patient's symptoms or findings on physical examination. Magnetic resonance imaging is used only for the evaluation of superior sulcus tumors or tumors that appear to involve the vertebral body. In the case of superior sulcus tumors, the coronal imaging provided by magnetic resonance imaging permits a more detailed evaluation of brachial plexus involvement than can be obtained with CT of the chest. Intervertebral foraminal extension and extradural spread are more readily appreciated with magnetic resonance imaging than with CT.

The radiographic findings are evaluated to determine the clinical T status (a measure of local invasiveness) and N status (a measure of systemic biological metastatic potential) of the tumor. All lung tumors are potentially curable with surgery if the mediastinal nodes are not involved. T3 tumors that involve the chest wall, diaphragm, or pericardium are also potentially curable with surgery. T4 tumors with only limited vertebral body involvement or limited involvement of the great vessels, heart, or trachea are also potentially curable with surgery.

Patients who present with a pleural effusion containing tumor cells, a superior sulcus tumor that extensively involves the brachial plexus more proximal to the T1 nerve root with loss of motor function of the affected limb, or a lesion with direct involvement of the esophagus are not considered candidates for surgery.

Nodal status is often assessed by measuring the cross-sectional diameter of the nodes under the mediastinal windows on CT. Contrast-enhanced CT is often helpful in differentiating mediastinal vascular structures from the surrounding nodes. Nodes 1 cm or larger in diameter are considered radiographically positive and often necessitate additional pathologic assessment prior to a major resection. It must be recognized, however, that 15% of nodes smaller than 1 cm may harbor micrometastatic disease and that 30% of nodes larger than 2 cm may be benign. Enlarged nodes can be biopsied by an interventional radiologist using transthoracic or transmediastinal needle biopsy or can be biopsied surgically through cervical mediastinoscopy, anterior mediastinotomy (Chamberlain procedure; used to evaluate prevascular and anteroposterior window nodes), or video-assisted thoracoscopic techniques.

Prior to surgery, all patients undergo spirometry testing with measurements taken before and after administration of a bronchodilator. Patients whose forced expiratory volume in 1 second (FEV_1) is less than 70% also undergo xenon ventilation-perfusion scanning, which permits estimation of the postresection FEV_1 on the basis of the regional distribution of the nuclear tracer. If the postresection FEV_1 is less than 40%, more detailed exercise oxygen consumption testing is performed before a final decision is made regarding whether a given patient is fit for surgery.

Patients with clinical stage I or II disease who have a predicted postresection FEV_1 of greater than 33% may undergo surgical resection. If the final pathologic stage is stage I, no further treatment is required, and patients are placed on a surveillance program after their first postoperative visit. Patients with positive mediastinal nodes on the final pathology report are offered radiation therapy to improve future local control; however, no survival advantage is seen with radiation therapy in this group.

Patients who are found on preoperative mediastinoscopy to have stage IIIA disease undergo brain and bone scans. If the disease is localized to the chest only, then combined treatment with neoadjuvant chemotherapy with a platinum-based regimen followed by radiation therapy is considered the standard of care. On rare occasions in patients with limited N2 disease (single-station, intranodal microscopic disease) documented by mediastinoscopy, surgery can be reconsidered after neoadjuvant chemotherapy and extensive restaging.

Patients with T3 and T4 tumors, a normal mediastinum, and no other symptoms undergo brain and bone scans prior to resection even if they have no symptoms of bone or brain involvement. The expected morbidity and mortality of the more extensive operation required to remove these lesions warrants this more detailed and costly evaluation prior to thoracotomy.

Patients with stage IIIB disease or metastatic disease undergo therapy based on their Zubrod performance status.

While most patients with stage IV disease (distant metastases) are treated with palliative intent only, patients with a solitary brain metastasis and a resectable lung lesion can still be cured with an aggressive surgical approach to both lesions.

Patients with stage I or II, completely resected non–small cell lung carcinoma have follow-up examinations every 6 months for the first year and then yearly thereafter with physical examination and chest radiography only. Examination of the supraclavicular fossa for nodal disease is perhaps the most important aspect of the follow-up physical examinations. Routine blood work, sputum cytology testing, and carcinoembryonic antigen testing are not performed. Other tests are performed only if symptoms develop or abnormalities are detected on physical examination.

Patients with stage III or IV non–small cell lung carcinoma have follow-up examinations every 2 to 3 months for the first 2 years and every 6 months thereafter. Chest radiography is performed at each follow-up visit. CT is done only if chest radiography demonstrates a change.

Clinical Guideline for Small Cell Lung Cancer

The staging system for small cell lung carcinoma has just 2 categories: limited-stage disease (involving the chest only) and extensive-stage disease (involving areas outside the chest—e.g., bone marrow, brain, or bones).

All patients with small cell carcinoma have their disease staged with a CT scan of the brain and a bone scan because the small cell histologic subtype has a much more aggressive biological behavior than the non–small cell subtype, with a greater propensity to metastasize.

The role of surgery in the treatment of small cell lung carcinoma is limited; surgery is rarely a component of the care of patients with this disease. Infrequently, a solitary pulmonary lesion is detected in an asymptomatic patient on a screening chest radiograph obtained for an unrelated reason. These solitary lesions are often resected and discovered to be small cell carcinoma on the final pathologic analysis. If, however, the pulmonary lesion is first sampled with a transthoracic needle biopsy and small cell subtype is either confirmed or suspected, mediastinoscopy is required prior to thoracotomy. Mediastinoscopy would be done even in the presence of a "normal" appearance on mediastinal CT imaging because small cell carcinoma typically spreads early to regional lymph nodes.

Treatment with a combination of cisplatin and etoposide is considered the standard of care for patients with small cell lung carcinoma, with radiation therapy considered for prophylactic cranial irradiation (even in patients with negative findings on CT of the brain), for treatment of mediastinal nodal disease, and for immediate palliation of cord compression or bone metastases.

Patients with small cell lung carcinoma are followed more closely than patients with non–small cell lung carcinoma—every 2 to 3 months for the first 2 years and every 6 months thereafter. Chest radiography is performed at each visit; CT scans are done only if chest radiography demonstrates a change.

CLINICAL PATHWAY FOR PATIENTS UNDERGOING PULMONARY RESECTION

Pathway Design and Implementation

In an effort to identify best practices and standardize the M. D. Anderson approach to pulmonary resection for lung cancer and to permit better measurement of outcomes in patients undergoing this procedure at M. D. Anderson, a multidisciplinary group from our institution met several times between October 1995 and December 1995 to develop a clinical pathway for pulmonary resection. All health care providers regularly involved in the care of lung cancer patients had an important role in crafting the pathway. The pathway development group therefore included thoracic surgeons, thoracic anesthesiologists, outpatient clinic nurses, operating room and recovery room nurses, inpatient floor nurses, social workers, case managers, surgical residents, advanced practice nurses, physician assistants, respiratory therapists, pharmacists, and dieticians.

During the pathway development process, each of the required steps in caring for patients undergoing pulmonary resection—including preoperative outpatient clinic visits and care delivered in the holding area of the operating room, the operating room itself, the postanesthesia care unit, and the inpatient telemetry unit—was identified within the overall plan of care, or clinical pathway. Each point on the pathway was evaluated to determine if it was necessary. Treatments and tests judged to be inappropriate, wasteful, or unnecessary were eliminated.

The final pathway packet included the pathway itself, outcomes documentation, preprinted physician order forms, patient informed consent forms, and patient educational materials. The pathway documents are maintained in a Lotus Notes database that can be accessed anytime from

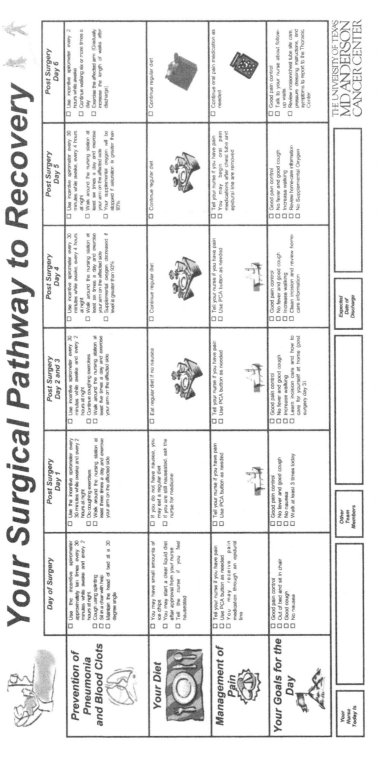

Figure 5-2. Patient "pathway to recovery" poster. Reprinted with permission from The University of Texas M.D. Anderson Cancer Center.

any computer within our institutional network. This database facilitates the maintenance and revision of all documents affiliated with the pathway. The purpose of the database is to track the patients on the pathway and serve as the single central source for printouts of standardized order and consent forms and preoperative educational materials designed for patients and their families.

We enlarged and laminated a "patient's version" of the pulmonary resection pathway and placed these posters strategically in each hospital room to remind patients of their daily goals (Figure 5–2). In addition to the posters that outline what to expect during each day of the hospital stay, patients are given handouts covering what to expect during surgery and recovery, use of the incentive spirometer, epidural pain control techniques, and other issues related to pathway-based care (Figure 5–3). Utilizing the patient's version of the pathway empowers patients and family members to participate in the plan of care. This approach is supported in the patient education literature and leads to setting clear patient expectations.

The pathway was implemented in January 1996. Before implementation of the pathway, extensive efforts were undertaken to ensure that all members of the health care team—attending physicians, residents, fellows, and nurses—understood the pathway and related documentation. Adherence to pathway-based care was stressed during fellows' and residents' rotations. In-service training on use of pathway documentation was held for all 3 nursing shifts. Posters describing how to document pathway-related events were developed and posted throughout the inpatient unit, the postanesthesia care unit, and the outpatient clinic.

As of December 2001, more than 1,900 patients had been treated on the pathway.

Pathway Procedures

Outpatient Clinic Visits

Once the decision has been made that a patient will undergo a pulmonary resection, the patient is enrolled on the pulmonary resection pathway. Enrollment is done in the outpatient clinic. When the patient is entered in the database, the computer system automatically generates order sets and standardized consent forms for surgery and use of blood products for inclusion in the medical record. Patient identifiers are automatically printed on each form.

Patient-specific educational materials are printed for the patient and his or her family members to review, including the pathway itself and information regarding the proper use of an incentive spirometer and the use of patient-controlled analgesia devices, including epidural catheters. The patient is also shown an educational video that describes the anesthesia consultation, what will occur in the holding area and the operating room, the use of telemetry monitors after surgery, recommended wound care practices and arm exercises, and the use of the chest tube drainage system.

Day of Surgery

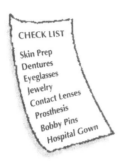

CHECK LIST
Skin Prep
Dentures
Eyeglasses
Jewelry
Contact Lenses
Prosthesis
Bobby Pins
Hospital Gown

holding area:
a patient waiting room
near the operating room

IV:
a small tube inserted into a
vein, through which you receive
medicine and fluids

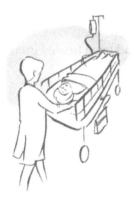

Getting ready for surgery

- Report for surgery as you were instructed.
- Put on a hospital gown. It is the only thing you can wear to the operating room.
- Do not wear anything that can come off during surgery, such as dentures or partial plates, eyeglasses or contact lenses, jewelry, bobby pins, hair clips, wigs, or any removable prosthesis, such as an artificial eye or leg.
- Go to the bathroom and empty your bladder.
- You may be given medicine to help you relax.
- You will be helped onto a stretcher and moved to the holding area.

In the holding area

- A blood pressure cuff will be put on your arm.
- An IV will be placed in a vein in your hand or arm.
- A nurse will ask you questions to verify any drug allergies or to discuss concerns you may have.

In the operating room

- You will come into the operating room on a stretcher. A nurse will help you move to the operating table.
- If you feel cold, ask for a blanket.
- Your family and friends may stay in the surgery waiting area. They are not allowed in the operating room.
- Staff will be wearing uniforms, masks, and caps.
- An ECG machine will monitor your heart rate.
- You will receive the anesthetic through your IV.
- After you are asleep, a tube will be put in your throat to help you breathe.

Figure 5–3. Patient education literature. Reprinted with permission from The University of Texas M. D. Anderson Cancer Center.

Anesthesia Consultation

Before surgery, patients are examined by a member of the Department of Anesthesia. A standard preoperative evaluation is performed, and preoperative blood work is done, including measurement of serum creatinine levels and a "type and screen" for blood. Electrocardiography is performed in patients over the age of 40 years and in all patients with a history of a cardiac disorder. A nurse or other health-care professional meets with the patient to explain the use of epidural pain management devices. These efforts are reinforced by all staff members of the thoracic service.

Clinical Preparation for Surgery

Elective admissions prior to the day of surgery have been eliminated from our standard of practice for patients undergoing pulmonary resection. Elderly and diabetic patients have their surgery scheduled for the beginning of the day. On the day of surgery, the epidural catheter is placed and intravenous access is obtained while the patient is in the holding area outside the operating room; this practice minimizes operating room time and personnel costs.

Operating Room

As part of the pulmonary resection pathway development process, the thoracic surgeons and the operating room nurses on the dedicated thoracic team conducted a detailed review of the use of operating room time and instruments. Their findings resulted in several practice changes that were incorporated into the final clinical pathway. The use of dedicated nursing teams has improved efficiency and optimized operating room utilization. The thoracotomy trays have been standardized so that there is no variation between surgeons. Specialty instruments that were rarely utilized were removed from the packs to expedite instrument counting and minimize set-up time. Skin preparation solutions were standardized, as were draping techniques. The use of perioperative antibiotics was standardized with the help of colleagues in the Department of Infectious Diseases. Finally, prophylaxis against deep venous thrombosis was also standardized.

In the operating room, patients with no history of gastroesophageal reflux are intubated initially with a laryngeal mask airway. This is a device that minimizes the trauma to the larynx associated with repeated endotracheal intubations and permits the initial bronchoscopy to be performed with full evaluation of the vocal cords and upper airway. The laryngeal mask airway is then replaced with a double-lumen endotracheal tube. Positioning and padding of the patient are routine and standardized. Surgical techniques differ among surgeons, but residents spend 1 to 2 months rotating on each surgeon's service so that they can learn his or her individual routine. Chest tube drainage systems and closure techniques are routine and vary little by surgeon. The epidural catheter is loaded with pain medication during the chest closure.

In virtually all cases, patients are extubated in the operating room and transported directly to the recovery room. Postoperative admission to the intensive care unit is very rare and is reserved for patients who have undergone concomitant chest wall resections or extensive procedures with replacement of large fluid volumes that necessitate overnight mechanical ventilation.

Recovery Room

Patients spend 2 to 3 hours in the recovery room, where the anesthesia pain service closely monitors pain control as patients awaken. A 24-hour, in-hospital anesthesia pain service monitors and adjusts the epidural dosing throughout the patient's hospital course to facilitate early ambulation and optimize pulmonary toilet. All patients have chest radiography with a portable radiography unit in the recovery room. Whether and how often radiographs are subsequently obtained is dictated by the patient's clinical condition and findings on daily physical examination. All patients are transferred to the telemetry unit when they are hemodynamically stable with acceptable chest tube drainage and adequate initial pain control.

Telemetry Unit and Remainder of Hospital Stay

The evening of surgery, patients are helped out of bed and are expected to spend at least 15 minutes in a chair and walk if possible. Incentive spirometry is started immediately after extubation. A dedicated thoracic respiratory therapist works daily with the patient, following the clinical pathway for decisions regarding the use of bronchodilators, oxygen weaning, and the periodic use of nasotracheal suctioning. Chest tubes are maintained on suction for the first 24 hours and then switched to water seal if there are no air leaks. In the telemetry unit, patients are continuously monitored with telemetry monitors to detect supraventricular arrhythmias (dysrhythmia) and with continuous oxygen saturation monitors. These units are portable and in potentially high-risk patients can be used even while patients are walking.

The clinical pathway clearly outlines the expected timeline for patient recovery, including benchmarks for walking, making the transition from clear liquids to solids, wound care, arm exercises, and discharge planning. Patients know ahead of time that they will be discharged the day the chest tubes are removed. Epidural catheters are maintained in place for most of the hospital stay. At least 6 to 12 hours prior to discharge, the catheter is removed, and oral analgesics are begun.

Analysis of Patient Outcomes and Costs Associated with Pathway-Based Care

Standardization of care through the use of clinical pathways facilitates analyses of trends in patient outcomes and costs over time and between health care providers. It is very important to analyze outcomes on a regular basis—for example, quarterly; such analysis requires a well-supported infrastructure, including several full-time employees and the software to support their efforts. A staffing model would be dependent on the number of pathways and usage of pathways in the facility. The interval between analyses and the specific trends analyzed can be determined on the basis of clinicians' requests or the importance of the specific clinical practice in question. Appropriate software should be in place prior to implementation of this type of analysis.

The outcomes that our multidisciplinary thoracic surgery team was interested in were readmission trends, 30-day mortality, and average cost per patient in each category of care. Data are presented here for the period covering the first 4 years after implementation of the pathway.

During the first 4 years after pathway implementation, the readmission rate was at or below 5% (Figure 5–4). This is an acceptable rate given that some of our patients have extensive lung resections, which are associated with a higher risk of postoperative complications that may require readmission. The multidisciplinary thoracic surgery team decided that a readmission rate for any single surgeon of greater than 5% would automatically trigger a detailed analysis of patients requiring readmission. This analysis would help the surgeon identify any opportunities for improving standard practice.

The 30-day mortality rate for patients undergoing pulmonary resection decreased over the first 4 years after pathway implementation (Figure 5–5). In the year 2000, the 30-day mortality rate was less than 1% and was considered acceptable by our thoracic surgery service.

In addition to monitoring patient outcomes, we also track the hospital charges associated with pathway-based care to determine where costs may be reduced. For example, in analyzing cost data, we identified respi-

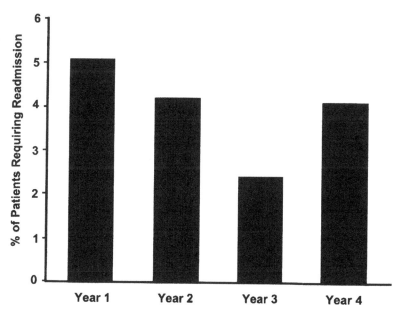

Figure 5–4. Proportion of patients undergoing pulmonary resection requiring readmission, years 1 to 4 after implementation of the pulmonary resection pathway.

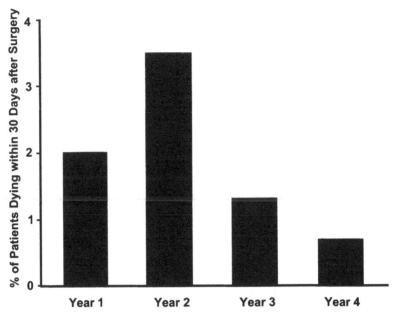

Figure 5–5. Proportion of patients treated with pulmonary resection dying within 30 days after surgery, years 1 to 4 after implementation of the pulmonary resection pathway.

ratory therapy services as expensive, and we have since transitioned many of these services to the nursing staff. Physician profiling by procedure helps physicians compare their own use of disposable instruments and suture material with that of their colleagues. Other physician practices profiled are the use of laboratory tests and the use of radiographs.

During the first 4 years after pathway implementation, total costs per pulmonary resection were higher than the costs for this procedure before pathway implementation. However, costs in certain categories of care, including surgery and diagnostic procedures, were close to costs before pathway implementation.

Analysis of Deviations from the Pathway

Twenty to 30% of patients undergoing pulmonary resection require individualized care that deviates from the standard of care as outlined in the pulmonary resection pathway. Deviations from the pathway can be attributed to one of 4 factors: patient, caregiver, system, or environment. Patient and caregiver factors are known as "people factors" and account for the majority of deviations from the pathway.

Examples of patient factors include patient refusal or inability to accomplish a given goal for walking. Examples of caregiver factors (a caregiver is defined as any health care professional who participates directly in a given patient's care) are a physician's or resident's delaying signing of the discharge orders, resulting in a hospital stay being prolonged by several hours, and a unit coordinator's forgetting to order a test. An example of a system factor would be a breakdown in the institution's electronic medical record that delays the scheduling of a chest radiograph. Environment factors are all other processes and structures that affect patient care—for example, procedure, room, or equipment availability and forces external to the hospital (Cole et al, 1996).

To better understand these deviations from pathway care, we developed a variance tracking form that is attached to each patient's chart. This form is used to record all deviations as they occur during the course of care, along with the reasons for these deviations. This form is scanned every couple of days, and the data are analyzed. The intent of our deviations tracking tool is to maximize compliance with the pathway and to monitor unexpected outcomes. Through a detailed, real-time evaluation of all deviations, we can get an accurate measurement of where improvements can be made and where efforts should be directed.

Analysis of deviations is essential for helping us determine where the pathway needs to be revised. On the basis of this type of analysis, we constantly scrutinize our definition of the optimal standard of care for our patients.

THE FUTURE

Our lung cancer guidelines and pathways will be revised in the future to reflect advances in the understanding of this disease and advances in technology.

Over the past few years, we have witnessed some minor changes to the staging system for lung cancer, introduction of newer drugs for stage IV disease, and randomized trials that have examined the use of preoperative chemotherapy for earlier-stage tumors. Surgical techniques, including the use of vascular grafting and techniques to resect tumors directly involving the spinal column and repair the resulting defects, have permitted us to redefine and extend the boundaries of lesions that may be resected for cure. All of these changes have been incorporated into revisions of our guidelines.

As newer tests and drugs become available, the standard initial evaluation of patients will change. With the advent of high-speed, low-dose CT scans, we envision that in the future the vast majority of lung cancers will be detected when they are in the 5- to 10-mm range.

KEY PRACTICE POINTS

- The purpose of using clinical practice guidelines and clinical pathways is to enhance, manage, and evaluate patient care while measuring and maintaining appropriate outcomes using a cost-effective approach.
- A clinical practice guideline is a framework for treating a specific disease entity and includes all treatment modalities supported by the medical literature, current practice standards, and expert opinion. Guidelines are often presented in the form of flowcharts.
- Clinical pathways are detailed, step-by-step descriptions of the various treatment options that form a practice guideline.
- Guidelines and pathways serve as valuable teaching tools that help residents and fellows learn best practices for patient care.
- The use of structured pathways can help trainees deliver optimal patient care with minimal unnecessary laboratory and radiographic testing.
- Use of structured pathways permits analysis of differences in patient outcomes and costs between physicians.
- Analysis of deviations from clinical pathways can indicate where pathways need to be changed.

Following the CT scan, patients will undergo a nuclear imaging staging procedure to determine whether distant metastases are present. If the findings are negative for distant metastases, patients will be referred directly to surgery, where biopsy and surgical treatment will be done at the same time after some form of exercise testing that will most likely differ from our present, static spirometric testing. Larger tumors that are still isolated to the chest will be treated with neoadjuvant chemotherapy prior to surgery. Patients with positive findings on nuclear screening will be referred to medical oncologists and may undergo chemotherapy, but probably with agents less toxic than those in use today.

Surgical pathways will be far simpler. The anesthetic agents will be better tolerated. Techniques will be developed for better postoperative pain control. Tissue sealants will be developed that will minimize the problem of postoperative air leaks that are often responsible for a prolonged hospital stay after pulmonary resection. Chest tubes will be removed within 12 to 24 hours, and patients will be monitored in a hotel environment with telemetry monitoring from a distance and with rehabilitation specialists rather than nurses helping to minimize the risk of perioperative pneumonia. Better oral analgesics will permit pain control without the ileus and gastrointestinal side effects that presently delay many discharges. Surveillance will continue with high-speed CT scanners, but the need for follow-up patient visits to the clinic will be minimized.

In the M. D. Anderson Thoracic Center, we now have more than 40 active research protocols for various stages and pathologic subtypes of lung cancer. It is often difficult for clinicians to remember all the specific inclusion and exclusion criteria for these research studies. In the near future, guidelines will be imbedded in our electronic medical record, and our computer system will facilitate decision analysis as the various data from the history and physical examination and radiographic workup of the patient are entered. This decision analysis will help physicians determine which patients may benefit from investigational studies and which patients should receive the standard of care as recognized by institutional or national guidelines. This decision tree analysis will be complicated and will require constant monitoring and updating as newer drugs and techniques become available. This will represent the best use of computers in the medical environment—to ensure that patients are always receiving the most appropriate and up-to-date care for their stage of disease.

Suggested Readings

Benson DS. *Measuring Outcomes in Ambulatory Care.* Chicago, Ill: American Hospital Publishing Inc; 1992.

Bohmer R. Critical pathways at Massachusetts General Hospital. *J Vasc Surg* 1998;28:373–377.

Butterworth J. Clinical pathways for the high-risk patient. *J Cardiothorac Vasc Anesth* 1997;11(2 Suppl 1):16–18.

Cabana MD, Rand CS, Powe NR, et al. Why don't physicians follow clinical practice guidelines? A framework for improvement. *JAMA* 1999;282:1458–1465.

Chen AY, Callender D, Mansyur C, et al. The impact of clinical pathways on the practice of head and neck oncologic surgery: The University of Texas M. D. Anderson Cancer Center experience. *Arch Otolaryngol Head Neck Surg* 2000;126:322–326.

Cole L, Lasker-Hertz S, Grady G, et al. Structured care methodologies: tools for standardization and outcomes measurement. *Nurs Case Manag* 1996;1:160–172.

Davis JT, Allen HD, Felver K, et al. Clinical pathways can be based on acuity, not diagnosis. *Ann Thorac Surg* 1995;59:1074–1078.

Donabedian A. *The Definition of Quality and Approaches to Its Assessment.* Ann Arbor, Mich: Health Administration Press; 1980:14–15. *Explorations in Quality Assessment and Monitoring,* vol 1.

Ellrodt G, Cook DJ, Lee J, et al. Evidence-based disease management. *JAMA* 1997;278:1687–1692.

Every NR, Hochman J, Becker R, et al, for the Committee on Acute Cardiac Care, Council on Clinical Cardiology, American Heart Association. Critical pathways: a review. *Circulation* 2000;101:461–465.

Gelinas MA, Fountain M. Management of cancer services: trends and opportunities. *Cancer Mgmt* 1997;6–15.

Ibarra V, Laffoon TA, Snyder M, et al. Clinical pathways in the perioperative setting. *Nurs Case Manag* 1997;2:97–104.

Jennings BM, Staggers N, Brosch LR. A classification scheme for outcome indicators. *Image J Nurs Sch* 1999;31:381–388.

Jones KR, Jennings BM, Moritz P, et al. Policy issues associated with analyzing outcomes of care. *Image J Nurs Sch* 1997;29:261–267.

Kaltenthaler E, McDonnell A, Peters J. Monitoring the care of lung cancer patients: linking audit and care pathways. *J Eval Clin Pract* 2001;7:13–20.

Kolb GR. Disease management is the future: breast cancer is the model. *Surg Oncol Clin N Am* 2000;9:217–232.

Lau C, Cartmill T, Leveaux V. Managing and understanding variances in clinical path methodology: a case study. *J Qual Clin Pract* 1996;16:109–117.

Pearson SD, Goulart-Fisher D, Lee TH. Critical pathways as a strategy for improving care: problems and potential. *Ann Intern Med* 1995;123:941–948.

Pearson SD, Kleefield SF, Soukop JR, et al. Critical pathways intervention to reduce length of hospital stay. *Am J Med* 2001;110:175–180.

Shulkin DJ, Ferniany IW. The effect of developing patient compendiums for critical pathways on patient satisfaction. *Am J Med Qual* 1996;11:43–45.

Strassner L. Scanner technology to manage critical path variance analysis. *Nurs Case Manag* 1997;2:141–147.

Teich JM, Glaser JP, Beckley RF, et al. The Brigham integrated computing system (BICS): advanced clinical systems in an academic hospital environment. *Int J Med Inf* 1999;54:197–208.

Tovar EA. Minimally invasive approach for pneumonectomy culminating in an outpatient procedure. *Chest* 1998;114:1454–1458.

Weingarten S. Critical pathways: what do you do when they do not seem to work? *Am J Med* 2001;110:224–225.

Wright CD, Wain JC, Grillo HC, et al. Pulmonary lobectomy patient care pathway: a model to control cost and maintain quality. *Ann Thorac Surg* 1997;64:299–302.

Zehr KJ, Dawson PB, Yang SC, et al. Standardized clinical care pathways for major thoracic cases reduce hospital costs. *Ann Thorac Surg* 1998;66:914–919.

6 TREATMENT OF EARLY-STAGE NON–SMALL CELL CARCINOMA OF THE LUNG

W. Roy Smythe

CHAPTER OVERVIEW

The purpose of this chapter is to address staging approaches and survival in early-stage (stages I and II) non–small cell lung carcinoma (NSCLC) and to review the recommended current and possible future treatment available for this disease. The discussions herein are based on published data from retrospective reviews and clinical trials available in the English-language literature, as well as symposia, unpublished data, and our institutional clinical experience at M. D. Anderson Cancer Center. Studies referenced in this manuscript were chosen on the basis of relevance to evaluation, staging, survival, and treatment in stage I and II NSCLC. The current best proven therapy for early-stage NSCLC is anatomic surgical resection, but overall survival is still somewhat disappointing. The expla-

Adapted from an article published in *Cancer Control: Journal of the Moffitt Cancer Center,* volume 8, number 4, 2001.

nation for these survival findings may lie in staging bias, and true stage-specific survival may be improved in the near future by the application of newer imaging modalities such as positron emission tomography. In addition to improvements in staging, neoadjuvant chemotherapy and other novel therapies may bring about changes in the current treatment algorithm and allow for improved survival as well.

INTRODUCTION

Of the more than 150,000 patients diagnosed with non–small cell lung carcinoma (NSCLC) in the United States each year, only a minority present with early-stage (stage I or II) disease as defined by the American Joint Committee on Cancer (AJCC) TNM staging system. In the latest National Cancer Institute Surveillance, Epidemiology, and End Results Program data analysis, 15% of patients diagnosed with NSCLC in the United States between 1989 and 1996 were found to have "localized" as opposed to "regional" (23%), "distant" (48%), or "unstaged" (14%) disease.

We are often somewhat heartened when a patient appears with a 1-cm peripheral lung cancer nodule without evidence of mediastinal or distant metastases rather than disseminated disease. Before stating that a "cure is certain," however, we must remember that a substantial proportion of patients treated for early-stage NSCLC eventually succumb to this aggressive neoplasm. Again according to Surveillance, Epidemiology, and End Results Program data, 5-year survival rates for patients with NSCLC improved only slightly between the mid-1970s and the mid-1990s, from 12.4% during the 1974–1979 reporting period to 14.1% during the 1989–1996 reporting period, the last period analyzed. In a review evaluating all recently published data regarding outcomes in patients with stage I or II NSCLC, Nesbitt et al (1995) estimated overall 5-year reported survival rates to be 64.6% for patients with stage I and 41.2% for patients with stage II disease. Naruke and colleagues and Mountain published 2 of the largest series to date evaluating postsurgical survival in patients with NSCLC (Naruke et al, 1988; Mountain, 1997). In these studies, survival was retrospectively assessed in 2,322 patients with stage I or II NSCLC (1997 AJCC TNM system designation) who were treated surgically. The 5-year survival rate for patients with T3N0M0 disease was 38% in the Mountain study and 33% in the Naruke study, and the survival rate in the most favorable subgroup (patients with T1N0M0 disease) was 67% in the Mountain study and 75% in the Naruke study (Table 6–1).

Clearly, we cannot promise a cure to patients with a diagnosis of NSCLC at any stage. However, there is no doubt that survival following treatment in patients with this disease is stage related and that patients with lower-stage disease have the best chance for cure. This fact underscores the importance of appropriate treatment of patients with earlier-stage disease, in whom the potential for a lost curative opportunity if inappropriate treatment is deliv-

Table 6–1.   Survival of Patients with Early-Stage NSCLC as Reported in the
Large Retrospective Reviews of Mountain and Naruke

	Mountain, 1997		Naruke, 1988	
TNM Subset	No. of Patients	5-Year Survival Rate, %	No. of Patients	5-Year Survival Rate, %
Stages I and II				
T1N0M0	511	67.0	245	75.5
T2N0M0	549	57.0	241	57.0
T1N1M0	76	55.0	66	52.5
T2N1M0	288	39.0	153	40.0
T3N0M0	87	38.0	106	33.3
Stage III				
T3N1M0	55	25.0	85	39.0
Any N2M0	344	23.0	368	15.1

Reprinted with permission from Smythe WR. Treatment of stage I and II non-small-cell lung cancer. *Cancer Control* 2001;8:318–325.

ered is greatest. The survival increase from 12.4% to 14.1% mentioned in the preceding paragraph may seem trivial, but it is important to remember that a 2% increase given 150,000 patients per year diagnosed with NSCLC translates into an additional 21,000 lives saved during this time period compared with what would have been expected 20 years earlier.

In this chapter, we will briefly address the "standard of care" for treatment of stage I and II NSCLC as supported by past experience. We will also make some predictions regarding how that standard may change in the near future and discuss means by which we may hope to further improve posttreatment survival in patients with early-stage NSCLC. Finally, we will discuss how newer screening modalities may or may not influence patient survival by altering the clinicopathologic staging biases that now exist in the diagnosis and treatment of NSCLC.

CONVENTIONAL PRETREATMENT PHYSIOLOGIC EVALUATION AND STAGING OF PATIENTS WITH CLINICAL STAGE I AND II DISEASE

All patients being considered for treatment of NSCLC should undergo a careful history and physical examination. An important goal should be the identification of occult problems that may lead to either a greater risk of postoperative complications or a need to more carefully evaluate for advanced or metastatic disease. Particular attention should be paid to the neurological history, including questions regarding the presence or absence of vertigo and headache, and to questions regarding new bone or joint pain as patient reports of such pain may lead to the discovery of metastases. Careful cardiac and respiratory histories should also be obtained as these organ systems are most frequently involved in postoperative complications following surgical resection for NSCLC. Patients should also be asked about head and neck symptoms (dysphagia, odynophagia, oropharyngeal pain, or bleeding) as this may lead to the discovery of a second or true primary (with pulmonary metastasis) aerodigestive malignancy.

Symptoms of any sort related to the primary malignancy can portend a poor prognosis in patients with stage I or II NSCLC. A review of patient records at M. D. Anderson Cancer Center revealed 33 patients with stage I or II NSCLC who experienced "precipitous" (within 9 months) recurrence after curative-intent anatomic resection with negative operative margins between 1988 and 1998. The only clinical variables that correlated with increased risk of recurrence compared to the risk in a control group (patients with the same stage of disease with no recurrence at 3 years) were weight loss ($P = .029$) and unusual histologic variants such as adenosquamous carcinoma (unpublished data).

The physical examination should rule out obvious sources of concern that would necessitate more involved evaluation, such as cardiac murmurs, carotid bruits, and respiratory findings out of proportion to the historical recollection of the patient (e.g., chronic obstructive pulmonary disease stigmata or wheezing). In addition, the physical examination is often the only reliable method for identifying unusual but well-known findings in NSCLC, such as supraclavicular nodal spread in apparently early disease or undiscovered skin malignancies representing primary disease with metastatic spread to the lung.

Routine imaging prior to staging should include posterior-anterior and lateral chest films as well as a computed tomography (CT) scan of the chest. The chest CT scan should include parenchymal as well as mediastinal windows to both evaluate the primary lesion and more carefully evaluate for the presence of enlarged mediastinal lymph nodes. This examination should also always include the upper abdomen to evaluate for occult adrenal and hepatic metastases.

Preoperative disease staging in patients with stage I and II disease is controversial and is rapidly evolving with the advent of positron emission tomography (PET) and other new techniques. CT reveals brain metastases in 3% to 5% of neurologically asymptomatic patients with NSCLC, although admittedly, some authors have demonstrated that the likelihood of brain metastases is less in patients with earlier-stage disease. Magnetic resonance (MR) imaging may be more sensitive than CT in the detection of brain metastases and in many centers is the test of choice for this evaluation. The bones are another common site for metastasis of NSCLC. A screening bone scan may reveal abnormalities in asymptomatic patients, and among patients with abnormalities detected, follow-up plain-film or MR imaging confirms metastatic disease in approximately 9% of cases

(Hillers et al, 1994). Although no careful study has been done to evaluate screening for occult metastatic disease in asymptomatic patients at all stages and although some have argued that such screening is not cost-effective, the M. D. Anderson approach is to screen all patients with NSCLC more extensive than clinical stage IA with both CT or MR imaging of the brain (especially if there are new neurological symptoms) and a whole-body bone scan. Patients with clinical stage IA disease without symptoms would have a low risk of bone or brain metastases, but if screening is not performed, the possibility of occult metastatic disease that could become manifest after surgical resection should be explained carefully to the patient during the pretreatment counseling session.

Pulmonary function testing, including spirometry and measurement of the diffusing capacity of the lung for carbon dioxide, are a routine part of the evaluation, even in patients with early-stage disease. It should be remembered that a lobectomy in a patient with an 8-mm NSCLC carries the same potential for functional compromise as a lobectomy in a patient with an 8-cm NSCLC—and perhaps even a greater potential for compromise since a greater number of functioning alveoli will be removed in the patient with the smaller tumor. Quantitative perfusion and exercise testing can be performed in patients in whom routine pulmonary function testing is inconclusive regarding the ability of a patient to tolerate an anatomic resection (e.g., patients with borderline pulmonary function on spirometry—i.e., a predicted forced expiratory volume in 1 second of less than 40% of predicted following resection).

SURGERY AS THE "STANDARD OF CARE"

Defining a standard of care for a given illness can be a daunting task. London has argued that even the Helsinki Accords, the document to which most around the world look for guidance in matters of human rights, is unclear in its description of "best proven therapeutic method" in discussions of research ethics with human subjects (London et al, 1999). The "standard of care" for one community may vary considerably from that of another, and this term should probably be replaced with "best proven method." In patients with stage I or II NSCLC without known metastatic disease or a reliable marker for metastases (similar to mediastinal nodal metastasis in patients with stage IIIA disease), modalities aimed at local control have been the mainstay of treatment. To date, neither adjuvant nor neoadjuvant treatment of any type, including radiation therapy and chemotherapy, has been shown to definitively improve the survival of patients with stage I or II disease. Therefore, at this time, the "best proven method" for treatment of patients with stage I or II NSCLC is aggressive treatment aimed at local control of the primary tumor—surgical resection, radiation therapy, or both.

Because of the relatively discrete nature of many early-stage NSCLCs, especially T1 tumors, there was a temptation in the past to perform sublobar or limited lung resection (i.e., "wedge resection" or "segmentectomy") for definitive local control. However, this approach has been shown to be inappropriate in patients physiologically tolerant of lobectomy because limited procedures are associated with higher rates of local recurrence and even possibly poorer survival. Multiple retrospective studies were reported between 1979 and 1990 that addressed the issue of limited versus full anatomic lung resection, but the results were far from conclusive and often conflicting regarding the true benefit of full anatomic resection. In 1995, however, the Memorial Sloan-Kettering group published a more convincing 12-year retrospective controlled study evaluating limited resection versus anatomic lobectomy or pneumonectomy in more than 500 patients. In this report, the 5- and 10-year survival rates were only 59% and 35%, respectively, in patients undergoing limited resection (n = 61), versus 77% and 70%, respectively, in patients undergoing lobectomy (n = 511) (Martini et al, 1995). Finally, that same year, a prospective, randomized trial was reported by the Lung Cancer Study Group in which lobectomy and limited resection were compared in patients with peripheral T1N0M0 NSCLC. In this study, more than 250 patients were randomly assigned to one approach or the other. The authors determined limited resection was associated with a 75% increase in the lung cancer recurrence rate directly attributable to a tripling of the local tumor recurrence rate. In addition, limited resection was associated with a 50% increase in deaths due to cancer (Ginsberg and Rubinstein, 1995).

Thoracoscopic resection of NSCLC has gained a measure of acceptance, and modest improvements in postoperative pain control and early return to work have been reported with this approach. Of course, thoracoscopic wedge resection suffers from the same potential oncologic problems as open limited resection via thoracotomy. Enthusiasm for thoracoscopic lobectomy in patients with NSCLC should be tempered by the following facts: the procedure can be technically difficult, a full mediastinal lymph node dissection is not reliably possible, careful palpation of the lung for occult extralobar metastatic disease is not always possible, and, finally, thoracoscopic lobectomy with an intercostal delivery incision may offer little postoperative pain advantage over a small muscle-sparing thoracotomy in this era of routine use of epidural and intravenous narcotic analgesics.

The increased risk of local recurrence with more limited resections seems somewhat intuitive when one simply considers the lobar anatomy and the prevailing lymphatic drainage patterns of the lung. Ishida et al (1990) demonstrated that 5% of patients with tumors measuring 1 to 2 cm and 12% of patients with tumors larger than 2 cm have N1 (hilar) nodal disease proximal to the primary lesion. Although it may be possible to remove most N2 (mediastinal) nodes at the time of a wedge resection, removal of N1 nodal tissue, which is often intraparenchymal at the hilum, requires a lobectomy. Sublobar resection would by definition leave behind pathologically detectable tumor in at least 5% to 12% of cases since intraparenchymal lymphatics proximal to N1 nodes are not evaluated (Ishida et al, 1990).

Whether a complete lymph node dissection (as opposed to lymph node sampling) is required at the time of resection in patients with early-stage NSCLC is also controversial. Some authors have suggested that for small peripheral NSCLCs, there is neither a staging nor a survival benefit conferred by performance of a complete mediastinal lymph node dissection rather than sampling or limited biopsy of hilar and mediastinal nodal stations at the time of tumor removal. However, others have questioned the ability of surgeons to discriminate, even in the operating room, between involved and uninvolved nodal regions. Takizawa et al (1998) found that in 157 patients undergoing surgical resection of 1.1- to 2.0-cm peripheral NSCLCs, 27 (17%) had nodal disease, and in 19 of 27 cases, there was no intraoperative finding that predicted this. Survival was directly correlated to the nodal stage, as expected: 5-year survival rates were 91% in patients with truly N0 disease and 30% in the 27 patients with N1 or N2 disease (Takizawa et al, 1998). Graham et al (1995) noted similar findings in 240 patients initially thought to have N0 or N1 disease; 46 (20%) were found on pathologic examination to have N2 disease, and no clinical stage subgroup was without this finding. Finally, in a report evaluating staging and survival in 337 patients with stage II or III NSCLC undergoing either mediastinal nodal sampling or complete nodal dissection, although staging accuracy was equivalent with the 2 approaches, more levels of N2 disease were noted in the dissection group, and these patients had improved survival (Keller et al, 2000). A large randomized study sponsored by the American College of Surgeons is currently evaluating this question in a more rigorous fashion. In addition to conventional nodal removal, many centers are currently working on a method to identify "sentinel" mediastinal lymph nodes in patients with NSCLC at the time of resection, making sampling more reliable. The current practice at M. D. Anderson is to perform a complete lymph node dissection at the time of primary tumor removal to obtain a more accurate pathologic stage. A more accurate pathologic stage may allow the clinician to have more meaningful discussions with the patient regarding posttreatment prognosis and in some cases may dictate additional treatment (see the section Postoperative Management later in this chapter).

Radiation Therapy versus Surgery

Although anatomic resection is the preferred treatment modality for local control of early-stage NSCLC, there is a subset of patients with early-stage disease who are either medically unfit for or refuse surgical treatment. These patients can benefit from radiation therapy or possibly from limited resection, as discussed in the previous section.

A number of reports have recently appeared in the literature describing effective radiation therapy as definitive therapy for patients with early-stage NSCLC. Morita et al (1997) compiled results from 10 Japanese hospitals for 149 patients with stage I NSCLC who were considered medically inoperable. The mean radiation dose administered was 64.7 Gy. The actuarial 3- and 5-year survival rates were 34.2% and 22.2%, respectively, and the 5-year survival rate was 31% in a subgroup of patients who underwent concomitant mediastinal nodal irradiation (Morita et al, 1997). Another study retrospectively examined outcomes in 103 patients with stage I and II NSCLC treated in the 1980s with "radical" radiation therapy (~60 Gy delivered with curative intent). In this study, overall survival rates at 3 and 5 years were only 35% and 14%, respectively; however, in a small subgroup of patients with T1 tumors and no history of antecedent weight loss, the survival rate at 5 years was 50% (Graham et al, 1995). An additional 71 patients receiving definitive radiation therapy for NSCLC secondary to medical contraindications to surgical resection were reported by the radiation therapy group here at M. D. Anderson. In this study, disease-specific 3-year survival rates following delivery of approximately 62 Gy were 47% and 42%, respectively, for T1 and T2 lesions, and the local control rates were 89% and 61%, respectively. Finally, as a possible harbinger of things to come in the field, a group of patients treated with proton-beam radiation therapy between 1994 and 1998 was recently reported by Bush et al (1999). In this study, the disease-free survival rate in patients with stage I disease at a median follow-up time of 2 years was 86%.

These studies and many similar reports suggest that at best a 30% 5-year survival rate should be expected in patients with stage I disease treated with definitive radiation therapy. Wedge resection via a minimal incision can lead to a 5-year survival rate of up to 50% in this same group of patients. Although these data argue for limited surgical resection in patients believed to be medically fit for surgery, the reader must take into account that medically inoperable patients reported in earlier papers on definitive radiation therapy often died of nononcologic causes, that disease-specific survival after definitive radiation therapy may approach that after wedge resection, and, finally, that the newer modalities of radiation therapy— such as proton-beam therapy, motion-gated approaches, transthoracic intratumoral treatment, and intensity-modulated radiation therapy—may yet prove to be superior to current surgical techniques.

CHEMOTHERAPY

The 2 approaches taken for administration of chemotherapy to patients with clinically resectable NSCLC have been preoperative (neoadjuvant) and postoperative (adjuvant).

The adjuvant chemotherapy approach has been rigorously studied and thus far has been shown to be of no significant benefit in patients with NSCLC regardless of stage. A meta-analysis was performed by the Non–Small Cell Lung Cancer Collaborative Group of England in 1995 examining the pooled results of 52 randomized trials in which adjuvant chemotherapy was utilized in patients with NSCLC. In this report, it was noted that chemotherapy engendered at best a 5% positive treatment effect (with platinum-based chemotherapy) and in some cases was detrimental to overall survival (when alkylating agents were used) (NSCLC Collaborative Group, 1995). Although past studies have not been positive, it is pertinent to note that these findings have yet to be retested with the more active chemotherapy combinations currently available.

The alternative approach, neoadjuvant chemotherapy, has been studied extensively as well, and in contrast has been shown in at least 2 small randomized trials (both of which were stopped early by review committees because of large positive effect in chemotherapy-treated groups) to be active in later-stage (IIIA) resectable NSCLC. These studies, undertaken on the basis of positive phase II trials performed by the Cancer and Leukemia Group B, the Southwest Oncology Group, and others, demonstrated a significant survival benefit for patients with stage IIIA disease undergoing surgical resection following "induction" platinum-based chemotherapy (Rosell et al, 1994; Roth et al, 1998). This approach in patients with potentially resectable stage IIIA NSCLC is currently being evaluated in the form of a cooperative-group national randomized trial.

These promising preliminary results with neoadjuvant chemotherapy, along with the well-known facts that patients with better performance status tend to enjoy better responses to chemotherapy and that a significant proportion of patients with stage I or II NSCLC eventually succumb to the disease, have led to initial efforts to evaluate the use of neoadjuvant chemotherapy in patients with early-stage NSCLC. In the past, one criticism of the use of chemotherapy in these patients was that the toxicity might well outweigh any beneficial effect and these patients can be cured in many cases with surgery alone. To evaluate this question more objectively, we compared surgical morbidity in 76 consecutive patients with NSCLC who underwent neoadjuvant chemotherapy and surgery at M. D. Anderson and 259 patients with NSCLC treated at M. D. Anderson with surgery alone. Interestingly, no significant differences were found in mortality, pulmonary morbidity, complications related to healing, length of stay, or re-admission rate (Figure 6–1) (Siegenthaler et al, 2001).

In a phase II study, Pisters et al (2000) assessed the feasibility of administering neoadjuvant chemotherapy to patients with early-stage NSCLC (IB through selected IIIA). In this study, termed "BLOT," for Bimodality Lung Oncology Team, 94 patients were treated with preoperative carboplatin (AUC = 6) and paclitaxel (225 mg/kg^2). Two cycles were administered prior to surgical resection. Fifty-six percent of the patients exhibited a major response, 96% completed planned preoperative chemotherapy, and 94% underwent a surgical procedure. No unexpected surgical or medical morbidity was noted (Pisters et al, 2000). As a result of these findings, a randomized trial comparing 3 courses of carboplatin and paclitaxel fol-

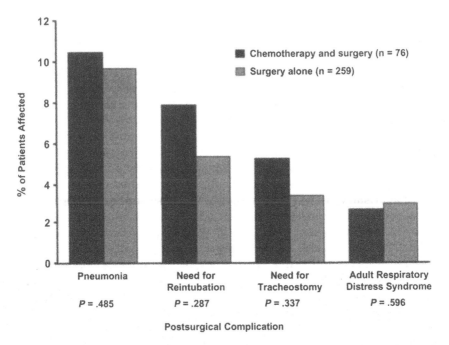

Figure 6–1. Postsurgical complications in patients with NSCLC treated at M. D. Anderson with and without neoadjuvant chemotherapy. Reprinted with permission from Smythe WR. Treatment of stage I and II non-small-cell lung cancer. *Cancer Control* 2001;8:318–325.

lowed by surgery versus surgery alone—the "BLOT or KNOT" trial (intergroup S9900) is now under way.

POSTOPERATIVE MANAGEMENT

In patients with early-stage NSCLC treated with surgery, a careful pathologic examination of the tumor specimen and the lymph nodes removed at the time of surgical resection of the primary tumor is extremely important. Occasionally a malignancy other than NSCLC is diagnosed, and this may dictate additional therapy or clinical evaluation (examples include small cell lung carcinoma or findings suggesting a metastatic lesion rather than a primary lung tumor). In addition, it is important to determine whether all the resection margins are negative for tumor involvement at the microscopic level and whether occult metastatic disease is present in the mediastinal lymph nodes. In the case of a microscopically positive margin, targeted postoperative adjuvant radiation therapy would be recommended as studies have shown that such treatment may improve survival. In the case of an occult lymph node metastasis, adjuvant mediastinal irradiation would be performed. Although postoperative mediastinal irradiation in patients with occult lymph node metastases has not been shown to improve survival, it is generally well tolerated and will reduce the local recurrence rate. This prevention of mediastinal local recurrence may have a significant impact on the patient's future quality of life.

Once general precautions regarding wound care, activity level, and use of oral pain medication have been reviewed and the patient has been discharged from the hospital, a 1-month follow-up visit is scheduled. At this visit, posterior-anterior and lateral chest roentgenography is performed, along with a complete blood cell count and a serum chemistry evaluation. During the history and physical examination, careful attention is paid to the status of wound healing and pain control. The roentgenograms are carefully evaluated for new effusions or infiltrates.

Subsequent follow-up visits for patients with early-stage NSCLC are scheduled at 6-month intervals for the first year and at 1-year intervals thereafter. Currently, posterior-anterior and lateral chest roentgenography, a complete blood cell count, and serum chemistry studies, including tests of liver function, are recommended as screening tests. The patient is counseled carefully regarding the early reporting of new symptoms suggesting recurrent disease, including neurological complaints (e.g., headaches, vertigo, or visual disturbances), persistent and severe bone pain, and respiratory symptoms (persistent cough or wheezing, hemoptysis, or chest wall pain). The future is likely to see the application of more sensitive measures of recurrence, such as high-resolution CT and PET; however, the routine use of these modalities in screening for recurrence will await stringent evaluation of the sensitivity and specificity of these modalities, evaluation of the true impact of early recurrence detection on prognosis, and cost-benefit analysis.

MEASUREMENT BIAS IN STAGING OF EARLY-STAGE NON–SMALL CELL LUNG CANCER

Data from multiple sources, including autopsy studies, PET evaluation of patients, and unconventional measures of micrometastasis suggest that a form of measurement bias is one of the reasons that a certain percentage of patients with stage I and II NSCLC succumb to recurrent disease. More simply stated, our conventional measures of metastatic disease—i.e., CT, MR imaging, and bone scans—are not sensitive enough to detect all disseminated disease, and a number of patients thought to have early-stage disease according to findings on clinical and pathologic evaluation actually harbor metastases and have their disease understaged. In autopsy studies, the discordance between clinical and autopsy diagnoses of malignant neoplasms has been reported to be as high as 44%. In addition, the most common reported site for a misdiagnosed or undiagnosed malignancy is the respiratory tract.

The increasing use of PET scanning as a pretreatment screening modality for NSCLC has also proved informative. In a recently published study evaluating PET as a screening method for patients deemed operable by clinical criteria, 11 of 102 patients were found to have metastatic disease undetected by conventional methods (Pieterman et al, 2000). Similar results have been reported by others, with most studies reporting metastatic disease in 11% to 14% of patients cleared for resection (stage IIIA or less) by conventional screening methods. In addition to an increase in the detection of distant metastases, virtually all of these studies have demonstrated an increase in the detection of unsuspected mediastinal and hilar nodal disease.

Finally, a number of recent studies have demonstrated that dissemination of cancer cells at detection levels much below even that of PET scanning can have an impact on the prognosis of patients with clinical early-stage NSCLC. Multiple authors have reported examinations of the bone marrow of "operable" patients with stage I to III disease for occult micrometastases. In these studies, monoclonal antibodies directed at epithelial cytokeratin antigens have demonstrated that 18% to 59% of patients with clinically operable stage I to III NSCLC harbor occult micrometastatic disease in the bone marrow and that this finding is directly correlated with survival, *exclusive of stage*. In a recent study by Passlick and colleagues (1999), 139 patients with NSCLC were evaluated with bone marrow biopsy and cytokeratin immunohistochemistry analysis at the time of a thoracic surgical procedure, and the median postsurgical follow-up time was 66 months. Among patients with stage I or II disease, micrometastases were detected in more than 48% of cases, and overall survival among node-negative patients was dramatically poorer in the bone-marrow-positive group. Findings parallel to those with bone marrow evaluation have been noted with immunohistochemical and polymerase chain reaction evaluation of lymph nodes deemed negative by conventional hematoxylin and eosin histopathologic examination in patients with surgically treated NSCLC. In a recent illustrative study, Maruyama et al (1997) evaluated 973 regional lymph nodes from 44 patients with pathologically staged stage I NSCLC. With use of a cytokeratin antibody, 70.5% of patients were found to have positive lymph nodes, and 19 and 12 patients were restaged as having N1 and N2 disease, respectively. The median survival time in these patients was statistically poorer than that of the rest of the patients in the study ($P = .004$) and was more in line with what was expected for the corrected stage category.

What about more sensitive methods of detecting true early disease, such as extremely sensitive screening methods that will be more likely to ensure that patients indeed have stage I disease? Results of the Early Lung Cancer Action Project, an effort to screen individuals at high risk for NSCLC on the basis of smoking history, were recently published. In this report, noncalcified nodules were noted in 233 of 1,000 patients, and 27 NSCLC tumors not discernible on plain film were found. Of these 27 lesions, 15 (56%) were 10 mm or less in size, and 26 were resectable (Henschke et al, 1999). Even though such studies provide hope that detection with sensitive screening techniques of "true" early-stage lesions may provide for improved survival, the jury is still out regarding both the clinical efficacy and the cost-effectiveness of large screening programs for NSCLC, even using the newer technologies at our disposal. Patz et al (2000) analyzed 510 patients with stage IA NSCLC measuring 0.27 to 3.0 cm treated surgically and found no significant relationship between tumor size and survival. The explanation for this may be that even NSCLCs less than 1 cm in diameter may exhibit vascular or lymphatic invasion in up to one third of cases.

Conclusions

Marcus Aurelius (121–180 A.D.) once stated that an individual should "look beneath the surface; let not the several quality of a thing nor its worth escape thee." As in many areas of medicine, the issues surrounding the treatment of patients with early-stage NSCLC—seemingly simple compared to those surrounding the treatment of patients with stage IIIA NSCLC, for example—are actually complex. A reasonable algorithm for the current treatment of stage I and II NSCLC, however, need not be so, and is presented in Figure 6–2.

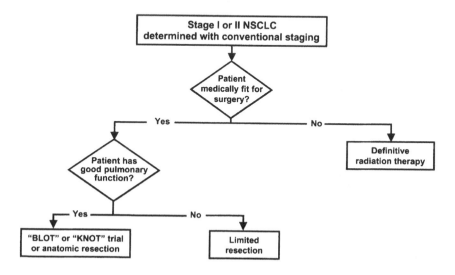

Figure 6–2. A proposed algorithm for treatment of clinical stage I or II NSCLC based on current (non-PET) staging techniques. Adapted from Smythe WR. Treatment of stage I and II non-small-cell lung cancer. *Cancer Control* 2001;8:318–325.

0114   W.R. Smythe

FUTURE DIRECTIONS

Future advances, including closed transthoracic radiation therapy, ther-
mal ablative therapy techniques, gene therapy, and others, may well sup-
plant the need to surgically resect early-stage NSCLCs to effect local control, and there is no doubt that the PET scan will eventually change the
way we stage this disease. In addition, the results of ongoing neoadjuvant and planned adjuvant trials utilizing newer, more active chemotherapeutic agents for NSCLC should be anxiously anticipated. One could
easily envision a future treatment algorithm based on these new technologies and findings (Figure 6–3), and we should be optimistic that the
prognosis of patients with stage I and II NSCLC will soon improve.

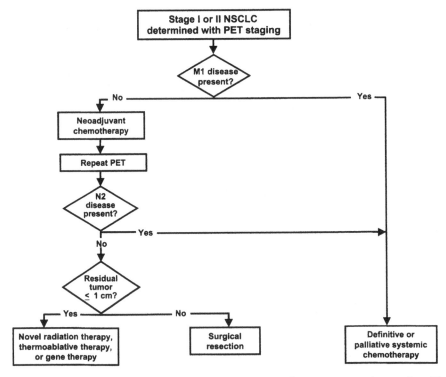

Figure 6–3. A possible future treatment algorithm for treatment of stage I or II
NSCLC based on PET staging, the possible effectiveness of neoadjuvant chemotherapy, and alternative novel local-control modalities for NSCLC. Adapted from
Smythe WR. Treatment of stage I and II non-small-cell lung cancer. *Cancer Control*
2001;8:318–325.

KEY PRACTICE POINTS

- Patients with apparent clinical early-stage NSCLC (AJCC stages I and II) may harbor asymptomatic distant metastases, and CT or MR imaging of the brain and a bone scan are recommended for all patients with clinical stage IB or more extensive disease. If full staging is not performed in a patient with stage IA disease, the small risk of occult metastatic disease should be carefully explained, and the patient should give informed consent to forego screening.

- Anatomic surgical resection (lobectomy or greater) is considered the current standard of care in patients with early-stage NSCLC who are medically fit to undergo surgery.

- A full mediastinal lymph node dissection should be performed in patients undergoing anatomic resection for clinical early-stage NSCLC to provide for more accurate pathologic staging and assessment of prognosis.

- In patients with early-stage NSCLC who are unable to tolerate an anatomic resection, wedge resection with negative surgical margins may be superior to radiation therapy alone. However, newer modes of radiation therapy may be shown to be of equivalent efficacy in the near future.

- One reason that so many patients with "early-stage" NSCLC eventually succumb to the disease is probably related to measurement bias in staging (i.e., understaging of patients). Newer staging modalities such as PET may allow for more accurate staging and drift of the survival numbers for early-stage NSCLC to a more favorable level. Clinicians should stay abreast of new developments and further verification of these modalities as accurate staging tools.

- As many patients with early-stage NSCLC will eventually succumb to the disease (usually distant rather than local recurrence), assessment of the utility of systemic chemotherapy in this patient population is crucial. Clinicians are urged to enroll patients in randomized trials such as intergroup S9900 to further evaluate the use of neoadjuvant chemotherapy in combination with surgical resection.

Suggested Readings

Bush DA, Slater JD, Bonnet R, et al. Proton-beam radiotherapy for early-stage lung cancer. *Chest* 1999;116:1313–1319.

Ginsberg RJ, Rubinstein LV. Randomized trial of lobectomy versus limited resection for T1 N0 non-small cell lung cancer. Lung Cancer Study Group. *Ann Thorac Surg* 1995;60:615–622.

Graham PH, Gebski VJ, Langlands AO. Radical radiotherapy for early nonsmall cell lung cancer. *Int J Radiat Oncol Biol Phys* 1995;31:261–266.

Henschke CI, McCauley DI, Yankelevitz DF, et al. Early Lung Cancer Action Project: overall design and findings from baseline screening. *Lancet* 1999;354:99–105.

Hillers TK, Sauve MD, Guyatt GH. Analysis of published studies on the detection of extrathoracic metastases in patients presumed to have operable non-small cell lung cancer. *Thorax* 1994;49:14–19.

Ishida T, Yano T, Maeda K, et al. Strategy for lymphadenectomy in lung cancer three centimeters or less in diameter. *Ann Thorac Surg* 1990;50:708–713.

Keller SM, Adak S, Wagner H, et al. Mediastinal lymph node dissection improves survival in patients with stages II and IIIa non-small cell lung cancer. Eastern Cooperative Oncology Group. *Ann Thorac Surg* 2000;70:358–365.

London L, Baldwin-Ragavan L, de Gruchy J. Revision of the Helsinki Declaration—ethical standards at risk? *S Afr Med J* 1999;89:812–813.

Martini N, Bains MS, Burt ME, et al. Incidence of local recurrence and second primary tumors in resected stage I lung cancer. *J Thorac Cardiovasc Surg* 1995; 109:120–129.

Maruyama R, Sugio K, Mitsudomi T, et al. Relationship between early recurrence and micrometastases in the lymph nodes of patients with stage I non-small-cell lung cancer. *J Thorac Cardiovasc Surg* 1997;114:535–543.

Morita K, Fuwa N, Suzuki Y, et al. Radical radiotherapy for medically inoperable non-small cell lung cancer in clinical stage I: a retrospective analysis of 149 patients. *Radiother Oncol* 1997;42:31–36.

Mountain CF. Revisions in the international system for staging lung cancer. *Chest* 1997;111:1710–1717.

Naruke T, Goya T, Tsuchiya R, et al. Prognosis and survival in resected lung carcinoma based on the new international staging system. *J Thorac Cardiovasc Surg* 1988;96:440–447.

Nesbitt JC, Putnam JB Jr, Walsh GL, et al. Survival in early-stage non-small cell lung cancer. *Ann Thorac Surg* 1995;60:466–472.

Non-Small Cell Lung Cancer Collaborative Group. Chemotherapy in non-small cell lung cancer: a meta-analysis using updated data on individual patients from 52 randomized trials. *BMJ* 1995;311:899–909.

Passlick B, Kubuschok B, Izbicki JR, et al. Isolated tumor cells in bone marrow predict reduced survival in node-negative non-small cell lung cancer. *Ann Thorac Surg* 1999;68:2053–2058.

Patz EF, Rossi S, Harpole DH, et al. Correlation of tumor size and survival in patients with stage IA non-small cell lung cancer. *Chest* 2000;117:1568–1571.

Pieterman RM, van Putten JWG, Meuzelaar JJ, et al. Preoperative staging of non-small-cell lung cancer with positron-emission tomography. *N Engl J Med* 2000;343:254–261.

Pisters KMW, Ginsberg RJ, Giroux DJ, et al. Induction chemotherapy before surgery for early-stage lung cancer: a novel approach. *J Thorac Cardiovasc Surg* 2000;119:429–439.

Rosell R, Gomez-Condina J, Camps C, et al. A randomized trial comparing preoperative chemotherapy plus surgery with surgery alone in patients with non-small-cell lung cancer. *N Engl J Med* 1994;330:153–158.

Roth JA, Atkinson EN, Fossella F, et al. Long-term follow-up of patients enrolled in a randomized trial comparing perioperative chemotherapy and surgery with surgery alone in resectable stage IIIA non-small-cell lung cancer. *Lung Cancer* 1998;21:1–6.

Siegenthaler MP, Pisters KM, Merriman KW, et al. Preoperative chemotherapy for lung cancer does not increase surgical morbidity. *Ann Thorac Surg* 2001;71: 1111–1112.

Takizawa T, Terashima M, Koike T, et al. Lymph node metastasis in small peripheral adenocarcinoma of the lung. *J Thorac Cardiovasc Surg* 1998;116:276–280.

7 SURGICAL TREATMENT OF LOCALLY ADVANCED NON–SMALL CELL LUNG CANCER

Stephen G. Swisher

CHAPTER OVERVIEW

Locally advanced (stage IIIA and IIIB) non–small cell lung cancer (NSCLC) includes a heterogeneous group of tumor types. The overall survival rate for patients with locally advanced NSCLC is poor (5% to 30% at 5 years) because of the high risk of both local-regional and distant recurrence. Nevertheless, some subsets of patients can be cured. A multidisciplinary approach with surgery, chemotherapy, and radiation therapy offers the best chance for cure. Surgical resection generally results in better local-regional control than does radiation therapy. However, this improved local-regional control must be balanced against the increased morbidity often associated with surgery. Furthermore, if the disease is advanced, in which case systemic recurrence is more likely, less emphasis may need to be placed on local-regional control, and radiation therapy may be preferable to surgery for control of the primary tumor.

Chemotherapy in patients with locally advanced NSCLC serves to target micrometastatic disease and thus complement the local-regional control provided by surgery and radiation therapy. However, chemotherapy has significant toxicity and has unclear benefits in certain subsets of patients. Patients with locally advanced NSCLC should be treated with aggressive multidisciplinary therapy in a manner that maximizes the chance for long-term cure while minimizing the overall risks of treatment.

INTRODUCTION

In 1997, lung cancer accounted for an estimated 160,000 deaths and 170,000 new cases of cancer in the United States (Parker et al, 1997). Though it receives less publicity than breast cancer or prostate cancer, lung cancer is the most common cause of cancer-related death in both men and women. Approximately 25% of all cancer deaths are attributable to lung cancer. The overall 5-year survival rate for patients with lung cancer is only 14%, primarily because the disease is usually advanced at presentation.

The most common type of lung cancer is non–small cell lung cancer (NSCLC), which accounts for about 75% of cases. Survival in patients with NSCLC is very stage dependent. Patients with early-stage (stage I and II) localized disease can be cured in many cases with surgery alone. For patients diagnosed with T1N0 disease, the 5-year survival rate with surgery alone approaches 60% to 70% (Nesbitt et al, 1995). Unfortunately, most patients present with locally advanced (stage IIIA or IIIB) or metastatic (stage IV) disease.

This chapter will try to define the subsets of patients with locally advanced NSCLC who are most likely to benefit from surgery. The chapter will also try to define how to optimize the timing and sequence of adjuvant and neoadjuvant radiation therapy and chemotherapy so as to maximize the therapeutic benefits of surgery while minimizing treatment-related side effects.

TREATMENT OPTIONS FOR LOCALLY ADVANCED
NON–SMALL CELL LUNG CANCER

The first thing to realize when treating patients with locally advanced NSCLC is that this category includes a wide variety of manifestations of disease (see the lung cancer staging system, which appears in chapter 1). Although all these different types of tumors are lumped together as stage III disease, some tumors within this group are best treated with surgery, and others are best treated without surgery (Table 7–1). The critical task from the clinician's standpoint is to recognize the different subsets so that appropriate multidisciplinary care can be tailored to the individual patient.

In deciding how to treat locally advanced NSCLC, it is helpful to consider the advantages and limitations of each of the conventional modalities of treatment—surgery, radiation therapy, and chemotherapy. Surgery and radiation therapy address primarily local-regional disease, while chemotherapy treats primarily systemic disease but has some local-regional effect.

Although surgery is probably more effective than radiation therapy in controlling local-regional disease, surgery is associated with increased morbidity and mortality and requires removal of noninvolved lung parenchyma. The benefit from the increased local-regional control afforded by surgery must therefore be balanced against the increased morbidity of the operation. Furthermore, if the disease is advanced, in which case systemic recurrence is more likely, less emphasis may need to be placed on local-regional control, and radiation therapy may be preferable to surgery for control of the primary tumor.

Even though many patients with locally advanced NSCLC have micrometastatic disease at presentation and ultimately develop metastatic disease, adequate local-regional control still has an effect on long-term survival. Kubota et al demonstrated in a randomized trial that patients with stage III disease treated with chemotherapy alone had far lower survival rates than patients treated with chemotherapy and radiation therapy because of the lack of local-regional control (Kubota et al, 1994).

Chemotherapy is aimed primarily at distant disease but in many instances can help improve local-regional control by sensitizing tumors to radiation (radiation-sensitizing chemotherapy) or downstaging tumors prior to surgery. Various studies have demonstrated improved survival with the addition of chemotherapy to radiation therapy (Schaake-Koning et al, 1992; Dillman et al, 1996; Sause et al, 2000) or surgery (Roth et al, 1998; Rosell et al, 1999).

Stage III disease is heterogeneous because in some subsets within this group long-term survival is dependent on local-regional control while in other subsets long-term survival is primarily dependent on control of dis-

**Table 7–1.   Role of Surgery in the Treatment of Patients with Locally
Advanced (Stage IIIA and IIIB) NSCLC**

Stage IIIA Non-Pancoast Tumors

T3N1   Surgery alone in physiologically fit patients.

T1–3N2   Induction chemotherapy followed by surgery may benefit patients who
are physiologically fit, do not have bulky adenopathy, or have a good
radiographic or histopathologic response to induction chemotherapy.

Stage IIIA Pancoast Tumors

T3N1   Surgery followed by postoperative chemoradiation in physiologically
fit patients.

T1–3N2   Because of poor long-term survival, these patients are best treated with
chemoradiation and no surgery (chapter 8).

Stage IIIB Non-Pancoast Tumors

T4N0–1   Surgery after induction chemotherapy may help a subset of patients
with local-regionally aggressive disease. Patients with malignant
pleural effusions (T4) should be treated nonsurgically with
chemoradiation because of poor long-term survival (chapter 8).

T4N2   Because of poor long-term survival, these patients are best treated with
chemoradiation and no surgery (chapter 8).

T1–4N3   Because of poor long-term survival, these patients are best treated with
chemoradiation and no surgery (chapter 8).

Stage IIIB Pancoast Tumors

T4N0–1   Surgery followed by postoperative chemoradiation may be beneficial
in physiologically fit patients treated at an experienced referral center.

T4N2   Because of poor long-term survival, these patients are best treated with
chemoradiation and no surgery (chapter 8).

T1–4N3   Because of poor long-term survival, these patients are best treated with
chemoradiation and no surgery (chapter 8).

tant disease. The traditional view is that stage IIIA disease is best treated
with surgery whereas stage IIIB disease is best treated with radiation therapy. However, as this chapter will show, that division is artificial and too
simplistic (Table 7–1).

In patients with locally advanced NSCLC, decisions regarding the use
of aggressive surgical resection are best made with a multidisciplinary approach in which patients are seen by thoracic surgeons, radiation oncologists, and medical oncologists and then discussed individually at a multidisciplinary conference. This multidisciplinary approach maximizes
the chance for long-term cure while minimizing the chance of treatment-
related morbidity.

Initial Assessment of Patients
with Locally Advanced Disease

Initial assessment of patients with stage III disease involves a careful history and physical examination, chest radiography, and computed tomography (CT) of the chest and upper abdomen. Because of the low yield in asymptomatic patients, bone scanning, CT of the brain, and magnetic resonance imaging of the brain are not done unless a patient has symptoms that suggest metastatic disease. Once a patient's disease has been staged clinically with noninvasive tests, a physiologic assessment should be performed to determine the patient's ability to tolerate different therapeutic modalities. In addition to a general evaluation of the patient's overall medical status, the physiologic assessment should include specific evaluation of the cardiovascular and respiratory systems. Cardiovascular screening should include a history and physical examination as well as chest radiography and electrocardiography. Patients with signs and symptoms of significant cardiac disease should undergo further noninvasive testing including exercise testing, echocardiography, or nuclear perfusion scans. Significant reversible cardiac problems should be addressed prior to treatment with chemotherapy, radiation therapy, or surgery.

The pulmonary reserve of lung cancer patients is commonly diminished because of tobacco use. Simple spirometry is an excellent initial screening test for quantifying a patient's pulmonary reserve and ability to tolerate surgical resection (Kearney et al, 1994). A predicted postoperative forced expiratory volume in 1 second (FEV_1) of less than 0.8 liters or less than 35% is associated with an increased risk of perioperative complications, respiratory insufficiency, and death. The predicted postoperative FEV_1 is estimated by subtracting the contribution of the lung to be resected from the preoperative FEV_1. In certain instances, the lung to be resected does not contribute much to the preoperative FEV_1 because of tumor, atelectasis, or pneumonitis. In such cases, postoperative FEV_1 can be predicted more accurately by performing a ventilation-perfusion scan and subtracting the exact contribution of the lung to be resected. In patients who are not candidates for surgery on the basis of spirometry criteria but are still believed to be candidates for surgery, oxygen consumption studies can be done that measure both respiratory and cardiac capacity (Walsh et al, 1994; Rao et al, 1995). A maximum oxygen consumption of more than 15 mL/min/kg indicates low risk, while a maximum oxygen consumption of less than 10 mL/min/kg indicates high risk (a mortality rate of greater than 30% in some series). Additional risk factors for complications after lung resection include a predicted postoperative diffusing capacity of the lung for carbon monoxide of less than 40%, maximum voluntary ventilation of less than 40%, and hypercapnia (> 45 mm CO_2) or hypoxemia (< 60 mm O_2) on preoperative arterial blood gas analysis (Ferguson et al, 1995). In conjunction with clinical assessment, these tests can help identify patients at high risk for complications during and after surgical resection. In patients with marginal pulmonary reserve, preoperative measures that can help minimize complications and improve performance on spirometry include training with an incentive spirometer, initiation of bronchodilators, weight reduction, good nutrition, and cessation of smoking for at least 2 weeks prior to surgery (Weiner et al, 1997).

TREATMENT OF PATIENTS WITH STAGE IIIA DISEASE

Stage IIIA NSCLC includes T1–3 tumors involving the ipsilateral mediastinal nodes (N2 disease) but not the contralateral mediastinal nodes (N3 disease). Stage IIIA NSCLC also includes T3 tumors (tumors that directly invade the chest wall, diaphragm, or proximal main bronchus) with N1 nodal involvement (Mountain, 1997). The basis for the division between stage IIIA disease and stage IIIB disease is the concept that stage IIIA disease is resectable with a standard operative approach (thoracotomy) whereas stage IIIB disease is not. However, there are subgroups of patients with stage IIIA disease who probably should not be treated with surgery. This section will describe which subsets of patients with stage IIIA disease are most likely to benefit from surgery.

T3N1 Disease

T3 tumors are tumors of any size that directly invade the chest wall, diaphragm, mediastinal pleura, or parietal pericardium or invade the main bronchus less than 2 cm distal to the carina but without carinal involvement or atelectasis of the entire lung. N1 nodal disease indicates metastasis to the ipsilateral peribronchial and/or ipsilateral hilar nodes and the intrapulmonary lymph nodes (Figure 7–1 and Table 7–2 and the lung cancer staging system, which appears in chapter 1). The most common type of T3N1 tumor is one that directly invades the chest wall and involves ipsilateral hilar nodes (Mountain and Dresler, 1997).

Because T3N1 tumors do not involve mediastinal nodes, surgery can improve the odds of long-term survival and is warranted in many cases. Pancoast (pulmonary sulcus) T3N1 tumors are similar in their behavior to non-Pancoast T3N1 tumors but are located in the apex of the lung, where anatomic constraints (the subclavian artery and vein, the brachial plexus, and the thoracic inlet) make surgery more difficult. Nevertheless, long-term survival is possible in patients with Pancoast T3N1 tumors if negative surgical margins can be achieved. Given the proximity of critical structures and the difficulty of negative margins with surgery alone, Pancoast tumors are usually treated with adjuvant radiation therapy or chemoradiation, whereas non-Pancoast tumors in certain instances may be treated with surgery alone.

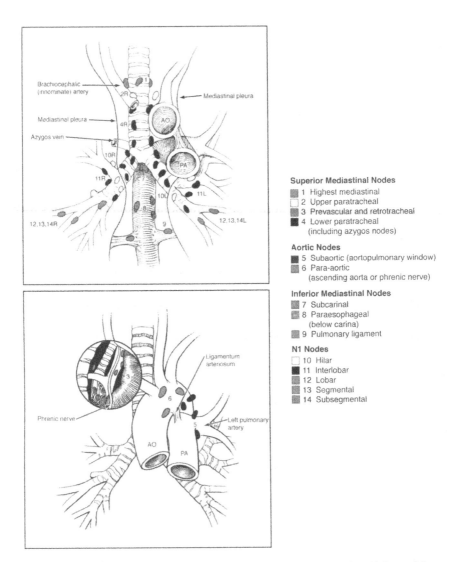

Figure 7–1. Regional lymph node stations for lung cancer staging. Adapted from Naruke T, Suemasu K, Ishikawa S. Lymph node mapping and curability of various levels of metastases in resected lung cancer. *J Thorac Cardiovasc Surg* 1976; 71:279–285; and American Thoracic Society. Clinical staging of primary lung cancer. *Am Rev Respir Dis* 1983;127:1–6. Copyright 1996, Mountain and Dresler. Reprinted with permission.

Table 7–2.   Lymph Node Map Definitions

N2 Nodes (All N2 nodes lie within the mediastinal pleural envelope.)

1   Highest mediastinal nodes: Nodes lying above a horizontal line at the upper rim of the brachiocephalic (left innominate) vein where it ascends to the left, crossing in front of the trachea at its midline.

2   Upper paratracheal nodes: Nodes lying above a horizontal line drawn tangential to the upper margin of the aortic arch and below the inferior boundary of number 1 nodes.

3   Prevascular and retrotracheal nodes: Prevascular and retrotracheal nodes may be designated 3A and 3P. Midline nodes are considered to be ipsilateral.

4   Lower paratracheal nodes: The lower paratracheal nodes on the right lie to the right of the midline of the trachea between a horizontal line drawn tangential to the upper margin of the aortic arch and a line extending across the right main bronchus at the upper margin of the upper lobe bronchus and contained within the mediastinal pleural envelope. The lower paratracheal nodes on the left lie to the left of the midline of the trachea between a horizontal line drawn tangential to the upper margin of the aortic arch and a line extending across the left main bronchus at the level of the upper margin of the left upper lobe bronchus, medial to the ligamentum arteriosum and contained within the mediastinal pleural envelope. Researchers may wish to designate the lower paratracheal nodes as No. 4s (superior) and No. 4i (inferior) subsets for study purposes; the No. 4s nodes may be defined by a horizontal line extending across the trachea and drawn tangential to the cephalic border of the azygos vein; the No. 4i nodes may be defined by the lower boundary of No. 4s and the lower boundary of No. 4, as described above.

Regional Lymph Node Classification

5   Subaortic (aortopulmonary window): Subaortic nodes are lateral to the ligamentum arteriosum or the aorta or left pulmonary artery and proximal to the first branch of the left pulmonary artery and lie within the mediastinal pleural envelope.

6   Para-aortic nodes (ascending aorta or phrenic): Nodes lying anterior and lateral to the ascending aorta and the aortic arch or the innominate artery, beneath a line tangential to the upper margin of the aortic arch.

7   Subcarinal nodes: Nodes lying caudal to the carina of the trachea, but not associated with the lower lobe bronchi or arteries within the lung.

8   Paraesophageal nodes (below carina): Nodes lying adjacent to the wall of the esophagus and to the right or left of the midline, excluding subcarinal nodes.

9   Pulmonary ligament nodes: Nodes lying within the pulmonary ligament, including those in the posterior wall and lower part of the inferior pulmonary vein.   *(continued)*

Table 7–2. *(continued)* **Lymph Node Map Definitions**

N1 Nodes (All N1 nodes lie distal to the mediastinal pleural reflection and within the visceral pleura.)

10   Hilar nodes: The proximal lobar nodes, distal to the mediastinal pleural reflection and the nodes adjacent to the bronchus intermedius on the right; radiographically, the hilar shadow may be created by enlargement of both hilar and interlobar nodes.

11   Interlobar nodes: Nodes lying between the lobar bronchi.
12   Lobar nodes: Nodes adjacent to the distal lobar bronchi.
13   Segmental nodes: Nodes adjacent to segmental bronchi.
14   Subsegmental nodes: Nodes around the subsegmental bronchi.

Reprinted with permission from Mountain CF, Dresler CM. Regional lymph node classification for lung cancer staging. *Chest* 1997;111:1719–1723.

Selection of Therapy

Because of their anatomic locations, T3N1 tumors often require technically challenging surgeries.

At M. D. Anderson Cancer Center, patients with T3N1 non-Pancoast tumors are assessed to determine whether they are physiologically fit enough to undergo surgical resection because their long-term survival will be determined in large part by the local-regional disease. Patients deemed unable to tolerate surgical resection are treated with radiation therapy.

Although surgery alone can cure some patients, systemic failure is still a major problem, and we are therefore treating patients with T3N1 non-Pancoast tumors in a multi-institutional randomized study (S9900) designed to evaluate the potential benefit of induction (preoperative) chemotherapy (paclitaxel and carboplatin) in this subgroup. In this trial, patients with T2–3N0 or T1–3N1 disease are randomly assigned to surgery alone or preoperative chemotherapy (paclitaxel and carboplatin) and surgery (Pisters et al, 2000). This study is a high-priority trial because it is a "proof of principle" study evaluating the potential benefit of induction chemotherapy in a group of patients who have poor outcomes with surgery alone.

Patients with T3N1 non-Pancoast tumors who are not eligible for or choose not to participate in this protocol are treated initially with surgery if this approach is technically and physiologically feasible. Chemotherapy is usually not given except in a protocol setting. Preoperative radiation therapy is not given, but postoperative radiation therapy is considered for patients with close or positive margins after surgery.

Patients with T3N1 Pancoast tumors are treated surgically as well. These tumors, however, are associated with a higher risk of local-regional failure because the anatomic constraints of the thoracic inlet (subclavian artery and vein, vertebral body, and brachial plexus) preclude a wide surgical margin. At M. D. Anderson, patients with T3N1 Pancoast tumors are treated in a phase II protocol evaluating the role of surgery and postoperative chemoradiation in this subgroup. After surgical resection, radiation therapy is delivered over 5 to 6 weeks. Patients receive 2 fractions per day, to a total dose of 60 Gy in patients with negative margins or 64.8 Gy in patients with positive margins, plus concurrent chemotherapy (cisplatin 50 mg/m^2 on days 1 and 8 and etoposide given by mouth 30 to 60 minutes prior to each administration of radiation therapy on days 1 through 5 and 8 through 12, with this chemotherapy cycle repeated starting on day 29). Prophylactic cranial irradiation (25 Gy in 10 fractions of 2.5 Gy) is given upon completion of chest irradiation because of the high risk of brain recurrences. Three additional cycles of chemotherapy are delivered after prophylactic cranial irradiation. Other institutions have successfully treated T3N1 Pancoast tumors with preoperative rather than postoperative chemoradiation (Rusch et al, 2001).

Although surgical resection of T3N1 Pancoast tumors is technically challenging, these tumors often have a local-regional recurrence pattern and can be cured in many instances with surgery. Given the rarity of T3N1 Pancoast tumors and the anatomic difficulties associated with resecting them, treatment is best performed at a referral center experienced with the multidisciplinary treatment of these difficult and rare tumors. The best opportunity for cure occurs when these tumors are approached from the time of diagnosis in a concerted, coordinated manner.

Operative Strategy

Non-Pancoast Tumors.   The most common type of T3N1 tumor is a tumor that invades the chest wall. Although chest wall invasion is not a contraindication to surgery, it necessitates a more extensive operation and makes assessment of the mediastinal nodes critical since mediastinal nodal involvement (N2 disease) is associated with markedly reduced long-term survival (Figure 7–1 and Table 7–2). Cervical mediastinoscopy should therefore be performed prior to chest wall resection in any patient with enlarged mediastinal or hilar lymph nodes on CT. Cervical mediastinoscopy can be performed immediately before the chest wall resection, with nodal status assessed using frozen section techniques.

For cervical mediastinoscopy, the patient is intubated with a single-lumen endotracheal tube, and bronchoscopy is performed to evaluate the presence of endobronchial disease. The patient is then placed in the supine position with the neck extended and a roll under the shoulder blades. A suprasternal incision is made, and the pretracheal plane is entered and then explored bluntly into the mediastinum. A cervical mediastinoscope is placed into the mediastinum, and lymph nodes from the lower and upper paratracheal regions (nodal stations 2R, 4R, 2L, and 4L) and subcarina (nodal station 7) (Figure 7–1 and Table 7–2) are biopsied. If the lymph nodes are positive, the procedure is terminated and the patient is evaluated for chemotherapy followed by surgery or radiation therapy for localregional control.

If the mediastinal lymph nodes are negative, chest wall resection and pulmonary resection can be performed in the same operative setting. A double-lumen endotracheal tube is placed to allow selective ventilation of the operative field. Bronchoscopy is used to confirm that the endotracheal tube is within the left main bronchus. The patient is then placed in the lateral decubitus position unless the tumor involves the anterior chest wall, in which case a supine position and an anterior approach through an inframammary or parasternal incision may be better. If a lateral decubitus position is chosen, a posterolateral incision is made with a muscle-sparing approach or with the standard approach (latissimus dorsi division) through the fifth intercostal space. This intercostal space should be adjusted so that the chest is entered without incision of the tumor.

Once the chest is entered, exploration is performed to rule out metastatic disease in other locations (e.g., pleural studding or pulmonary metastases). The surgeon also assesses whether the patient can tolerate the chest wall and pulmonary resection that will be required to remove the tumor. Partial resection of the tumor with residual positive margins is not beneficial for the patient, and it must be decided early whether the operation is technically and physiologically feasible.

If a decision is made to proceed with the operation, the chest wall is resected at least 1 to 2 ribs above and below the tumor. The chest wall is divided anteriorly initially with rib shears with ligation of the intercostal vessels. Superior and inferior margins can then be divided with cautery, with rib shears used to divide the posterior rib attachments. In some cases, posterior extension requires disarticulation of the rib from the transverse process using an osteotome. Paravertebral tissue should be resected if it lies close to the tumor. In rare cases, unexpected vertebral involvement is noted. In these cases, we work in conjunction with our neurosurgeons, who are available as needed, to ensure a negative margin with either partial or total vertebrectomy (see the description of surgery for Pancoast T4N0–1 tumors under the heading Operative Strategy in the section Treatment of Patients with Stage IIIB Disease).

Once the chest wall resection is complete, the pulmonary resection is performed. A lobectomy is usually required, although in some cases a pneumonectomy will be required because of the extent of the tumor. Segmentectomies or wedge resections are performed only if findings on the patient's pulmonary function tests indicate that the patient cannot tolerate an anatomic resection. Once the pulmonary resection is complete, the specimen is removed en bloc from the operative field. A complete mediastinal lymph node dissection is then performed, with removal of the nodes at stations 4, 7, 8, 9, 10, and 11 on the right side and 5, 6, 8, 9, 10, and 11 on the left side (Figure 7–1 and Table 7–2). Chest tubes or Blake drains are then placed, and a decision is made regarding the need for chest wall reconstruction.

If the chest wall defect is larger than the patient's hand, reconstruction is usually performed, especially if the defect is not covered by the scapula. The chest wall may be reconstructed with Marlex mesh alone or with methyl methacrylate to give the reconstructed chest wall increased rigidity for both cosmetic and functional reasons. The edges of the mesh are approximated to the surrounding ribs with nylon sutures brought through holes placed in the rib or around adjoining ribs. The wound is then closed in the usual fashion, with a subcutaneous Blake drain placed if a muscle-sparing approach has been utilized. Postoperative management should focus on early extubation and pulmonary toilet, with removal of the chest tubes once all air leaks have ceased and drainage is less than 300 mL per day.

Pancoast Tumors.   T3N1 Pancoast tumors are treated with an approach similar to that used for T3N1 non-Pancoast tumors, with cervical mediastinoscopy performed first. If the lymph nodes are negative, surgical resection proceeds through an extended posterolateral incision extending up through the trapezius muscle between the scapula and paravertebral muscles. This incision allows access to the apex of the chest so that the apical tumor can be resected. A rib spreader can be placed under the scapula and on the superior aspect of the sixth rib so that the scapula is elevated to allow exposure of the upper ribs. An anterior incision is made with rib shears, although particular care must be taken with division of the first rib to avoid injury to the subclavian artery, subclavian vein, or brachial plexus. The anterior and middle scalene muscle attachments to the first rib are divided as well to allow the resected first rib to be removed once the posterior attachments are divided. After the anterior attachments to the vertebral body are divided, the ribs are disarticulated from the transverse processes posteriorly with a Cobb elevator. The nerve roots and intercostal vessels are ligated as each rib is disarticulated to avoid the bleeding and cerebrospinal fluid leaks that may result from avulsion. The first rib is divided posteriorly after the C8 and T1 nerve roots have been identified. It is critical to identify these nerve roots so that the C8 nerve is not inadvertently resected, resulting in a dysfunctional clawed hand. If unexpected involvement of the brachial plexus is discovered, this disease is not resected because of the high risk of resulting functional problems; instead, the disease is treated with postoperative radiation therapy.

Once the chest wall resection is complete, an en bloc anatomic lung resection (lobectomy or pneumonectomy) is performed with mediastinal lymph node dissection. Because anatomic resection is associated with improved local control (Ginsberg et al, 1995), a wedge or segmental resection is performed only if the pulmonary function tests indicate that the patient cannot tolerate a more extensive pulmonary resection. Reconstruction of the chest wall is rarely required because the scapula usually covers the defect. If the tumor involves the fourth rib, however, the chest wall may need to be reconstructed with Marlex mesh to prevent the edge of the scapula from catching on the fifth rib. Postoperative care emphasizes early extubation and pulmonary toilet, with removal of the chest tubes once the lung has sealed and drainage is less than 300 mL per day.

Postoperative Treatment

Patients with T3N1 tumors are at high risk for both systemic and local-regional recurrence.

At M. D. Anderson, patients with T3N1 non-Pancoast tumors treated outside a protocol setting are not given postoperative chemotherapy. Radiation therapy is given only if the surgical margins are involved or close or a large number of unsuspected involved ipsilateral mediastinal or subcarinal nodes are found on the final pathologic examination. Patients with T3N1 non-Pancoast tumors treated in a protocol setting are enrolled in the randomized S9900 trial, in which one group is treated with preoperative chemotherapy (paclitaxel and carboplatin) and the other group is treated with surgery only (Pisters et al, 2000). No postoperative chemotherapy or radiation therapy is delivered.

Patients with T3N1 Pancoast tumors are treated in the M. D. Anderson phase II protocol ID 92–038, in which surgical resection is followed by postoperative chemoradiation because of the high risk of local-regional recurrence and the difficulty of achieving wide surgical margins because of anatomic constraints in the apex of the lung.

After surgery, patients with T3N1 Pancoast and non-Pancoast tumors have follow-up clinic visits 1 month after surgery, at 6-month intervals for 4 visits, and then yearly thereafter. The limited treatment options for recurrent NSCLC have limited the cost-effectiveness of aggressive radiologic surveillance after surgical resection. However, there is an increased incidence of second primary lung cancers in patients treated for NSCLC (3% per year), and annual or semiannual chest radiography may help detect these lesions. Any patient who develops symptoms in the interim between scheduled follow-up examinations should also be evaluated aggressively for recurrence or a new primary tumor (Walsh et al, 1995).

T1–3N2 Disease

T1–3 tumors are tumors of any size that may invade the chest wall or diaphragm but do not invade the mediastinum, heart, great vessels, trachea, esophagus, vertebral body, or carina. N2 nodal disease indicates involvement of the ipsilateral but not contralateral mediastinal and/or subcarinal lymph nodes (see Figure 7–1, Table 7–2, and the lung cancer staging system, which appears in chapter 1).

Although surgery in patients with T1–3N2 NSCLC can eliminate the known disease in both the primary site and the lymph nodes, the presence of mediastinal nodal disease is associated with a high risk of metastatic recurrence following surgical resection (Mountain and Dresler, 1997). The outcome of this group of patients is dictated more by the systemic disease (N2 and micrometastatic) than by the local-regional problems, and consequently, improved survival requires effective systemic treatment (chemotherapy) as well as local-regional treatment (surgery or radiation therapy). Multiple randomized trials have demonstrated that induction chemotherapy with surgery (Roth et al, 1998; Rosell et al, 1999) or radiation therapy (Schaake-Koning et al, 1992; Dillman et al, 1996; Sause et al, 2000) results in a significant survival advantage, and this group of patients should therefore be treated with systemic therapy as well as local-regional treatment for maximal therapeutic benefit.

Patients with T1–3N2 Pancoast tumors have a very poor prognosis. Several series have shown that N2 involvement in Pancoast tumors is associated with no long-term survivors (Anderson et al, 1986; Attar et al, 1998). Therefore, except in a protocol setting, surgery is usually not performed for T1–3N2 Pancoast tumors; patients with these lesions are treated with chemotherapy and radiation therapy alone. It is important, however, that the involvement of N2 nodes be documented pathologically because enlarged nodes on CT do not always harbor neoplasm.

Selection of Therapy

Because of the mediastinal lymph node involvement, T1–3N2 tumors have a high propensity to harbor occult micrometastatic disease, and thus local-regional treatment alone (i.e., radiation therapy or surgery alone) is associated with poor long-term survival rates, in the range of 10% to 20% (Andre et al, 2000). The addition of induction chemotherapy to surgery or radiation therapy is associated with an increase, albeit modest, in long-term survival rates, to 15% to 30% (Roth et al, 1998; Rosell et al, 1999). Chemotherapy is therefore essential in this group of patients. What has not yet been defined completely, however, is the optimum local-regional therapy (i.e., surgery or radiation therapy or both). In an effort to answer this critical question, we have tried to enroll patients in a randomized intergroup study (RTOG 93–09) evaluating chemoradiation versus chemoradiation and surgery. However, accrual of patients to this study has been very slow because of patients' and physicians' reluctance to rely on random assignment to determine whether surgery is performed. In addition, the advent of newer, less toxic chemotherapy combinations that can be given concurrently with radiation therapy has made the traditional cisplatin, etoposide, and concurrent radiation therapy delivered in the study less interesting (Choy et al, 1994; Gressen and Curran, 2001).

Among patients with T1–3N2 non-Pancoast tumors who do not wish to be treated on protocol, we try to identify those patients who have a good chance for long-term survival. These patients are then targeted for the more aggressive approach of induction chemotherapy and surgery as opposed to induction chemotherapy and radiation therapy. Criteria that are used to help identify patients to be treated with surgery include young age and good physiologic condition. In addition, patients with only microscopic involvement of a few lymph node stations as opposed to bulky mediastinal nodal involvement tend to be favored (Luzzi et al, 2000; Maurel et al, 2000). Another criterion that can identify patients who may benefit from surgery is good response to induction chemotherapy (Bueno et al, 2000). In patients whose N1 and N2 nodes become negative after induction chemotherapy (30%), the 5-year survival rate is about 35%, opposed to 9% if the N2 or N1 nodes remain positive. In addition, patients who have a significant pathologic response to treatment also have markedly increased long-term survival. We have a tendency to treat these patients with surgery because we believe that they may benefit from the increased local-regional control provided by surgery.

Patients with a poor long-term survival, usually because of metastatic recurrence, probably do not benefit from the increased local-regional control of surgery versus radiation therapy. Patients with poor performance status who have lost significant amounts of weight, reflecting systemic disease, also seldom benefit from surgery and the resulting improved local-regional control. These patients should probably be treated with the less morbid approach of radiation therapy to maximize quality of life while minimizing treatment-related morbidity.

Patients with T1–3N2 Pancoast tumors have an extremely poor prognosis (0% 5-year survival) (Anderson et al, 1986; Attar et al, 1998) and should not be treated surgically except perhaps in a protocol setting. The poor prognosis of this group of patients places them in the unresectable category better treated with chemoradiation rather than surgery (see chapter 8).

Operative Strategy

In patients with T1–3N2 disease, the primary lung tumor is resected in the standard fashion with a posterolateral thoracotomy and an anatomic lung resection (pneumonectomy or lobectomy). Removal of the whole lung was previously the most commonly performed operation for NSCLC; it now accounts for only 20% of all resections. Although pneumonectomy results in a more complete resection than parenchyma-conserving techniques (lobectomy), pneumonectomy comes at the cost of greater surgery-associated mortality (4%–10%) and morbidity without clear survival benefits. Given that patients treated with lobectomy and pneumonectomy have similar survival and that lobectomy is associated with lower morbidity and mortality rates, lobectomy is the preferred method of resection. The advent of sleeve lobectomies and bronchoplasty procedures in which portions of the main bronchus are removed without loss of the distal lung have further decreased the need for pneumonectomy. Segmentectomy and nonanatomic resection (wedge resection and lumpectomy) are associated with increased local recurrence rates compared with lobectomy (Ginsberg et al, 1995). The general consensus remains that these procedures should be performed only in high-risk patients with minimal pulmonary reserve who could not tolerate a lobectomy.

It is important to perform a mediastinal lymph node dissection after resection of the primary tumor because patients with T1–3N2 disease are known to harbor metastatic disease in the lymph nodes. Lymph node dissection on the right side is begun by exposing the azygos vein and incising the mediastinal pleura superiorly. The boundaries of the dissection are the subclavian vein superiorly, the trachea posteriorly, the azygos vein inferiorly, and the vena cava anteriorly. The vagus and phrenic nerves are identified and serve as landmarks—the lymph node dissection proceeds within these structures. Lymph nodes resected from the right should include nodes at levels 10, 4, 3, and 2 as well as the subcarinal (7), paraesophageal (8), and inferior pulmonary ligament nodes (9) (Figure 7–1 and Table 7–2). On the left side, the aorta is within the field and serves as a landmark guiding resection of the para-aortic (6) and subaortic (5) lymph nodes after incision of the mediastinal pleura. When these lymph nodes are being resected, it is important to identify and preserve the vagus nerve and the recurrent laryngeal nerve, which arise at the level of the aortic arch near the ligamentum arteriosum. The subcarinal (7) and inferior pulmonary ligament nodes (9) should also be resected. The morbidity of mediastinal lymph node dissection is low when the procedure is done by experienced surgeons. Possible complications include bleeding or damage to the recurrent laryngeal nerve or lymphatic duct. Once the nodes have been resected, chest tubes are placed, and the chest and overlying muscles are closed. Postoperative care emphasizes adequate pain control and pulmonary toilet. The chest tubes are removed once the air leaks have sealed and the drainage is less than 300 mL per day.

Because of the poor prognosis of patients with T1–3N2 Pancoast tumors, most of these patients are treated nonsurgically with chemoradiation (see chapter 8).

Postoperative Treatment

Patients with T1–3N2 non-Pancoast tumors are at high risk for primarily systemic recurrence. However, patients are not treated with postoperative chemotherapy because of the lack of evidence from randomized trials regarding a benefit for adjuvant chemotherapy. If, after discussion with a medical oncologist, a patient wishes to undergo adjuvant chemotherapy, it is delivered in an off-protocol setting. Radiation therapy is given only if the margins are involved or close or a large number of involved N2 nodes are found on the final pathologic examination. Patients with T1–3N2 non-

Pancoast tumors that have been resected have follow-up clinic visits 1 month after surgery, at 6-month intervals for 4 visits, and yearly thereafter.

TREATMENT OF PATIENTS WITH STAGE IIIB DISEASE

Stage IIIB NSCLC encompasses tumors involving the contralateral mediastinal nodes (N3 disease) and T4 tumors, which by definition invade the mediastinum, heart, great vessels, trachea, esophagus, vertebral body, or carina or have separate tumor nodules in the same lobe or are associated with a malignant pleural effusion (Mountain, 1997).

Patients with contralateral mediastinal nodal involvement are better treated with chemoradiation rather than surgery because of the high propensity of such tumors to metastasize (see chapter 8). However, patients with T4 tumors with minimal nodal involvement (N0 or N1 disease) may benefit from surgery because these tumors are often more local-regionally than systemically aggressive. Survival rates of up to 30% have been reported for resected T4N0–1 tumors (Tsuchiya et al, 1994; Mitchell et al, 1999; Rendina et al, 1999). However, T4 tumors associated with N2 or N3 nodal involvement or malignant pleural effusions are probably better treated without surgery since their biological behavior is more systemic.

In this section, we will focus on operative strategies for T4N0–1 tumors. All other subsets of stage IIIB disease will be discussed in chapter 8.

Both patients with T4N0–1 non-Pancoast tumors and patients with T4N0–1 Pancoast tumors can benefit from extended surgical resections (Dartevelle et al, 1993; Macchiarini et al, 1994; Tsuchiya et al, 1994; Gandhi et al, 1999; Mitchell et al, 1999; Rendina et al, 1999). Given the proximity of critical structures and the difficulty of achieving negative margins with surgery alone, most T4N0–1 non-Pancoast tumors are treated initially with induction chemotherapy in an attempt to downstage the tumor and improve the chance of obtaining negative microscopic margins at surgery. At our institution, Pancoast tumors are treated initially with surgery; this is followed by postoperative chemoradiation to treat any residual microscopic disease. Patients with T4N0–1 tumors must be physiologically fit to tolerate the extended surgical resections required, and preoperative pulmonary function tests are needed.

Selection of Therapy

T4N0–1 non-Pancoast tumors are usually treated with 2 to 3 courses of induction chemotherapy. The most commonly used regimen is paclitaxel and carboplatin, but other regimens—including cisplatin and navelbine or gemcitabine and navelbine—are equally effective at downstaging tumors and treating potential micrometastatic disease (Macchiarini et al, 1994; Pisters et al, 2000). At M. D. Anderson, we tend not to give preoperative radiation therapy because it is associated with an increased risk of wound healing problems (especially at bronchial margins) after surgery and because the dose that can be delivered before surgery is lower than the dose that can be delivered after (45 Gy vs 66 Gy). If the final pathologic margins after surgery are involved, postoperative radiation therapy is delivered to reduce the risk of local-regional recurrence.

Patients with T4N0–1 Pancoast tumors are treated in a phase II study evaluating surgical resection followed by postoperative chemoradiation. After surgery, radiation therapy is delivered over 5 to 6 weeks. Patients receive 2 fractions per day, to a total dose of 60 Gy in patients with negative margins or 64.8 Gy in patients with positive margins, plus concurrent chemotherapy (cisplatin 50 mg/m^2 on days 1 and 8 and etoposide given by mouth 30 to 60 minutes prior to each administration of radiation therapy on days 1 through 5 and 8 through 12, with this chemotherapy cycle repeated starting on day 29). Prophylactic cranial irradiation (25 Gy in 10 fractions of 2.5 Gy) is given on completion of chest irradiation because of the high risk of brain recurrences. Three additional cycles of chemotherapy are delivered after prophylactic cranial irradiation. This aggressive approach has resulted in long-term survival in a fraction of patients in whom negative pathologic margins can be obtained (Gandhi et al, 1999). Because of the complexity of this operation, careful coordination between the medical oncologists, surgical oncologists, and radiation oncologists is required. These rare tumors should be treated at an experienced referral center to ensure the maximum chance for overall success.

Operative Strategy

Surgery for T4N0–1 non-Pancoast tumors is usually performed after induction chemotherapy. In some cases, the preoperative chemotherapy has significantly downstaged the tumor (Figure 7–2). Nevertheless, the original extent of the tumor must be kept in mind to avoid leaving behind tissue that may still contain microscopic deposits of viable tumor. To help ensure complete resection, scans showing the original extent of the tumor are displayed in the operating room during surgery. The main T4 tumors approached surgically are tumors that invade the carina, vertebral body, or atrium. Resection of the vertebral body will be discussed in the discussion of Pancoast tumors.

Invasion of the carina is rare and should be approached surgically only if all the mediastinal nodes are negative on cervical mediastinoscopy. All carinal resections should focus on minimizing the tension on airway anastomoses by developing a pretracheal plane without interrupting the lateral blood supply of the trachea. The hilum can also be mobilized with an inferior hilar release of the pericardium on either side, and a suprahyoid laryngeal release can be performed if necessary. After surgery, all patients are put in cervical flexion, with a stitch secured from the chin to the ante-

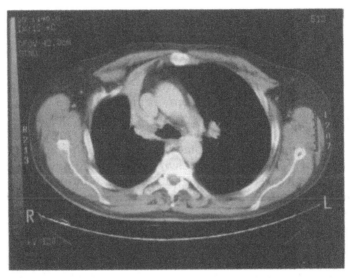

A

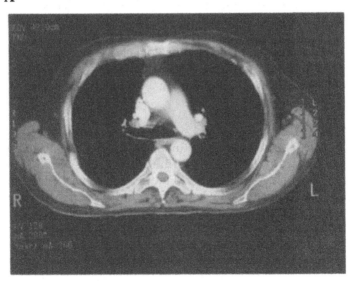

B

Figure 7–2. Downstaging of a T4N0 tumor involving the carina with preoperative chemotherapy. Images are from before (A) and after (B) 3 courses of paclitaxel and carboplatin. Right upper lobe sleeve resection with preservation of the right middle and lower lobe was subsequently performed. The patient was alive without evidence of disease 3 years after surgery.

rior chest wall to prevent inadvertent cervical extension. This stitch is left in place until the end of the first postoperative week. The carina is resected and reanastomosed with simple interrupted 4–0 Vicryl sutures. After creation of the anastomosis, an intercostal muscle pedicle is used to buttress the suture line. After surgery, attempts are made to remove the endotracheal tube early on and maintain adequate pulmonary toilet. Repeated bronchoscopic procedures may be required to help clear secretions in the resected tracheal airway.

Defining the optimal management of T4N0–1 Pancoast tumors that invade the spine or subclavian arteries is controversial. Invasion of these structures was traditionally considered a contraindication to surgery because of the difficulty of the operation and poor long-term results if negative pathologic margins were not obtained (Anderson et al, 1986; Attar et al, 1998). For long-term survival to be achieved, it is critical to obtain a true negative margin and not just shave the tumor off the adjoining structure. Since vertebral invasion is common with Pancoast tumors, at M. D. Anderson we have drawn upon our experience with metastatic spinal tumors to learn how to approach T4 Pancoast tumors with vertebral invasion. These tumors are treated with a combination of transthoracic vertebrectomy, reconstruction with methyl methacrylate, and spinal fixation with locking plate and screw constructs (Gandhi et al, 1999). All operations are begun with cervical mediastinoscopy to rule out mediastinal nodal involvement. If the mediastinal nodes are not involved according to frozen section techniques, surgical resection proceeds through a posterolateral thoracotomy with an extension over the vertebrae if posterior fixation is required. In certain cases, an anterior cervical approach is used in addition to the posterior approach to dissect the tumor free of the cervical and vascular structures, perform vascular reconstructions if needed, or divide the anterior portion of the chest wall. The posterolateral incision allows the involved ribs to be disarticulated and resected en bloc with the involved chest wall and lung parenchyma. The involved vertebrae are then resected separately by the neurosurgery team according to the amount of vertebral involvement.

In patients with only neural foramina or transverse process involvement, the transverse processes are drilled out with a high-speed diamond-burr power drill. The nerve root sleeve is then visualized and ligated at the nerve root proximal to the dorsal root ganglion. Tumor involving the surrounding osseous elements is ablated with additional resection using the high-speed diamond-burr drill. If there is significant extension of the tumor into the spinal canal or gross invasion of the proximal transverse process, facet joints, or lamina, a multilevel laminectomy is performed with a posterior midline extension of the thoracotomy incision. This allows visualization of the thecal sac as well as the ipsilateral nerve roots involved with tumor. After nerve root transection and removal of the main specimen, the remainder of the involved vertebral body is removed using a combination of the high-speed diamond-burr power drill, curettes of various sizes, and a Cavitron ultrasonic aspirator. The vertebrectomy defect is repaired with methyl methacrylate using a chest tube strut. Anterior fixation is achieved with an anterior cervical locking plate and screw construct. In extensive resections and multilevel laminectomies, additional posterior segmental fixation is done by using hooks, rods, and Wisconsin spinous process wires (in selected cases) several levels above and below the laminectomy site. Posterior fusion is obtained dorsally with an allograft and Grafton, a fusion promoter.

This complex approach is performed with multidisciplinary coordination between the neurosurgery and thoracic surgery teams and allows negative margins to be obtained in the maximum number of patients. After surgery, patients are extubated early and put immediately in active rehabilitation. This extensive operation has allowed resection of T4N0–1 Pancoast tumors that were formerly believed to be unresectable. Long-term survival is possible when negative pathologic margins are achieved.

Postoperative Treatment

T4N0–1 non-Pancoast NSCLCs are treated with postoperative radiation therapy if margins are involved. Postoperative chemotherapy is not typically administered since preoperative chemotherapy has already been given and many patients are less able to tolerate postoperative chemotherapy. Long-term survival can be achieved in up to 30% of these patients with this aggressive multidisciplinary approach.

T4N0–1 Pancoast tumors are treated with postoperative chemoradiation to minimize the chance of local-regional recurrences. Delivery of radiation postoperatively as opposed to preoperatively as advocated by some groups (Rusch et al, 2001) allows a larger dose of radiation to be delivered because surgery has already been performed. These tumors require a coordinated multidisciplinary approach to maximize the chance for cure.

Future Directions

In the future, the advent of novel biological agents may provide additional therapeutic treatment options for patients with locally advanced NSCLC, and molecular diagnostic markers may allow more accurate means of assessing which patients with locally advanced NSCLC would receive the greatest benefit from surgery or other forms of treatment.

Acknowledgement

The author is grateful to Debbie Smith for assistance with the preparation of this manuscript.

KEY PRACTICE POINTS

- Locally advanced (stage IIIA and stage IIIB) NSCLC encompasses a very heterogeneous group of tumor types.

- The initial assessment to determine whether a patient is fit for surgery should include an assessment of the patient's physiologic reserves with a thorough physical examination, history, cardiac evaluation, and pulmonary function testing.

- Surgical resection is beneficial in subsets of patients with locally advanced NSCLC in which the possibility of improved local-regional control outweighs the potential increased morbidity of surgery.

- Subsets of non-Pancoast tumors for which surgery may be beneficial include T3N1 tumors (surgery alone in physiologically fit patients); T1–3N2 tumors (induction chemotherapy followed by surgery in patients who are physiologically fit, do not have bulky adenopathy, or have a good radiographic or histologic response to induction chemotherapy); and T4N0–1 tumors (surgery after induction chemotherapy in a subset of patients with local-regionally aggressive disease).

- T4N2 and T1–4N3 non-Pancoast tumors and T4 non-Pancoast tumors associated with malignant pleural effusions are best treated nonsurgically because of the poor long-term survival (chapter 8).

- Subsets of Pancoast tumors for which surgery may be beneficial include T3N1 and T4N0–1 tumors (surgery followed by postoperative chemoradiation to minimize the chance of local-regional recurrence).

- T1–4N2–3 Pancoast tumors and T4 Pancoast tumors associated with malignant pleural effusions are best treated nonsurgically because of the poor long-term survival (chapter 8).

SUGGESTED READINGS

Anderson TM, Moy PM, Holmes EC. Factors affecting survival in superior sulcus tumors. *J Clin Oncol* 1986;4:1598–1603.

Andre F, Grunenwald D, Pignon JP, et al. Survival of patients with resected N2 non-small-cell lung cancer: evidence for a subclassification and implications. *J Clin Oncol* 2000;18:2981–2989.

Attar S, Krasna MJ, Sonett JR, et al. Superior sulcus (Pancoast) tumor: experience with 105 patients. *Ann Thorac Surg* 1998;66:193–198.

Bueno R, Richards WG, Swanson SJ, et al. Nodal stage after induction therapy for stage IIIA lung cancer determines patient survival. *Ann Thorac Surg* 2000;70:1826–1831.

Choy H, Akerley W, Safran H, et al. Phase I trial of outpatient weekly paclitaxel and concurrent radiation therapy for advanced non-small-cell lung cancer. *J Clin Oncol* 1994;12:2682–2686.

Dartevelle PG, Chapelier AR, Macchiarini P, et al. Anterior transcervical-thoracic approach for radical resection of lung tumors invading the thoracic inlet. *J Thorac Cardiovasc Surg* 1993;105:1025–1034.

Dillman RO, Herndon J, Seagren SL, et al. Improved survival in stage III non-small-cell lung cancer: seven-year follow-up of Cancer and Leukemia Group B (CALGB) 8433 trial. *J Natl Cancer Inst* 1996;88:1210–1215.

Ferguson MK, Reeder LB, Mick M. Optimizing selection of patients for major lung resection. *J Thorac Cardiovasc Surg* 1995;109:275–281.

Gandhi S, Walsh GL, Komaki R, et al. A multidisciplinary surgical approach to superior sulcus tumors with vertebral invasion. *Ann Thorac Surg* 1999; 68:1778–1784.

Ginsberg RJ, Rubinstein LV, for the Lung Cancer Study Group. Randomized trial of lobectomy versus limited resection for T1 N0 non-small cell lung cancer. *Ann Thorac Surg* 1995;60:615–622.

Gressen EL, Curran WJ Jr. Effectiveness of radiation therapy on non-small-cell lung cancer. *Clinical Lung Cancer* 2001;2:182–194.

Kearney DJ, Lee TH, Reilly JJ, et al. Assessment of operative risk in patients undergoing lung resection. Importance of predicted pulmonary function. *Chest* 1994;105:753–759.

Kubota K, Furuse K, Kawahara M, et al. Role of radiotherapy in combined modality treatment of locally advanced non-small-cell lung cancer. *J Clin Oncol* 1994;12:1547–1552.

Luzzi L, Paladini P, Ghiribelli C, et al. Assessing the prognostic value of the extent of mediastinal lymph node infiltration in surgically-treated non-small cell lung cancer (NSCLC). *Lung Cancer* 2000;30:99–105.

Macchiarini P, Chapelier AR, Monnet I, et al. Extended operations after induction therapy for stage IIIb (T4) non-small cell lung cancer. *Ann Thorac Surg* 1994;57:966–973.

Maurel J, Martinez-Trufero J, Artal A, et al. Prognostic impact of bulky mediastinal lymph nodes (N2>2.5 cm) in patients with locally advanced non-small-cell lung cancer (LA-NSCLC) treated with platinum-based induction chemotherapy. *Lung Cancer* 2000;30:107–116.

Mitchell JD, Mathisen DJ, Wright CD, et al. Clinical experience with carinal resection. *J Thorac Cardiovasc Surg* 1999;17:39–52.

Mountain CF. Revisions in the International System for Staging Lung Cancer. *Chest* 1997;111:1710–1717.

Mountain CF, Dresler CM. Regional lymph node classification for lung cancer staging. *Chest* 1997;111:1719–1723.

Nesbitt JC, Putnam JB Jr, Walsh GL, et al. Survival in early-stage non-small cell lung cancer. *Ann Thorac Surg* 1995;60:466–472.

Parker SL, Tong T, Bolden S, et al. Cancer statistics, 1997. *CA Cancer J Clin* 1997;47:5–27.

Pisters KM, Ginsberg RJ, Giroux DJ, et al, for the Bimodality Lung Oncology Team. Induction chemotherapy before surgery for early-stage lung cancer: a novel approach. *J Thorac Cardiovasc Surg* 2000;119:429–439.

Rao V, Todd TR, Kuus A, et al. Exercise oximetry versus spirometry in the assessment of risk prior to lung resection. *Ann Thorac Surg* 1995;60:603–608.

Rendina EA, Venuta F, De Giacomo T, et al. Sleeve resection and prosthetic reconstruction of the pulmonary artery for lung cancer. *Ann Thorac Surg* 1999; 68:995–1001.

Rosell R, Gomez-Codina J, Camps C, et al. Preresectional chemotherapy in stage IIIA non-small-cell lung cancer: a 7-year assessment of a randomized controlled trial. *Lung Cancer* 1999;26:7–14.

Roth JA, Atkinson EN, Fossella F, et al. Long-term follow-up of patients enrolled in a randomized trial comparing perioperative chemotherapy and surgery with surgery alone in resectable stage IIIA non-small-cell lung cancer. *Lung Cancer* 1998;21:1–6.

Rusch VW, Giroux DJ, Kraut MJ, et al. Induction chemoradiation and surgical resection for non-small cell lung carcinomas of the superior sulcus: initial results of Southwest Oncology Group Trial 9416 (Intergroup Trial 0160). *J Thorac Cardiovasc Surg* 2001;121:472–483.

Sause W, Kolesar P, Taylor S IV, et al. Final results of phase III trial in regionally advanced unresectable non-small cell lung cancer: Radiation Therapy Oncology Group, Eastern Cooperative Oncology Group, and Southwest Oncology Group. *Chest* 2000;117:358–364.

Schaake-Koning C, van den Bogaert W, Dalesio O, et al. Effects of concomitant cisplatin and radiotherapy on inoperable non-small cell lung cancer. *N Engl J Med* 1992;326:524–530.

Tsuchiya R, Asamura H, Kondo H, et al. Extended resection of the left atrium, great vessels, or both for lung cancer. *Ann Thorac Surg* 1994;57:960–965.

Walsh GL, Morice RC, Putnam JB Jr, et al. Resection of lung cancer is justified in high-risk patients selected by exercise oxygen consumption. *Ann Thorac Surg* 1994;58:704–710.

Walsh GL, O'Connor M, Willis KM, et al. Is follow-up of lung cancer patients after resection medically indicated and cost-effective? *Ann Thorac Surg* 1995; 60:1563–1570.

Weiner P, Man A, Weiner M, et al. The effect of incentive spirometry and inspiratory muscle training on pulmonary function after lung resection. *J Thorac Cardiovasc Surg* 1997;113:552–557.

8 Nonsurgical Treatment of Early-Stage and Locally Advanced Non–Small Cell Lung Cancer

Ritsuko Komaki

CHAPTER OVERVIEW

Approximately half of all patients with early-stage or locally advanced non–small cell lung cancer are treated with radiation therapy either because their medical condition makes them unable to safely undergo surgery or because their tumor is considered unresectable. In medically inoperable patients with stage I lesions, radiation therapy is usually given without chemotherapy because adjuvant chemotherapy in these patients has not been shown to improve outcomes. Patients with stage II or III non–small cell lung cancer who cannot be treated surgically are treated with radiation therapy with or without chemotherapy depending on their performance status, weight loss, and medical conditions.

Introduction

As discussed in chapters 6 and 7, surgery offers the best chance for local control in patients with early-stage non–small cell lung cancer (NSCLC) and is beneficial in patients with locally advanced (stage IIIA and IIIB) NSCLC in whom the possibility of improved local control outweighs the potential for increased morbidity. However, approximately half of all patients with early-stage or locally advanced NSCLC are treated nonsurgically (with radiation therapy with or without chemotherapy) either because they are unable to tolerate surgical resection (this group includes patients with stage I, II, and III disease) or because their tumor is considered unresectable (this group includes patients with stage III disease). This chapter will describe treatment options for patients with early-stage or locally advanced NSCLC who cannot be treated successfully with surgery.

Pretreatment Workup

An adequate staging workup for patients with NSCLC currently includes computed tomography (CT) of the chest and fluorodeoxyglucose–positron emission tomography (PET) scanning. Careful attention to the mediastinum is critical in making the diagnosis of mediastinal lymph node involvement. If CT of the chest reveals questionable lymph nodes, such as lymph nodes 1 to 2 cm in diameter, mediastinoscopy is recommended. If the PET scan shows increased uptake and CT of the mediastinal lymph nodes is negative, whether mediastinoscopy should be done or not is fairly controversial. Other components of the workup for metastatic disease are described in chapter 3.

The pretreatment workup should also include tests and examinations designed to determine the patient's fitness for surgery. Very poor performance status and significant weight loss are considered contraindications to surgery. Patients considered medically unfit for surgery include those with poor lung function (a forced expiratory volume in 1 second [FEV_1] less than 1.2 liters or less than 35% of the predicted value; a predicted postoperative FEV_1 less than 1.03 liters or less than 33% of predicted; or an alveolar-arterial difference in partial pressure of oxygen greater than 45 mg), a recent myocardial infarction, or a bleeding tendency (Kupelian et al, 1996).

Stage I Lesions

In patients with clinical stage I disease who are medically unfit for surgery, radiation therapy can be given with curative intent. These patients are usually not treated with concurrent chemotherapy because their comorbid conditions prevent aggressive treatment. Adjuvant chemotherapy in addition to radiation therapy in this population has not been shown to improve outcomes because patients' comorbid conditions interfere with long-term assessment of treatment efficacy.

Radiation therapy is usually delivered with 6- to 18-MV photons. Since these patients have very poor lung function, the margins around the gross tumor volume (GTV) should be minimal to avoid pulmonary complications after completion of radiation therapy. After treatment planning with contrast material and respiratory gating, the contour of the GTV is drawn. The clinical target volume (CTV) is drawn at 5 mm outside the GTV for squamous cell carcinoma and at 8 mm outside the GTV for adenocarcinoma to ensure coverage of subclinical disease extension. The gating for respiration motion reduces the planning target volume (PTV), which encompasses the CTV plus a margin around it. Usually respiratory gating reduces the PTV from 15 to 20 mm beyond the CTV down to about 5 mm beyond the CTV. If a lesion is attached to the vertebral body or located at the apex of the lung, gating is not necessary since the lesion usually does not move beyond 10 mm with respiration (Figure 8–1). Dose and volume constraints differ depending on the normal organ tissue surrounding the tumor. If respiratory gating is not done because of unpredictable respiration patterns, the motion of the tumor has to be checked under fluoroscopy, and we must take much larger mar-

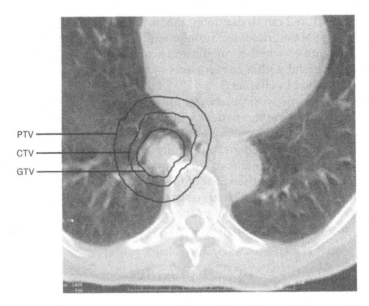

Figure 8–1. Radiation therapy target volumes in an 80-year-old man with a T1 lesion in the right lower lobe, severe asthma, and chronic obstructive pulmonary disease with FEV_1 of 35%. GTV, gross tumor volume; CTV, clinical target volume; PTV, planning target volume. No respiratory gating was used.

gins—up to 3 cm, depending on the motion of the tumor. Fluoroscopy is sometimes a poor predictor of tumor motion because the anteroposterior and rotational motions can be significant. Furthermore, stage I lesions are not well visualized under fluoroscopy. Ideally, in the future, PET or CT will better define the GTV and CTV.

Radiation doses for T1 or T2 lesions are usually 60 Gy or higher. To find the maximum tolerated dose with 3-dimensional conformal treatment, the Radiation Therapy Oncology Group (RTOG) 93–11 trial (Table 8–1) has been investigating dose escalation for small lesions ($< 25\%$ of the total lung volume). Doses up to 90 Gy have been tolerated, although long-term effects, such as cardiac damage, have started to appear. Whether a dose of 90 Gy results in better tumor control than that seen with lower doses (< 70 Gy) is not yet known. Patients with stage I disease who cannot be treated with surgery usually have clinically staged disease; thus, survival comparisons between these patients and surgically treated patients are difficult. Several surgical series have demonstrated that 24% to 37% of patients with clinical T1N0 or T2N0 disease have their disease upstaged on pathologic examination after surgery, which explains the poor results in clinically staged patients who are treated with radiation therapy alone. We analyzed patients with stage I disease who were treated with radiation therapy alone between 1980 and 1990 at M. D. Anderson Cancer Center (Kupelian et al, 1996). Nineteen patients had clinical stage T1N0 NSCLC,

Table 8–1. Schema for Radiation Therapy Oncology Group Trial 93–11, a Phase I/II Dose Escalation Study Using 3-Dimensional Conformal Radiation Therapy in Patients with Inoperable NSCLC*

Group 1 ($< 25\%$ of total lung volume receives > 20 Gy)

   Dose level 1: 70.9 Gy in 33 fractions over 7–8 weeks (closed 1/8/98)
   Dose level 2: 77.4 Gy in 36 fractions over 7–8 weeks (closed 9/23/98)
   Dose level 3: 83.8 Gy in 39 fractions over 8–9 weeks (closed 12/20/99)
   Dose level 4: 90.3 Gy in 42 fractions over 9–10 weeks (opened 12/20/99)

Group 2 (25% to $< 37\%$ of total lung volume receives > 20 Gy)

   Dose level 5: 70.9 Gy in 33 fractions over 7–8 weeks (closed 6/14/99)
   Dose level 6: 77.4 Gy in 36 fractions over 7–8 weeks (opened 6/14/99)
   Dose level 7: 83.8 Gy in 39 fractions over 8–9 weeks

Group 3 ($\geq 37\%$ of total lung volume receives > 20 Gy)

   Dose level 8: 64.5 Gy in 30 fractions over 6–7 weeks (closed 7/1/99)
   Dose level 9: 70.9 Gy in 33 fractions over 7–8 weeks (closed 7/1/99)
   Dose level 10: 77.4 Gy in 36 fractions over 7–8 weeks (closed 7/1/99)

* All patients must have a completed 3-dimensional plan prior to entering this protocol. Total lung volume is defined as the total volume of both lungs minus the PTV. Only 1 dose level per stratification group will open at a time. Dose prescription is to the ICRU 50 reference point.

and 26 patients had clinical stage T2N0 NSCLC. The median total dose of radiation was 63 Gy, and 80% of the patients received doses higher than 60 Gy. Responses were documented with chest radiography, and in 60% of the patients, the maximum response was seen within 6 months after completion of radiation therapy. The median follow-up time was 36 months. Disease-specific survival rates at 3 years were 49% for patients with T1 disease and 47% for patients with T2 disease. Local control rates at 3 years were 89% for T1 lesions and 61% for T2 lesions (Figure 8–2). The significant prognostic factors for better disease-free survival were Karnofsky performance status score of 70 or higher, tumor size of 5 cm or smaller, and radiation therapy dose of 50 Gy or greater. The significant prognostic factors for better local control were tumor size of 4 cm or less, radiation therapy dose of 60 Gy or greater, and complete response according to chest radiography within 6 months after completion of radiation therapy. Coverage of the nodal drainage area with elective radiation therapy did not affect survival or local control. No lethal complications were seen, and documented symptomatic radiation pneumonitis occurred in only 7% of the patients (Kupelian et al, 1996).

At M. D. Anderson, we usually treat stage I tumors with 66 Gy delivered at 2 Gy per fraction 5 days per week without inhomogeneity correction.

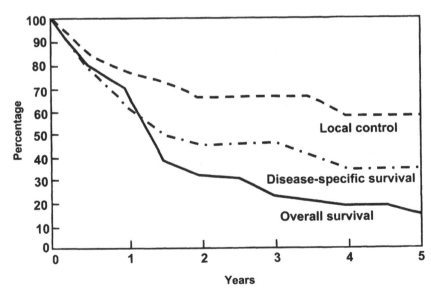

Figure 8–2. Overall survival, disease-specific survival, and local control rates for 45 patients with clinical stage I NSCLC treated with radiation therapy alone. Reprinted from *International Journal of Radiation Oncology Biology and Physics*, volume 36, number 3, Kupelian PA, Komaki R, Allen P, Prognostic factors in the treatment of node-negative non-small cell lung carcinoma with radiotherapy alone, pages 607–613, 1996, with permission from Elsevier Science.

STAGE II AND III LESIONS

Radiation Therapy Alone

In dose escalation studies done in the 1970s and 1980s, a standard dose of radiation therapy for stage II or III NSCLC that could not be treated surgically was set at 60 Gy over 6 weeks given at 2 Gy per fraction without any break (Perez et al, 1980, 1986) (Table 8–2). These studies were done in the pre-CT and pre-PET era. The total dose was escalated from 40 Gy given as split-course or continuous radiation therapy up to 60 Gy given as continuous radiation therapy. The best option in terms of primary tumor control was found to be 60 Gy in 6 weeks; the 3-year local control rate with this regimen was thought to be more than 60%. With CT scanning or biopsies after radiation therapy, we now know that the local control rate is actually much lower.

In an attempt to increase rates of local control and cure without increasing late reactive normal tissue damage, the RTOG performed a dose escalation trial using twice-daily radiation therapy, 1.2 Gy per fraction (RTOG 83–11) (Cox et al, 1990). This trial demonstrated improved survival and local control with doses of at least 69.6 Gy. There was no survival advantage with doses higher than 69.6 Gy without the use of 3-dimensional conformal radiation therapy.

The radiation therapy technique for stage III disease that cannot be treated surgically used to involve more generous margins, such as a 20- to 25-mm margin around the GTV. For upper-lobe lesions, the supraclavicular lymph nodes were usually covered with elective nodal radiation therapy fields. For lower-lobe lesions, the lower mediastinal lymph nodes and the subcarinal area were usually covered. In most cases, contralateral hilar and mediastinal lymph nodes were covered by a 15- to 20-mm margin beyond the lateral border of the vertebral body. For upper-lobe and midlobe lesions, subcarinal lymph nodes were irradiated electively with the fields designed to extend 50 mm below the carina.

Table 8–2.   Outcomes in Radiation Therapy Oncology Group Trial 73–01, a Prospective Randomized Study of Various Radiation Doses and Fractionation Schedules in the Treatment of Inoperable Non-Oat-Cell Carcinoma of the Lung (N = 365)

Regimen	Complete Response Rate	3-Year Rate of Local or Distant Recurrence	Median Survival Time	3-Year Local Failure Rate
20 Gy over 1 week x 2	8%	44%	8 mo	44%
40 Gy over 4 weeks	21%	49%	10 mo	52%
50 Gy over 5 weeks	20%	39%	9 mo	42%
60 Gy over 6 weeks	24%	33%	11 mo	33%
				(P = .02)

Sources: Perez et al, 1980 and 1986.

Around 1998, by using 3-dimensional conformal radiation therapy and
respiratory gating, we started to use a much tighter margin. We usually set
the CTV at 5 to 8 mm beyond the GTV and set the PTV at 10 to 15 mm beyond the CTV when respiratory gating is done. When patients have atelectasis, magnetic resonance imaging and PET help to distinguish tumor
from atelectasis. However, if the patient has a totally collapsed lung and
the tumor is endobronchial, we usually do endobronchial brachytherapy
to open up the main bronchial obstruction. Endobronchial techniques are
described later in this chapter. After expansion of the lung, we usually
give 60 Gy of external-beam radiation over 6 weeks.

Combined Chemotherapy and Radiation Therapy

Because of the poor outcomes in patients with stage II or III NSCLC treated
with radiation therapy alone, the Cancer and Leukemia Group B conducted a trial designed to determine the value of adding chemotherapy to
this treatment. In this trial, 155 patients with stage III NSCLC with good
performance status and weight loss of less than 5% were randomly assigned to treatment with 2 cycles of vinblastine and cisplatin followed by
radiation therapy (60 Gy in 6 weeks) or radiation therapy alone (60 Gy in 6
weeks) (Dillman et al, 1990) (Table 8–3). Patients who were treated with induction chemotherapy followed by radiation therapy had a median survival of 13.8 months, compared to 9.7 months for patients treated with radiation therapy alone ($P = .04$). The 2-year survival rate was significantly
better among the patients who received induction chemotherapy (26% vs
13%; $P = .006$). A reanalysis of the results of this study after a longer follow-
up time (Dillman et al, 1996) showed a 5-year survival rate of 19% for patients treated with induction chemotherapy, compared to 7% for those who
received radiation therapy alone.

In RTOG trial 88–08 (Sause et al, 1995), 452 patients with stage III
NSCLC with good performance status and weight loss of less than 5%

Table 8–3. Outcomes in Cancer and Leukemia Group B Trial Comparing
Induction Chemotherapy plus High-Dose Radiation Therapy
versus Radiation Therapy Alone in Patients with Stage III
NSCLC

Outcome	Chemotherapy and Radiation Therapy (N = 78)	Radiation Therapy Alone (N = 77)
Survival rate		
1-Year	55%	44%
2-Year	26%	13%
5-Year	19%	7%
Median survival time	13.8 months	9.7 months

Source: Dillman et al, 1990 and 1996.

Table 8–4. Schema for Radiation Therapy Oncology Group Trial 88–08: Effect of Chemotherapy on Failure Patterns in Patients with Unresectable NSCLC Treated with Radiation Therapy

Stratification criteria

    Histology: squamous vs other
    Karnofsky performance status: 70–80 vs 90–100
    Stage: II vs IIIA vs IIIB

Arm 1 (conventional radiation therapy)

    60 Gy in daily 2.0-Gy fractions over 6 weeks

Arm 2 (chemotherapy followed by conventional radiation therapy)

    Vinblastine weekly for 6 weeks
    Cisplatin on days 1 and 29
    Conventional radiation therapy beginning on day 50

Arm 3 (hyperfractionated radiation therapy)

    69.6 Gy in twice-daily 1.2-Gy fractions over 6 weeks

were randomly assigned to treatment with conventional radiation therapy alone, hyperfractionated radiation therapy alone, or chemotherapy followed by conventional radiation therapy. Treatment details are given in Table 8–4. The median survival in the group that received chemotherapy was 13.8 months, compared to 11.4 months among the patients who received hyperfractionated radiation therapy. The 2-year survival rate was 32% among the patients who received combined treatment versus 19% among the patients who received hyperfractionated radiation therapy ($P = .003$).

RTOG trial 91–06 was a phase II trial in which patients received a combination of the most effective radiation therapy regimen identified in RTOG trial 83–11 (a total dose of 69.6 Gy) and concurrent oral etoposide and intravenous cisplatin (Lee et al, 1996). Eligibility criteria included unresectable NSCLC, good performance status, and weight loss less than 5%. Among the 76 patients enrolled, the 2-year survival rate was 40%, and the median survival was 19.7 months (Lee et al, 1996). This median survival was better than the median survival of 10.3 months in RTOG trial 83–11 (twice-daily radiation therapy alone) (Table 8–5) (Komaki et al, 1997b). However, acute esophagitis was significantly more common among the patients treated with twice-daily radiation therapy and concurrent chemotherapy.

At M. D. Anderson, RTOG trial 92–04 was activated in 1992 to compare 2 combinations of chemotherapy and radiation therapy in patients with inoperable stage II or III NSCLC, a Karnofsky performance status score of 70 or higher, and minimal weight loss (Komaki et al, 1997a, in press). Treatment details are given in Table 8–6. The arm-1 treatment (induction chemotherapy followed by concurrent chemoradiation) was based on previous RTOG

Table 8–5. Survival among Patients Treated with Hyperfractionated
Radiation Therapy with Concurrent Chemotherapy
(RTOG Trial 91–06) or Hyperfractionated Radiation Therapy
Alone (RTOG Trial 83–11)

Outcome	RTOG 91-06	RTOG 83-11
Survival rate		
Baseline	100%	100%
6 months	82%	72%
12 months	67%	48%
18 months	51%	29%
24 months	36%	22%
Median survival time	18.9 months	10.6 months
Dead patients/total patients	57/76	194/203
		Log-rank P = .014

Table 8–6. Schema for Radiation Therapy Oncology Group Trial 92–04,
a Randomized Phase II Study of 2 Chemotherapy and Radiation
Therapy Combinations for Patients with Locally Advanced,
Inoperable NSCLC and Favorable Characteristics

Stratification criteria

Stage: II vs IIIA vs IIIB
Cell type: squamous vs nonsquamous
Karnofsky performance status: 90–100 vs 70–80

Arm 1 (induction chemotherapy followed by concurrent chemoradiation)

Vinblastine: 5 mg/m^2 weekly IV bolus, weeks 1–5
Cisplatin: 100 mg/m^2 IV days 1 and 29; 75 mg/m^2 days 50, 71, and 92
Radiation therapy: starting on day 50, a total of 63 Gy given in 34 fractions
of 2 Gy in 7 weeks

Arm 2 (immediate concurrent chemoradiation)

Cisplatin: 50 mg/m^2 IV days 1 and 8
Etoposide: 50 mg twice daily during the first 2 weeks of each radiation
therapy cycle
Radiation therapy: starting on day 1, a total of 69.6 Gy given in 58 twice-daily
fractions of 1.2 Gy in 6 weeks

studies (Sause et al, 1992, 1995). A total of 168 patients were enrolled, and
163 patients were eligible for analysis. Eighty-one patients were treated
with induction chemotherapy followed by concurrent chemoradiation (arm
1), and 82 patients were treated with immediate concurrent chemoradiation
(arm 2). The rate of acute esophagitis was significantly higher in arm 2 (37%)
than in arm 1 (3%) (P < .0001). Also, the rate of late chronic esophageal complications was significantly higher in arm 2 (17% vs 4%; P = .003). The com-

plete response rates were 37% in arm 1 and 42% in arm 2. There was a significant difference in time to in-field progression favoring arm 2 (45% in arm 1 vs 26% in arm 2 at 2 years and 49% in arm 1 vs 30% in arm 2 at 4 years) (P = .009). The median overall survival times were 16.4 months in arm 1 and 15.5 months in arm 2 (P = .88). There was no significant survival difference between the 2 arms at 2 years or 4 years.

RTOG trial 94–10, the results of which were published in 2000, was designed to compare concomitant versus sequential chemotherapy and thoracic radiation therapy in patients with inoperable stage II or III NSCLC with a Karnofsky performance status score higher than 70 and weight loss less than 5% (Komaki et al, 2000b). In this trial, patients were randomly assigned to receive sequential chemotherapy and radiation therapy (vinblastine and cisplatin for 2 cycles followed by 63 Gy in 7 weeks) (arm 1); chemotherapy (vinblastine and cisplatin) with concurrent once-daily radiation therapy (63 Gy in 7 weeks) (arm 2); or chemotherapy (oral etoposide and cisplatin) with concurrent twice-daily radiation therapy (69.6 Gy in 1.2-Gy twice-daily fractions in 6 weeks) (arm 3). Treatment details are given in Table 8–7. Radiation therapy was given using conventional techniques rather than 3-dimensional conformal radiation therapy techniques.

Table 8–7. Schema for Radiation Therapy Oncology Group Trial 94–10, a 3-Arm Phase III Study of Concomitant versus Sequential Chemotherapy and Thoracic Radiation Therapy for Patients with Locally Advanced, Inoperable NSCLC

Stratification criteria

Stage: II vs IIIA vs IIIB
Karnofsky performance status 90–100 vs 70–80

Arm 1 (chemotherapy followed by once-daily radiation therapy)

Vinblastine: 5 mg/m^2 intravenous bolus weekly for first 5 weeks
Cisplatin: 100 mg/m^2 given intravenously over 30–60 minutes, days 1 and 29
Radiation therapy: 63 Gy in 34 daily fractions over 7 weeks (1.8 Gy x 25 fractions, then 2.0 Gy x 9 fractions) beginning day 50

Arm 2 (concurrent chemotherapy and once-daily radiation therapy)

Vinblastine: 5 mg/m^2 intravenous bolus weekly for first 5 weeks
Cisplatin: 100 mg/m^2 given intravenously over 30–60 minutes, days 1 and 29
Radiation therapy: 63 Gy in 34 daily fractions over 7 weeks (1.8 Gy x 25 fractions, then 2.0 Gy x 9 fractions) beginning day 1

Arm 3 (concurrent chemotherapy and twice-daily radiation therapy)

Etoposide: 50 mg by mouth twice daily x 10 only on radiation therapy days 1–5 and 8–12 (75 mg/day if body surface area < 1.7 m^2)
Cisplatin: 50 mg/m^2 intravenously over 30–60 minutes on days 1, 8, 29, and 36
Radiation therapy: 69.6 Gy in 58 twice-daily 1.2-Gy fractions (at least 6 hours apart) over 6 weeks beginning day 1

A total of 610 patients were enrolled, many of them from M. D. Anderson. Median survival was 17 months in patients treated with concurrent chemoradiation with daily fractionation; 16 months in patients treated with concurrent chemoradiation with twice-daily fractionation; and 14.6 months in patients treated with sequential chemotherapy followed by daily radiation therapy (Komaki et al, 2000b). Rates of acute grade 3 or higher nonhematologic side effects were significantly more common among the patients treated with concurrent chemoradiation with twice-daily fractionation (63%) than among those treated with concurrent chemoradiation with once-daily fractionation (50%) ($P = .011$) or sequential therapy (31%) ($P < .001$).

At present, patients at M. D. Anderson with NSCLC with good performance status and minimal weight loss are treated with once-daily fractionation with vinblastine and cisplatin or weekly paclitaxel and carboplatin.

We are conducting an ongoing randomized study in which all patients receive a total tumor dose of 63 Gy in 1.8-Gy daily fractions with concurrent paclitaxel and carboplatin with or without shark cartilage as an anti-angiogenic agent. All patients receive 2 cycles of paclitaxel and carboplatin as induction chemotherapy before concurrent chemotherapy and radiation therapy. A total of 756 evaluable patients will be required to permit detection of a 25% difference in median survival.

Superior Sulcus Tumors

Patients with superior sulcus tumors that cannot be treated surgically should be considered candidates for curative or palliative radiation therapy with or without chemotherapy. Ahmad and colleagues (1984) reported on 48 patients with superior sulcus tumors treated with radiation therapy alone using either cobalt 60 or cesium 137 teletherapy up to a total tumor dose of 50 to 60 Gy over 5 to 6 weeks. The actuarial 3-year survival rate was 28%, and the actuarial 5-year survival rate was 21%. There were no severe complications among the patients treated with radiation therapy alone except for some fibrotic changes in 1 patient that were recognized in the radiographs but did not cause any symptoms.

Van Houtte and colleagues (1984) reported on 31 patients with superior sulcus tumors treated with external-beam high-energy radiation therapy up to a total tumor dose of 20 to 70 Gy. The overall 5-year survival rate was 18%. Doses below 50 Gy and bone invasion were associated with a higher local recurrence rate.

Komaki and colleagues (1981) reported on 36 patients with inoperable superior sulcus tumors who were treated with external-beam radiation therapy between 1963 and 1977 at the Medical College of Wisconsin. Local control correlated positively with larger field size and longer median survival. All patients who survived beyond 2 years had local tumor control, and no patient survived beyond 2 years if treatment failed locally (i.e., if local disease was never controlled or if the patient had a local recurrence). Between 1978 and 1983, an additional 32 patients with inoperable superior sulcus tumors were studied (Komaki et al, 1987). Relief of pain was achieved in 91% of the patients who presented with pain. Three fourths of the patients with Horner's syndrome responded to radiation therapy. The disease-free survival rates were 65% at 12 months, 38% at 24 months, 25% at 36 months, and 15% at 48 months. Again, no patient survived beyond 2 years if treatment failed locally. The brain was the most common site of distant metastases after the completion of radiation therapy. At a minimum follow-up time of 2 years, brain metastases had occurred in 23 (34%) of 68 patients (Komaki et al, 1987).

Treatment strategies combining high-dose radiation therapy ($\geq$ 66 Gy) with chemotherapy for patients with unresectable or node-positive (N2) superior sulcus tumors should be further investigated (Komaki et al, 2000a).

ENDOBRONCHIAL AND ENDOTRACHEAL LESIONS

Endobronchial and endotracheal lesions can cause life-threatening symptoms, including shortness of breath, postobstructive pneumonitis, and hemoptysis. Endobronchial brachytherapy has been used to deliver high radiation doses to these relatively accessible tumors either as a component of potentially curable therapy or, more commonly, in the palliative setting after external-beam radiation therapy has failed to control the disease. Occasionally, patients who present with a completely obstructed (Figure 8–3) or par-

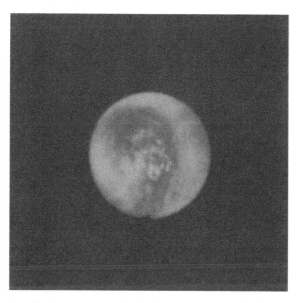

Figure 8–3. Exophytic endobronchial lesion obstructing the bronchus.

tially obstructed airway due to an endobronchial lesion or with hemoptysis due to bleeding from endotracheal or endobronchial lesions can be treated with curative intent with a combination of external-beam radiation therapy and endobronchial brachytherapy.

At M. D. Anderson, irradiation of endobronchial lesions is usually done using high-dose-rate brachytherapy with remote afterloading catheters using a single iridium 192 source attached to a stainless steel cable. Iridium 192 has an active length of 3.5 mm and an active diameter of 0.06 mm (Figure 8–4). The source has an activity of approximately 270 GBq (10 Ci) at the time of installation and is replaced roughly every 3 months since the half-life of this isotope is 74 days. The machine permits positioning of the source within the catheter along a 24-cm path at 2.5-mm intervals. The total dose and corresponding time of administration are determined before treatment is administered. We usually give 15 Gy at a distance of 6 mm from the center of the catheter, which takes approximately 5 to 20 minutes depending on the activity of the source and the number of catheters used. Usually, pa-

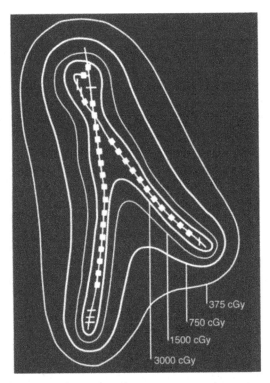

Figure 8–4. Isodose curves delivering 15 Gy at a distance of 6 mm from the center of sources. From Komaki R, Garden AS, Cundiff JH, et al. Endobronchial radiotherapy. In: Roth J, Cox JD, Hong WK, eds. *Lung Cancer.* 2nd ed. Blackwell Science; 1998:190, with permission.

KEY PRACTICE POINTS

- In patients with early-stage or locally advanced NSCLC that is technically resectable, it is important to determine the patient's physical fitness for surgery.

- In patients with early-stage or locally advanced NSCLC who are unable to tolerate surgical resection, radiation therapy with or without chemotherapy can be curative.

- For patients with unresectable NSCLC, the combination of radiation therapy and chemotherapy is a standard treatment.

- Concurrent chemoradiation therapy is a standard treatment for patients with NSCLC with good performance status and minimal weight loss.

- When concurrent chemoradiation therapy is delivered with curative intent, it is critical to reduce the volume of normal tissue irradiated by using 3-dimensional conformal and respiratory gating techniques.

tients are sedated for bronchoscopy. A catheter is inserted into the area partially obstructed by the endobronchial lesion. After confirmation of the catheter location, the bronchoscope is removed, and the catheter is secured at the nostril with adhesive tape. Then the patient is brought to the radiation oncology department, and the location of the catheter is reconfirmed using orthogonal films. The dummy source is removed, and the actual iridium source is placed in the catheter.

We have reported on 175 patients treated with high-dose-rate endobronchial brachytherapy at M. D. Anderson (Kelly et al, 2000). Ninety percent of them also received external-beam radiation therapy. Most of the 175 patients received 30 Gy at 6 mm by endobronchial brachytherapy, which was divided into 2 fractions over 2 weeks. Of the 115 patients (66%) who experienced improvement in symptoms, 32% had a significant improvement. Repeated bronchoscopy demonstrated an objective response rate of 78%. Patients who had significant improvement in symptoms after endobronchial brachytherapy survived significantly longer than patients with no change or worsening symptoms (7 months vs 4 months; $P =$ .0032) (Kelly et al, 2000).

Suggested Readings

Ahmad K, Fayos JV, Kirsch MM. Apical lung carcinoma. *Cancer* 1984;54:913–917.

Cox JD, Azarnia N, Byhardt RW, et al. A randomized phase I/II trial of hyperfractionated radiation therapy with total doses of 60.0 Gy to 79.2 Gy: possible survival benefit with greater than or equal to 69.6 Gy in favorable patients with Radiation Therapy Oncology Group stage III non-small-cell lung carcinoma:

report of Radiation Therapy Oncology Group 83–11. *J Clin Oncol* 1990; 8:1543–1555.

Dillman RO, Herndon J, Seagren SL, et al. Improved survival in stage III non-small-cell lung cancer: seven-year follow-up of Cancer and Leukemia Group B (CALGB) 8433 trial. *J Natl Cancer Inst* 1996;88:1210–1215.

Dillman RO, Seagren SL, Propert KJ, et al. A randomized trial of induction chemotherapy plus high dose radiation versus radiation alone in stage III non-small-cell lung cancer. *N Engl J Med* 1990;323:940–945.

Kelly JF, Delclos ME, Morice RC, et al. High-dose-rate endobronchial brachytherapy effectively palliates symptoms due to airway tumors: the 10-year M. D. Anderson Cancer Center experience. *Int J Radiat Oncol Biol Phys* 2000;48:697–702.

Komaki R, Derus SB, Perez-Tamayo C, et al. Brain metastasis in patients with superior sulcus tumors. *Cancer* 1987;59:1649–1653.

Komaki R, Morice RC, Walsh GL. High-dose-rate remote afterloading endobronchial chemotherapy. In: Roth JA, Cox JD, Hong WK, eds. *Lung Cancer.* 2nd ed. Malden, Mass: Blackwell Science; 1998:163–179.

Komaki R, Putnam JB Jr, Walsh G, et al. The management of superior sulcus tumors. *Semin Surg Oncol* 2000a;18:152–164.

Komaki R, Roh J, Cox JD, et al. Superior sulcus tumors: results of irradiation of 36 patients. *Cancer* 1981;48:1563–1568.

Komaki R, Scott C, Ettinger D, et al. Randomized study of chemotherapy/radiation therapy combinations for favorable patients with locally advanced inoperable nonsmall cell cancer: Radiation Therapy Oncology Group (RTOG) 92–04. *Int J Radiat Oncol Biol Phys* 1997a;38:149–155.

Komaki R, Scott C, Lee JS, et al. Impact of adding concurrent chemotherapy to hyperfractionated radiotherapy for locally advanced non-small cell lung cancer (NSCLC): comparison of RTOG 83–11 and RTOG 91–06. *Am J Clin Oncol* 1997b;20:435–440.

Komaki R, Seiferheld W, Curran W, et al. Sequential vs. concurrent chemotherapy and radiation therapy for inoperable non-small cell lung cancer (NSCLC): analysis of failures in a phase III study (RTOG 9410). *Int J Radiat Oncol Biol Phys* 2000b;48(suppl 1):113.

Komaki R, Seiferheld W, Ettinger D, et al. Randomized phase II chemotherapy and radiation therapy trial for patients with locally advanced inoperable non-small cell lung cancer (NSCLC): long-term follow-up of RTOG 92–04. *Int J Radiat Oncol Biol Phys.* In press.

Kupelian PA, Komaki R, Allen P. Prognostic factors in the treatment of node-negative non-small cell lung carcinoma with radiotherapy alone. *Int J Radiat Oncol Biol Phys* 1996;36:607–613.

Lee JS, Scott C, Komaki R, et al. Concurrent chemoradiation therapy with oral etoposide and cisplatin for locally advanced inoperable non-small-cell lung cancer. Radiation Therapy Oncology Group protocol 91–06. *J Clin Oncol* 1996;14:1055–1064.

Perez CA, Bauer M, Edelstein S, et al. Impact of tumor control on survival in carcinoma of the lung treated with irradiation. *Int J Radiat Oncol Biol Phys* 1986;12:539–547.

Perez CA, Stanley K, Rubin P, et al. A prospective randomized study of various irradiation doses and fractionation schedules in the treatment of inoperable non-oat-cell carcinoma of the lung. Preliminary report by the Radiation Therapy Oncology Group. *Cancer* 1980;45:2744–2753.

Sause WR, Scott C, Taylor S, et al. Phase II trial of combination chemotherapy and radiation in non-small-cell lung cancer, Radiation Therapy Oncology Group 88–04. *Am J Clin Oncol* 1992;15:163–167.

Sause WT, Scott C, Taylor S, et al. Radiation Therapy Oncology Group (RTOG) 88–08 and Eastern Cooperative Oncology Group (ECOG) 4588: preliminary results of a phase III trial in regionally advanced, unresectable non-small-cell lung cancer. *J Natl Cancer Inst* 1995;87:198–205.

Van Houtte P, MacLennan I, Poulter C, et al. External radiation in management of superior sulcus tumors. *Cancer* 1984;54:223–227.

9 TREATMENT OF PATIENTS WITH ADVANCED NON–SMALL CELL LUNG CANCER

Ralph Zinner

CHAPTER OVERVIEW

In the past decade, chemotherapy has been firmly established as a relevant treatment strategy for patients with advanced non–small cell lung cancer (NSCLC) and good performance status. In the 1990s, existing platinum-based regimens were shown to double 1-year survival rates, to approximately 20%, as compared to survival rates in patients treated with best supportive care; later, chemotherapy doublets consisting of third-generation agents in combination with platinum agents were shown to further improve 1-year survival rates, to 30% to 40%. Although chemotherapy causes side effects, symptoms are usually relieved and quality of life is usually improved in patients with advanced NSCLC treated with chemotherapy. In 5 phase III trials reported in 2000 and 2001, comparisons of several chemotherapy doublets comprised of a platinum paired with a third-generation agent showed that these regimens have quite similar impacts on overall survival and quality of life. Thus, in selecting one regimen versus another, issues of toxicity, convenience of administration, and cost should be the dominant considerations. Third-generation agents improve survival, symptoms, and quality of life in patients 70 years of age or older as well as in younger patients. Two large randomized trials reported in 2000 showed that second-line therapy with docetaxel improves overall survival compared with survival after alternate chemotherapy (vinorelbine or ifosfamide) or best supportive care, establishing docetaxel as a standard in this setting. In the near future, some of the numerous biological therapeutics under preclinical and clinical study may be found to further extend survival and improve quality of life in patients with good performance status and may be shown to be reasonable treatment options for patients with poorer performance status.

INTRODUCTION

Lung cancer is the leading cause of cancer-related death in the United States and Europe. It is estimated that 169,500 people were newly diagnosed with and 157,000 people died of lung cancer in the United States in 2001 (Greenlee et al, 2000). Eighty percent of all cases of lung cancer are non–small cell lung cancer (NSCLC). Despite advances in the control of local disease, more people die from lung cancer than from breast cancer, prostate cancer, and colon cancer combined. This is in part because one third of patients with lung cancer present with metastatic disease. In addition, most patients treated with definitive therapy for local disease have a relapse, at which point they usually have disease that can no longer be eradicated. The focus of this chapter is systemic therapy for patients with clinically evident systemic disease either at presentation or at relapse.

GOALS OF THERAPY

Systemic therapy is the mainstay of treatment in patients with NSCLC with distant metastatic disease (stage IV disease) or malignant pleural effusion (stage IIIB disease). Unfortunately, the 5-year survival rate with systemic therapy remains less than 5%. Until the 1990s, it was unclear whether there was a survival benefit from chemotherapy in patients with advanced disease. The natural history of metastatic NSCLC is grim, with a median survival time of about 5 to 6 months and a 1-year survival rate of 10%.

Meta-analyses published in the 1990s indicated that treatment with platinum-based regimens as opposed to best supportive care (BSC) in chemonaive patients increases lifespan about 6 weeks and doubles the 1-year survival rate to about 20% (Rapp et al, 1988; NSCLC Collaborative Group, 1995). In addition, despite the known risk of side effects of chemotherapy, in patients with sufficient performance status (PS), chemotherapy palliates symptoms.

Further increases in overall survival in patients with good PS were achieved in the 1990s through incorporation of third-generation chemotherapeutics into platinum-based regimens. Phase III studies showed that this strategy resulted in median survival times of about 8 to 10 months and 1-year survival rates of about 30% to 40% (Schiller et al, 2000; Fossella, 2001; Kelly et al, 2001a; Rodriguez et al, 2001; Scagliotti et al, 2001; Van Meerbeeck et al, 2001). Moreover, 2 recent phase II studies (Fossella et al, 2000; Shepherd et al, 2000) demonstrated a survival advantage and improved symptom control and quality of life when docetaxel was used as second-line therapy.

Currently, the goals of chemotherapy in the setting of advanced NSCLC are palliation of symptoms, improvement in quality of life, and prolongation of survival. Since the survival benefit from chemotherapy is minimal, physicians need to balance the potential benefits of therapy with the known risks of side effects and need to adequately discuss treatment options with patients.

SELECTION OF PATIENTS FOR TREATMENT AND SELECTION OF REGIMENS

In patients with advanced NSCLC, one of the most important predictors of benefit is PS. In general, first-line chemotherapy is indicated in patients with a PS score of 0 or 1, is considered on a case-by-case basis for patients with a PS score of 2, and is rarely indicated in patients with a PS score of 3. In decisions regarding the most appropriate type of chemotherapy for individual patients, both PS and age are taken into account.

The bulk of the data available from phase III studies of chemotherapy in patients with advanced NSCLC derive from patients with a PS score of 0 or 1; few patients with a PS score of 2 were enrolled in these trials. Patients with a PS score of 2 typically are less likely to respond to therapy, live fewer months, and are more likely to suffer side effects from chemotherapy. In a retrospective study of 1,960 patients with advanced NSCLC, patients with PS scores of 0 and 2 had median survival times of 9.4 and 3.3 months, respectively (Jiroutek et al, 1999). In a Southwest Oncology Group retrospective study of 2,531 patients with advanced NSCLC, patients with PS scores of 0 or 1 versus 2 had median survival times of 6.4 and 3.4 months, respectively (Albain et al, 1991). In both studies, PS was found to be a significant independent prognostic factor. In addition, patients with poorer PS have an increased risk of side effects from chemotherapy (Schiller et al, 2000). Since patients with a PS score of 2 have short median survival times even with treatment and have worse side effects from treatment, standard platinum-based doublets cannot be recommended without reservation in these patients. In all cases, the risk of harm and the relatively small chance of benefit are clearly communicated to the patient. For patients with a PS score of 2, weekly regimens, such as single-agent vinorelbine on days 1 and 8 on a 3-week schedule or gemcitabine 1,000 mg/m^2 days 1 and 8 on a 3-week schedule, can be considered. These agents are relatively well tolerated, and there is the added benefit of increased ability to titrate the dose if side effects occur. Weekly regimens of carboplatin plus paclitaxel and taxotere are under investigation in a number of clinical trials and may offer similar advantages.

Patients with a PS score of 3 are treated with supportive care and palliative local treatments—radiation therapy and, in some cases, palliative surgery. Rarely, patients with a PS score of 3 are treated with gentle chemotherapeutics as described above for patients with a PS score of 2 with the proviso that the patient is informed of the risks and the fact that benefit is not likely.

Since older patients are more likely to have comorbid conditions and can have a less robust physical condition overall, monotherapy with gemcitabine or vinorelbine is often used (Table 9–1). Perrone and colleagues observed an increase in 1-year survival, improved quality of life, and minimal toxicity with the addition of vinorelbine 30 mg/m^2 days 1 and 8 on a 3-week cycle to BSC compared to BSC alone in patients with good PS who were 70 years of age or older (Perrone et al, 1998). Frasci and colleagues demonstrated improved survival when gemcitabine was added to vinorelbine (Frasci et al, 2000), but in a larger study done by Gridelli and colleagues (2001), this doublet was more toxic than vinorelbine alone, resulting in a significantly higher incidence of leukopenia and neutropenia; was more costly; and did not prolong survival as compared to vinorelbine or gemcitabine alone. Therefore, vinorelbine and gemcitabine are not administered in combination to elderly patients.

Though older patients often have comorbid conditions, those with good PS may be able to tolerate regimens used for younger patients. This is an issue of substantial concern since 30% of patients with NSCLC are 70 years of age or older. Since few patients aged 70 years or older are treated in clinical trials, less information is available for these patients than for younger patients. Two of 3 recent retrospective studies showed no increase in risk or decrease in benefit with platinum-containing combinations in patients 70 years or older with good PS compared to patients younger than 70 years (Rosvold et al, 1999; Hensing et al, 2001). One study showed a trend towards greater morbidity (Kelly et al, 2001b). Thus, patients with good PS who are 70 years of age or older are often offered treatment with platinum-based regimens. However, since patients substantially older than 70 years were not studied separately, possibly because there were too few of these patients to treat them as a separate subset, use of platinum-containing regimens in these patients requires special caution, and these patients are often treated with single-agent vinorelbine or gemcitabine.

Table 9-1. Chemotherapy in Older Patients

Study and Treatment Regimen	No. of Patients	Response Rate	Median Survival Time	1-Year Survival Rate	P for Survival
Perrone (ELVIS) (1998)					
Vinorelbine + best supportive care	80	20%	27 weeks	27%	
Best supportive care	81	—	21 weeks	5%	.04
Frasci (2000)					
Vinorelbine	60	15%	18 weeks	13%	
Vinorelbine + gemcitabine	60	22%	29 weeks	30%*	.01
Gridelli (MILES) (2001)					
Vinorelbine	233	18.5%	37 weeks	41%	
Gemcitabine	233	17.3%	28 weeks	26%	
Vinorelbine + gemcitabine	232	20%	32 weeks	31%	

* Projected.

TIMING AND DURATION OF CHEMOTHERAPY

Chemotherapy should be initiated while the patient still has a good PS (American Society of Clinical Oncology [ASCO] clinical practice guidelines, 1997). Since advanced NSCLC typically has a rapid natural course, delay in initiation of treatment risks deterioration in PS and should typically be minimized.

The optimal duration of any one regimen remains to be determined. The 1997 ASCO clinical practical guidelines recommend 2 to 8 cycles of chemotherapy for patients with advanced NSCLC. However, until recently, no data on duration of therapy in patients with advanced NSCLC had been published or presented. In a recent phase III study (Smith et al, 2001), patients were randomly assigned to either 3 or 6 courses of mitomycin, vinblastine, and cisplatin (MVP). There was no difference in survival between the 2 treatments, and quality-of-life parameters were the same or improved in patients randomly assigned to receive only 3 courses.

In a study reported at the 2001 ASCO meeting, patients were randomly assigned to receive 4 cycles of carboplatin plus paclitaxel (limited therapy) versus the same regimen until progression (continuous therapy) (Peterman et al, 2001; Socinski et al, 2001). The median number of treatments was 4 for both arms, with 42% of patients in the continuous-therapy arm receiving more than 4 cycles. Median survival times in the limited-therapy and continuous-therapy arms, respectively, were 6.6 and 8.5 months. The 1- and 2-year survival rates in the limited-therapy arm were 28.5% and 15%, respectively; the corresponding rates in the continuous-therapy arm were 34% and 11%. There was no significant difference between the 2 arms with respect to survival. Quality-of-life scores were similar between the 2 arms. Therapy beyond 4 cycles increased neurotoxicity. In another study reported at the 2001 ASCO meeting, patients with stage IIIB or IV disease received induction mitomycin, ifosfamide, and cisplatin, and patients who responded to this regimen were randomly assigned to receive or not receive weekly vinorelbine for 6 months as maintenance therapy (Depierre et al, 2001). Patients randomly assigned to receive maintenance vinorelbine had no improvement in survival, and this treatment induced additional toxicity. There is anecdotal evidence at M. D. Anderson Cancer Center that some patients have further shrinkage of tumors with vinorelbine beyond 8 courses and that this therapy is well tolerated. However, such therapy cannot be considered a standard and must be approached with great care on a case-by-case basis.

The results of these studies on the optimal duration of chemotherapy need to be interpreted with caution. One study used MVP, an older regimen; another used sequential MVP followed by vinorelbine, which is problematic since vinorelbine has minimal second-line activity. It will be interesting to learn whether the results of the third study—of carboplatin plus paclitaxel—are corroborated by future studies. While we await the results of additional studies designed to address the optimal duration of therapy and performed using current regimens, patients are generally treated according to the 1997 ASCO recommendations—i.e., with 2 to 8 cycles, with the number of cycles determined by the patient's ability to tolerate therapy; relief of symptoms; and response to the regimen.

Workup before Therapy

In patients with advanced NSCLC, the workup at presentation and at recurrence should include a complete history and physical examination; blood cell count with differential and platelet counts; liver function tests (measurement of bilirubin, alkaline phosphatase, aspartate aminotransferase, alanine aminotransferase, and lactate dehydrogenase levels); chest radiography; and computed tomography of the chest. Other tests, such as magnetic resonance imaging of the brain or bone scanning, should be done as suggested by symptoms, findings on physical examination, or earlier test results to determine the diagnosis and stage. The role of positron emission tomography in ruling out distant metastases is still being defined. However, in the setting of mediastinal lymph node–positive disease, positron emission tomography may be especially useful in ruling out distant metastatic disease.

Selection of Agents

First-Line Treatment

For chemonaive younger patients with good PS, first-line treatment at M. D. Anderson consists of one of several doublets made up of a platinum compound paired with a third-generation agent. These regimens are the best studied and most clearly established. They build upon the demonstrated survival advantage offered by platinum compounds. Studies supporting the current approach to first-line treatment are outlined in this section.

At least 4 randomized studies have compared monotherapy using a third-generation agent with BSC as first-line therapy (Perrone et al, 1998; Anderson et al, 2000; Ranson et al, 2000; Roszkowski et al, 2000) (Table 9–2). All 4 agents—docetaxel, paclitaxel, gemcitabine, and vinorelbine—resulted in improved quality of life and symptom relief, improved survival, or both. A fifth trial (Crawford et al, 1996) showed the superiority of vinorelbine over an earlier-generation nonplatinum chemotherapeutic.

Trials comparing third-generation single agents (vinorelbine, irinotecan, and gemcitabine) with old-line platinum-containing doublets show that the 2 approaches result in similar survival outcomes (Le Chevalier et al, 1994, 2001; Manegold et al, 1997; Perng et al, 1997) (Table 9–3). How-

Table 9-2.   Single-Agent Third-Generation Agents versus Best Supportive Care as First-Line Therapy

Study and Treatment Regimen	No. of Patients	Response Rate	Median Survival Time	1-Year Survival Rate	2-Year Survival Rate	P for Survival	Quality of Life	Symptoms Improved with Chemotherapy?
Roszkowski (2000)								
Docetaxel + BSC	137	13%	6.0 months	25%	12%	.026	Better	Yes
BSC	70	—	5.7 months	16%	0%			
Ranson (2000)								
Paclitaxel + BSC	79	16%	6.8 months	20%–41%		.037	Better	Yes
BSC	78	—	4.8 months	18%–39%				
Anderson (2000)								
Gemcitabine + BSC	150	19%	5.7 months	25%		.84	Better	Yes
BSC	150	—	5.9 months	22%				
Perrone (ELVIS) (1998)*								
Vinorelbine + BSC	80	20%	6.2 months	27%			Better	Yes
BSC	81	—	4.8 months	5%		.04		
Crawford (1996)								
Vinorelbine	143	12%†	6.9 months	25%		.03		
5-FU + leucovorin	68	3%	5.1 months	16%				—

BSC indicates best supportive care; 5-FU, fluorouracil; and NR, not reported.
* All patients at least 70 years of age.
† No P value reported.

R. Zinner

Table 9-3. Third-Generation-Agent Monotherapy versus Cisplatin plus the Same Monotherapy or an Older-Generation Agent

Study and Treatment Regimen	No. of Patients	Response Rate	Median Survival Time	1-Year Survival Rate	P for Survival
		Phase III Studies			
Le Chevalier (1994, 2001)					
Vinorelbine	206	14%* (P = .001)	7.2 months	30%	.01*
Cisplatin + vindesine	200	19% (P = .02)	7.6 months	27%	.04†
Cisplatin + vinorelbine	206	30%†	9.2 months	35%	
Depierre (1994)					
Vinorelbine	119	16%	7.4 months	NR	
Cisplatin + vinorelbine	121	43% (P = .0001)	7.6 months	NR	.48
Komiya (2000)					
Irinotecan	129	21%	10.6 months	42%	
Cisplatin + vindesine	126	32%	10.6 months	38%	
Cisplatin + irinotecan	130	44% (P = .0004)	11.5 months	47%	.145
		Phase II Studies			
Manegold (1997)					
Gemcitabine	71	18%	6.6 months		
Cisplatin + etoposide	75	15%	7.6 months		
Perng (1997)					
Gemcitabine	27	19%	8.5 months		
Cisplatin + etoposide	26	21%	11.1 months		

NR indicates not reported.
* Cisplatin and vinorelbine versus vinorelbine alone.
† Cisplatin and vindesine versus cisplatin and vinorelbine.
Adapted from vol 1 no 4 Lung Cancer.

ever, third-generation single agents are probably inferior to the same agent combined with a platinum, notwithstanding the equivalence seen in the Depierre study (Depierre et al, 1994; Le Chevalier et al, 1994; Komiya et al, 2000). Therefore, third-generation monotherapy appears to be superior to BSC, perhaps equivalent to a platinum–early-generation doublet but likely inferior to platinum–third-generation doublets.

Studies have shown that doublets consisting of vinorelbine, gemcitabine, or tirapazamine plus cisplatin are associated with longer survival times than single-agent cisplatin (Wozniak et al, 1998; Gatzemeier et al, 2000; Sandler et al, 2000; von Pawel et al, 2000) (Table 9–4). Although the paclitaxel combination was not associated with improved survival in the Gatzemeier study, it was relatively well tolerated as compared with high-dose single-agent cisplatin.

Doublets composed of platinum compounds plus third-generation agents are generally better tolerated than older cisplatin-containing combinations and tend to result in modest improvement in survival (Belani et al, 1998; Giaccone et al, 1998; Martoni et al, 1998; Cardenal et al, 1999; Crino et al, 1999; Bonomi et al, 2000; Komiya et al, 2000; Takiguchi et al, 2000; Kunitoh et al, 2001; Le Chevalier et al, 2001) (Table 9–5). Of the 11 trials listed in Table 9–5, two showed significant improvement in survival with third-generation doublets, and 3 others showed a trend towards improvement in survival. These 5 trials used vinorelbine, paclitaxel, gemcitabine, docetaxel, and irinotecan. In addition, 4 other trials showed better tolerability if not an obvious survival advantage with third-generation regimens compared to older regimens. One trial showed neither improved survival nor improved tolerability (Belani et al, 1998), and one trial showed a trend toward inferior survival (Danson et al, 2001). Therefore, 9 of 11 trials showed at least a trend toward better survival or tolerability with the use of third-generation–platinum doublets.

Though few of the initial phase III trials investigating combinations of platinum compounds and third-generation agents used carboplatin, this drug has become a standard part of the armamentarium against advanced NSCLC. Carboplatin is a cisplatin analogue but differs from cisplatin in its side effect profile. The primary side effect of carboplatin is myelosuppression, and carboplatin has lesser ototoxicity, renal toxicity, and neurotoxicity than cisplatin. In an early 5-arm randomized trial, carboplatin produced the best median survival time (Bonomi et al, 1989).

At least 5 trials have compared different platinum compound–third-generation-agent doublets (Schiller et al, 2000; Fossella, 2001; Kelly et al, 2001a; Rodriguez et al, 2001; Scagliotti et al, 2001; Van Meerbeeck et al, 2001) (Table 9–6). Unlike earlier phase III trials in which third-generation agents were combined with cisplatin, many of the trials shown in Table 9–6 replaced cisplatin with carboplatin. With the exception of the TAX 326 trial, the doublets examined in each study yielded similar response, toxicity, and overall survival outcomes.

Table 9–4. Third-Generation Agents plus Platinum versus Single-Agent Platinum Compounds

Study and Treatment Regimen	No. of Patients	Response Rate	Median Survival Time	1-Year Survival Rate	P for Survival	Quality of Life	Side Effects Worse Than with Other Regimen
Wozniak (1998)							
Cisplatin	209	12%	6 months	20%		NR	
Cisplatin + vinorelbine	206	26% (P = .0002)	8 months	36%	.0018		Neutropenia
Sandler (2000)							
Cisplatin	262	11.1%	7.6 months	28%		NR	
Cisplatin + gemcitabine	260	30.4% (P<.0001)	9.1 months	39%	.004		Neutropenia and thrombocytopenia
Gatzemeier (2000)							
Cisplatin (100 mg/m^2)	207	17%	8.6 months	36%		Same	Ototoxicity, N/V, nephrotoxicity
Cisplatin 80 mg/m^2 + paclitaxel 175 mg/m^2	207	26% (P = .028)	8.1 months	30%	.862		
Von Pawel (2000)							
Cisplatin	219	13.7%	6.4 months	23%		NR	
Cisplatin + tirapazamine	218	27.5% (P <.001)	8.4 months	34%	.0078		

NR indicates not reported; N/V, nausea and vomiting.

In the TAX 326 trial, a significant improvement in overall survival was detected in the cisplatin-docetaxel arm compared to the cisplatin-vinorelbine arm. However, this difference was only 0.9 months and was detectable because this was a large study. The ECOG 1594 study, which also included a cisplatin-docetaxel arm, did not show a survival advantage in that arm, though the drug combinations to which cisplatin-docetaxel was compared were not the same in the ECOG 1594 study as in the TAX 326 study.

In a statistical analysis of the 5 trials that compared different platinum–third-generation doublets plus the MILES study (Gridelli et al, 2001; see Table 9–1), it was calculated that the odds were 51% that one of the 14 comparisons in these studies would have a positive P value by chance alone (Evans and Lynch, 2001). In the TAX 326 study, the P value for the survival difference was barely significant at .047. Taken together, these data show that it is reasonable to use docetaxel together with a platinum compound in the first-line setting. However, it would be premature to conclude that docetaxel-containing regimens are superior to other platinum–third-generation doublets in the first-line setting.

Of note, the TAX 326 study was not designed to compare the carboplatin-docetaxel arm with the cisplatin-docetaxel arm. However, this result, combined with the preliminary survival results from the phase III pan-European study showing median survival times and 1-year survival rates of 9.8 months and 38% for cisplatin-paclitaxel and 8.5 months and 33% for carboplatin-paclitaxel (Gatzemeier et al, 2000; see Table 9–4) raises the question whether cisplatin may offer a slight survival advantage. Though ECOG 1594 (Schiller et al, 2000) did not show a benefit with cisplatin-paclitaxel compared to carboplatin-paclitaxel, these 2 arms were not truly a direct comparison since the paclitaxel was delivered differently in each arm—over 24 hours when combined with cisplatin and over 3 hours when combined with carboplatin. If there is a survival advantage with cisplatin compared to carboplatin, it is most likely quite small and of minimal clinical significance in advanced NSCLC. Such a survival difference, should it exist, might be more meaningful in stage III disease where slight improvements in efficacy may be translated into larger cure fractions (Evans and Lynch, 2001).

These studies in advanced NSCLC comparing various platinum compound–third-generation-agent doublets indicate that carboplatin can substitute for cisplatin and indicate that any of the third-generation agents studied are reasonable choices. Vinorelbine, paclitaxel, gemcitabine, and docetaxel have been extensively validated. Irinotecan and tirapazamine can be considered but are less validated.

Since platinum agents account for much of the toxicity from third-generation–platinum doublets, there is interest in developing nonplatinum-containing regimens. Third-generation agents as monotherapy

R. Zinner

Table 9-5. Third-Generation Platinum-Containing Doublets versus Second-Generation Platinum-Containing Doublets

Study and Treatment Regimen	No. of Patients	Response Rate	Median Survival Time	1-Year Survival Rate	P for Survival	Quality of Life	Side Effects Worse Than with Other Regimen
Le Chevalier (2001)						NR	
Vinorelbine	206	14% (P = .00)	7.2 months	30%	.01		
Cisplatin + vindesine	200	19% (P = .02)	7.4 months	27%	.04		Neurotoxicity
Cisplatin + vinorelbine	206	30%	9.2 months	35%			Neutropenia
Bonomi (2000)							
Cisplatin + etoposide	193	12%	7.6 months	32%			
Cisplatin + paclitaxel (135 mg/m^2)	190	25% (P = .002)*	9.5 months	37%	.090*	Same	Neutropenia
Cisplatin + paclitaxel (250 mg/m^2)	191	28% (P = .001)†	10.0 months	40%	.097† .048‡	Same	Myalgias, neuro-toxicity, possible cardiac toxicity
Komiya (2000)							
Irinotecan	129	21%	10.6 months	42%			
Cisplatin + vindesine	126	32%	10.6 months	38%			
Cisplatin + irinotecan	130	44% (P = .0004)	11.5 months	47%	.145		
Cardenal (1999)							
Cisplatin + etoposide	65	22%	7.2 months	26%			
Cisplatin + gemcitabine	69	41% (P < .02)	8.7 months	32%	.18	Same	
Kunitoh (TAX-JP-301) (2001)							
Cisplatin + vindesine	151	32%	9.7 months	43%			Hematologic
Cisplatin + docetaxel	151	56% (P = .01)	11.3 months	48%	.245	Favorable	Gastrointestinal
Giaccone (1998)							
Cisplatin + teniposide	162	28%	9.9 months	41%			Hematologic, arthralgias
Cisplatin + paclitaxel	155	41% (P = .018)	9.7 months	43%	.971	Better	Myalgias, neurotoxicity, hypersensitivity

Table 9-5. (continued)   Third-Generation Platinum-Containing Doublets versus Second-Generation Platinum-Containing Doublets

Study and Treatment Regimen	No. of Patients	Response Rate	Median Survival Time	1-Year Survival Rate	P for Survival	Quality of Life	Side Effects Worse Than with Other Regimen
Crino (1999)							
Cisplatin + mitomycin/ ifosfamide	152	26%	9.6 months	34%			Alopecia
Cisplatin + gemcitabine	155	38% (P = .029)	8.6 months	33%	.877	Same	Thrombocytopenia
Martoni (1998)						NR	
Cisplatin + epirubicin	95	33%	10.5 months				Myelosuppression, alopecia
Cisplatin + vinorelbine	103	27%	9.6 months				
Takiguchi (2000)						NR	
Cisplatin + vindesine	101	22%	11.5 months	48%			Neutropenia
Cisplatin + irinotecan	98	29%	10.4 months	43%	.760		Diarrhea
Belani (1998)						NR	
Cisplatin + etoposide	179	14%	9.1 months	37%			Vomiting, myalgias
Carboplatin + paclitaxel	190	22% (P = .059)	7.7 months	32%	NR¶		Neurotoxicity
Danson (2001)							
Carboplatin + gemcitabine	145	31%	7.3 months		.273		Hematologic
Cisplatin + mitomycin C + ifosfamide OR cisplatin + mitomycin C +vinblastine	151	34%	8.5 months				

* For cisplatin and etoposide versus cisplatin and paclitaxel 135 mg/m².
† For cisplatin and etoposide versus cisplatin and paclitaxel 135 mg/m².
‡ When both paclitaxel arms combined compared with etoposide arm.
¶ P not reported for response or survival. Data from Schiller et al, 2000.

Table 9–6. Comparisons between Different Platinum–Third-Generation-Agent Doublets

Study and Treatment Regimen	No. of Patients	Response Rate	Median Survival Time	1-Year Survival Rate	P for Survival	Quality of Life	Side Effects Worse Than with Other Regimen
SWOG 9509 (Kelly, 2001a)							
Cisplatin + vinorelbine	202	28%	8 months	36%		Same	Leukopenia, neutropenia, N/V, patients quit study because of toxicity
Carboplatin + paclitaxel	206	25%	8 months	38%	—		Neuropathy
ECOG 1594 (Schiller, 2000)						NR	
Cisplatin + paclitaxel	292	21.3%	7.8 months	31%			Cardiac, renal
Cisplatin + gemcitabine	288	21%	8.1 months	36%	—		Platelets, anemia, weakness
Cisplatin + docetaxel	293	17.3%	7.4 months	31%	—		Hypersensitivity reactions, renal
Carboplatin + paclitaxel	290	15.3%	8.2 months	35%			N/V, renal
EORTC 8975 (Van Meerbeeck, 2001)						NR	
Cisplatin + paclitaxel	153	31%	8.1 months	35.5%			
Cisplatin + gemcitabine	158	36%	8.8 months	32.6%	.9*		
Gemcitabine + paclitaxel	157	27%	6.9 months (P = .08)	26.5%	.09†		

Table 9–6. (continued) Comparisons between Different Platinum–Third-Generation-Agent Doublets

Study and Treatment Regimen	No. of Patients	Response Rate	Median Survival Time	1-Year Survival Rate	P for Survival	Quality of Life	Side Effects Worse Than with Other Regimen
TAX 326 (Fossella, 2001; Rodriguez, 2001)							
Cisplatin + vinorelbine	404	NR	10.1 months	42% (14%)‡			Anemia, N/V, weight loss
Cisplatin + docetaxel	408	NR	11.3 months	47% (21%)‡¶	.047‡¶	Better	
Carboplatin + docetaxel	404	NR	9.1 months	38% (16%)‡**	NS‡**	Better	
ILCP (Scagliotti, 2001)						NR	
Cisplatin + vinorelbine	201	31%	9.5 months	37%			
Cisplatin + gemcitabine	205	30%	9.8 months	37%			
Carboplatin + paclitaxel	201	32%	9.9 months	43%			

NR indicates not reported; N/V, nausea and vomiting.
* For cisplatin and paclitaxel versus cisplatin and gemcitabine.
† For cisplatin and paclitaxel versus gemcitabine and paclitaxel.
‡ Two-year survival is shown in parentheses.
¶ Cisplatin and docetaxel versus cisplatin and vinorelbine.
** Carboplatin and docetaxel versus cisplatin and vinorelbine.

may play an important role in the treatment of chemonaive older patients, as discussed earlier in the chapter (Table 9–1). However, in younger chemonaive patients, a third-generation monotherapeutic appears to be inferior to the same drug in combination with a platinum (Table 9–3).

However, there has been interest in the development of nonplatinum-containing doublets as a means of improving toxicity profiles without sacrificing survival benefit. Of 3 trials presented at ASCO in 2000 and 2001 that compared nonplatinum-containing doublets to platinum-containing doublets (Table 9–7), one showed parity or improvement with the non-platinum-containing doublet (Kosmidis et al, 2000), another showed parity (Alberola et al, 2001), and a third showed a trend towards a worse outcome with the nonplatinum-containing doublet (Van Meerbeeck et al, 2001). In addition, there is not a clear advantage to the use of nonplatinum doublets over nonplatinum monotherapy, as demonstrated by the conflicting results of the Frasci and Gridelli trials in patients older than 70 years (Table 9–1). Therefore, though initial results with nonplatinum-containing regimens are intriguing, platinum-containing regimens remain the first choice at present.

There is also interest in improving survival through the addition of an additional third-generation agent to an established platinum–third-generation doublet to make a triplet (Table 9–8). At present, there is not an obvious survival advantage to this approach. In one study (Comella et al, 2000), improved survival and no increase in toxicity was seen in the triplet arm compared with one of the doublets. A larger study (Alberola et al, 2001) showed no survival advantage but increased toxicity in the triplet arm. Thus, at present, triplet chemotherapy is considered investigational.

Taken together, the data thus far support the use of doublets composed of either cisplatin or carboplatin together with paclitaxel, docetaxel, gemcitabine, or vinorelbine—and possibly irinotecan—in the first-line treatment of patients with advanced NSCLC. Since there are no obvious differences between the available doublets with respect to survival or toxicity, issues of toxicity, convenience, and cost relevant to the individual patient are the dominant considerations in selecting the most appropriate regimen.

Second-Line Treatment

As of this writing, docetaxel is the only agent approved by the US Food and Drug Administration for second-line therapy in patients with advanced NSCLC. This approval is based on the results of 2 recent phase III studies, the TAX 317 and TAX 320 studies, both of which showed improved survival in patients with NSCLC previously treated with platinum (Fossella et al, 2000; Shepherd et al, 2000) (Table 9–9).

Table 9–7. Non-Platinum-Containing Doublets versus Platinum-Containing Doublets

Study and Treatment Regimen	No. of Patients	Response Rate	Median Survival Time	1-Year Survival Rate	P
Kosmidis (2000)					
Carboplatin + paclitaxel	165	29%	10.7 months	41%	
Gemcitabine + paclitaxel	164	37%	12.3 months	51%	.047
		(P = .17)			
GEPC 98–02 (Alberola, 2001)					
Cisplatin + gemcitabine	166	43%	8.7 months	35%	
Cisplatin + gemcitabine + vinorelbine	176	38%	7.9 months	31%	
Gemcitabine + vinorelbine followed by vinorelbine or ifosfamide	175	26%	8.1 months	35%	
EORTC 8975 (Van Meerbeeck, 2001)					
Cisplatin + paclitaxel	153	31%	8.1 months	35.5%	
Cisplatin + gemcitabine	158	36%	8.8 months	32.6%	.9*
		(P = .3)*			
Gemcitabine + paclitaxel	157	27%	6.9 months	26.5%	.09†
		(P = .5)†			

* Cisplatin and paclitaxel versus cisplatin and gemcitabine.
† Cisplatin and paclitaxel versus gemcitabine and paclitaxel.

Table 9-8. Third-Generation Cisplatin-Containing Triplets versus Third-Generation Cisplatin-Containing Doublets

Study and Treatment Regimen	No. of Patients	Response Rate	Median Survival Time	1-Year Survival Rate	P for Survival
Comella (2000)					
Cisplatin + gemcitabine + vinorelbine	69	47%	10.4 months	45%	NR
Cisplatin + gemcitabine	70	30%	9.2 months	40%	.0058*
Cisplatin + vinorelbine	68	25%	7.8 months	34%	
GEPC 98–02 (Alberola, 2001)					
Cisplatin + gemcitabine	166	43%	8.7	35%	
Cisplatin + gemcitabine + vinorelbine	176	38%	7.9	31%	
Gemcitabine + vinorelbine followed by vinorelbine + ifosfamide	175	26%	8.1	35%	

NR indicates not reported.
* Triplet therapy versus cisplatin and vinorelbine.

Table 9–9.   Docetaxel as Second-Line Therapy

Study and Treatment Regimen	No. of Patients	Response Rate	Median Survival Time	1-Year Survival Rate	P for Survival
(TAX 320) (Fossella, 2000)					
Docetaxel 100 mg/m^2	125	10.8%	7 months	21%	NR
Docetaxel 75 mg/m^2	125	6.7%	5.7 months	32%	.025*
Vinorelbine or ifosfamide	123	0.8%	5.6 months	19%	
(TAX 317) (Shepherd, 2000)					
BSC	51		4.9 months	28%	.780
Docetaxel 100 mg/m^2 + BSC	49	6%	5.9 months	19%	
BSC	49		4.6 months	12%	.010
Docetaxel 75 mg/m^2 + BSC	55	6%	7.5 months	37%	

* For docetaxel 75 mg/m^2 versus vinorelbine or ifosfamide.

In TAX 317, patients were initially randomly assigned to treatment with docetaxel 100 mg/m^2 every 3 weeks or BSC. Eligibility requirements included receipt of at least 1 previous platinum-based regimen and PS score of 0 to 2. Patients who had previously been treated with a taxane were excluded. The initial docetaxel dose was too toxic as observed in the first 49 patients treated. The dose was then reduced to 75 mg/m^2 for the rest of the patients. For all patients, treatment with docetaxel was associated with a survival advantage ($P = .047$). However, this survival advantage was especially pronounced in patients treated at 75 mg/m^2, in whom median survival time and 1-year survival rates were 7.5 months and 37%, versus 4.6 months and 11% for BSC ($P = .01$ for overall survival). In addition, treatment with docetaxel improved quality of life as compared to BSC.

The TAX 320 study differed from the TAX 317 study in the following ways: the control arm was either vinorelbine or ifosfamide, determined by the treating physician; the patients were randomly assigned to either 75 mg/m^2 or 100 mg/m^2; and previous paclitaxel exposure was permitted. Patients who received 75 mg/m^2 had a significantly improved 1-year survival rate as compared to the rate in patients in both control arms. Previous paclitaxel exposure did not affect the likelihood of response or survival. Patients treated at 75 mg/m^2 who had disease that was refractory to platinum compounds had survival similar to that of patients who had disease not refractory to platinum compounds. In the 100 mg/m^2 and vinorelbine and ifosfamide treatment groups, there was a trend towards higher survival in the patients whose disease was not refractory to platinum-based regimens.

Data from a number of phase II trials show conflicting evidence regarding the activity of gemcitabine, paclitaxel, and irinotecan in the second-line setting, and no phase III trial results are available that assess whether survival or quality of life is improved with these regimens (Fossella, 2000). Therefore, at present, for patients with a PS score of 0 or 1, docetaxel is recommended as second-line therapy in patients who did not receive this agent as first-line therapy. For patients with a PS score of 2, second-line chemotherapy, like first-line chemotherapy, should be offered with caution if at all. Patients with good PS who have recurrent disease after first- or second-line docetaxel should be encouraged to enter a clinical trial assessing novel therapeutics.

BIOLOGICALS

The progress made through third-generation chemotherapy is real but modest. Study of additional combinations of third-generation agents may further improve survival and tolerability. However, we are reaching a therapeutic plateau.

There is increased hope that through the use of new classes of therapeutics, new ground will be broken in the fight against NSCLC. These classes of medicines, like currently available chemotherapeutics, are often designed around molecular targets. However, the new therapies are designed to interact with new classes of such targets, including receptors, signal transducers, and the genes identified as important in cancer. In addition, support tissues, such as tumor blood vessels, are increasingly being targeted. In addition to new targets, novel tools are available to reach and alter the targets, such as monoclonal antibodies, genes, and vaccines, among others.

Some of these agents are already standard of care in other cancer types. A prominent example in a solid tumor is the use of trastuzumab (Herceptin) in Her2/neu-overexpressing breast cancer. Phase II trials of Herceptin in NSCLC are under way at a number of centers. Other phase II trials of new agents for treatment of NSCLC have recently been reported and indicate that some of these agents have activity against NSCLC.

In 2000, a randomized phase II study of carboplatin plus paclitaxel with or without the monoclonal antibody inhibitor of vascular endothelial growth factor (VEGF) (an anti-angiogenic agent) showed promise of improved overall survival, although there was an increased risk of pulmonary hemorrhage in patients with squamous cell histology (DeVore et al, 2001; Johnson et al 2001). A phase III study of anti-

VEGF antibody in metastatic NSCLC of nonsquamous cell histology is now under way.

ZD1839 (Iressa), an epidermal growth factor receptor (EGFR) tyrosine kinase inhibitor, is well tolerated and active as a single agent in multiple solid tumor types. Phase I studies have shown that Iressa is well tolerated and active against NSCLC (Baselga et al, 2000; Ferry et al, 2000). Iressa is also well tolerated in combination with carboplatin and paclitaxel (Miller et al, 2001). A phase III randomized trial of Iressa in combination with carboplatin and paclitaxel as first-line therapy in advanced NSCLC recently completed accrual. OSI-774 (Tarceva), another EGFR tyrosine kinase inhibitor, was associated with a response rate of 12.3% in heavily pretreated patients with NSCLC (Perez-Soler et al, 2001). A phase III randomized trial of carboplatin and paclitaxel with or without Tarceva in the treatment of chemonaive advanced NSCLC is accruing patients.

In a phase I/II trial, ISIS-3521, an antisense inhibitor of protein kinase C-alpha, combined with carboplatin and paclitaxel in the treatment of advanced NSCLC was associated with a median survival time of 15.9 months (Yuen et al, 2001). A phase III trial of carboplatin and paclitaxel with or without ISIS-3521 is under way.

CONCLUSIONS

Most patients diagnosed with NSCLC ultimately develop clinically apparent disseminated disease, which is presently incurable. In the 1990s, studies showed that doublets consisting of platinum compounds plus third-generation agents improved survival, relieved symptoms, improved quality of life, and were superior to earlier-generation platinum regimens, and these doublets have become the standard of care in younger patients with good PS. Multiple recent studies demonstrate that no single doublet is clearly superior. Therefore, toxicity, convenience of administration, and cost are the principle considerations in choosing a regimen. Patients 70 years of age or older with good PS may benefit from the same regimens as younger patients, although patients much older than 70 years have not been adequately evaluated in clinical studies and may best benefit from single-modality therapies, such as vinorelbine or gemcitabine.

There clearly remains a great need to improve therapy for all patients with advanced NSCLC. Since a large array of new and promising biologicals are in various stages of clinical development, the opportunity to enroll patients in clinical trials has never been better. Though the third-generation doublets and third-generation monotherapy described in this chapter can be considered standard, there is merit in the idea of shifting thinking such that treatment in clinical trials is considered an appropriate first therapeutic choice for these patients.

KEY PRACTICE POINTS

- Chemotherapy doublets consisting of platinum compounds plus third-generation agents are the current standard of care for patients with advanced NSCLC who have good PS (a PS score of 0 or 1) and are less than 70 years of age.
- The wide variety of platinum–third-generation doublets studied to date have similar survival profiles; therefore, in the choice of doublets, the prime considerations are toxicity, convenience of administration, and cost.
- Nonplatinum-containing doublets and chemotherapy triplets have shown promise in some clinical trials but are not yet established.
- In newly diagnosed younger patients with good PS, there is evidence that treatment beyond 3 to 4 courses of platinum-containing regimens produces no survival benefit but increases the incidence of side effects.
- Maintenance therapy with vinorelbine has not been demonstrated to offer benefit. However, there are anecdotal accounts of benefit from treatment sustained beyond 8 courses. Therefore, this practice, though not standard, can be considered on a case-by-case basis.
- Older patients with good PS may benefit from the regimens used in younger patients, but patients who are much older than 70 years have not been fully evaluated in clinical studies and may best benefit from monotherapy with third-generation agents, such as vinorelbine and gemcitabine.
- Docetaxel at 75 mg/m^2 every 3 weeks is the standard of care as second-line treatment, including in patients previously treated with paclitaxel.
- Opportunities for enrollment in clinical trials of promising new agents have never been better and should be emphasized whenever treatment is being considered.

SUGGESTED READINGS

Albain KS, Crowley JJ, Hutchins L, et al. Predictors of survival following relapse or progression of small cell lung cancer. Southwest Oncology Group Study 8605 report and analysis of recurrent disease data base. *Cancer* 1993;72:1184–1191.

Albain KS, Crowley JJ, LeBlanc M, et al. Survival determinants in extensive-stage non-small-cell lung cancer: the Southwest Oncology Group experience. *J Clin Oncol* 1991;9:1618–1626.

Alberola V, Camps C, Provencia M, et al. Cisplatin/gemcitabine (CG) vs cisplatin/gemcitabine/vinorelbine (CGV) vs sequential doublets of gemcitabine/vinorelbine followed by ifosfamide/vinorelbine (GV/IV) in advanced non-small cell lung cancer (NSCLC): results of a Spanish Lung Cancer Group phase III trial (GEPC/98–02). *Proc Am Soc Clin Oncol* 2001;42. Abstract 1229.

American Society of Clinical Oncology. Clinical practice guidelines for the treatment of unresectable non-small-cell lung cancer. Adopted on May 16, 1997 by the American Society of Clinical Oncology. *J Clin Oncol* 1997;15:2996–3018.

Anderson H, Hopwood P, Stephens RJ, et al. Gemcitabine plus best supportive care (BSC) vs BSC in inoperable non-small cell lung cancer—a randomized trial with quality of life as the primary outcome. UK NSCLC Gemcitabine Group. Non-Small Cell Lung Cancer. *Br J Cancer* 2000;83:447–453.

Baselga J, Herbst R, LoRusso P, et al. Continuous administration of ZD1839 (Iressa), a novel oral epidermal growth factor receptor tyrosine kinase inhibitor (EGFR-TKI), in patients with five selected tumor types: evidence of activity and good tolerability. *Proc Am Soc Clin Oncol* 2000. Abstract 686.

Belani CP, Natale RB, Lee JS, et al. Randomized phase III trial comparing cisplatin/etoposide versus carboplatin/paclitaxel in advanced and metastatic non-small cell lung cancer (NSCLC). *Proc Am Soc Clin Oncol* 1998;39. Abstract 1751.

Bonomi PD, Finkelstein DM, Ruckdeschel JC, et al. Combination chemotherapy versus single agents followed by combination chemotherapy in stage IV non-small-cell lung cancer: a study of the Eastern Cooperative Oncology Group. *J Clin Oncol* 1989;7:1602–1613.

Bonomi P, Kim K, Fairclough D, et al. Comparison of survival and quality of life in advanced non-small-cell lung cancer patients treated with two dose levels of paclitaxel combined with cisplatin versus etoposide with cisplatin: results of an Eastern Cooperative Oncology Group trial. *J Clin Oncol* 2000;18:623–631.

Breathnach OS, Freidlin B, Conley B, et al. Twenty-two years of phase III trials for patients with advanced non–small-cell lung cancer: sobering results. *J Clin Oncol* 2001;19:1734–1742.

Cardenal F, Lopez-Cabrerizo MP, Anton A, et al. Randomized phase III study of gemcitabine-cisplatin versus etoposide-cisplatin in the treatment of locally advanced or metastatic non-small-cell lung cancer. *J Clin Oncol* 1999;17:12–18.

Comella P, Frasci G, Panza N, et al. Randomized trial comparing cisplatin, gemcitabine, and vinorelbine with either cisplatin and gemcitabine or cisplatin and vinorelbine in advanced non-small-cell lung cancer: interim analysis of a phase III trial of the Southern Italy Cooperative Oncology Group. *J Clin Oncol* 2000;18:1451–1457.

Crawford J, O'Rourke M, Schiller JH, et al. Randomized trial of vinorelbine compared with fluorouracil plus leucovorin in patients with stage IV non-small-cell lung cancer. *J Clin Oncol* 1996;14:2774–2784.

Crino L, Scagliotti GV, Ricci S, et al. Gemcitabine and cisplatin versus mitomycin, ifosfamide, and cisplatin in advanced non-small-cell lung cancer: a randomized phase III study of the Italian Lung Cancer Project. *J Clin Oncol* 1999;17:3522–3530.

Danson A, Clemons M, Middleton M, et al. A randomised study of gemcitabine with carboplatin (GC) versus mitomycin, vinblastine and cisplatin (MVP) or mitomycin C, ifosfamide and cisplatin (MIC) as first line chemotherapy in advanced non-small cell lung cancer (NSCLC). Presentation at the 37th Annual Meeting of the American Society of Clinical Oncology, May 12–15, 2001; San Francisco, CA. Abstract 1285.

Depierre A, Chastang C, Quoix E, et al. Vinorelbine versus vinorelbine plus cisplatin in advanced non-small cell lung cancer: a randomized trial. *Ann Oncol* 1994;5:37–42.

Depierre A, Quoix E, Mercier M, et al. Maintenance chemotherapy in advanced non-small cell lung cancer (NSCLC): a randomized study of vinorelbine (V) versus observation (OB) in patients (Pts) responding to induction therapy (French Cooperative Oncology Group). *Proc Am Soc Clin Oncol* 2001;42. Abstract 1231.

DeVore RF, Fehrenbacher L, Herbst RS, et al. A randomized phase II trial comparing rhumab VEGF (recombinant humanized monoclonal antibody to vascular endothelial cell growth factor) plus carboplatin/paclitaxel (CP) to CP alone in patients with stage IIIB/IV NSCLC. *Proc Am Soc Clin Oncol* 2001;41. Abstract 1896.

Evans TL, Lynch TJ Jr. Lung cancer. *Oncologist* 2001;6:407–414.

Ferry D, Hammond L, Ranson M, et al. Intermittent oral ZD 1839 (Iressa), a novel epidermal growth factor receptor tyrosine kinase inhibitor (EGFR-TKI), shows evidence of good tolerability and activity: final results from a phase I study. *Proc Am Soc Clin Oncol* 2000. Abstract 5E.

Fossella F. Second-line chemotherapy for non-small cell lung cancer. In: Pass H, Mitchell J, Johnson D, et al, eds. *Lung Cancer: Principles and Practice.* 2nd ed. Philadelphia, Pa: Lippincott Williams & Wilkins; 2000:903–909.

Fossella F. Docetaxel + cisplatin (DC) and docetaxel + carboplatin (DCb) vs vinorelbine + cisplatin (VC) in chemotherapy-naïve patients with advanced and metastatic non-small cell lung cancer (NSCLC): results of a multicenter, randomized phase III study. ECCO—The European Cancer Conference, 2001. Abstract 562 (information from slide presentation).

Fossella FV, DeVore R, Kerr RN, et al. Randomized phase III trial of docetaxel versus vinorelbine or ifosfamide in patients with advanced non-small-cell lung cancer previously treated with platinum-containing chemotherapy regimens. The TAX 320 Non-Small Cell Lung Cancer Study Group. *J Clin Oncol* 2000;18:2354–2362.

Frasci G, Lorusso V, Panza N, et al. Gemcitabine plus vinorelbine versus vinorelbine alone in elderly patients with advanced non-small-cell lung cancer. *J Clin Oncol* 2000;18:2529–2536.

Gatzemeier U, von Pawel J, Gottfried M, et al. Phase III comparative study of high-dose cisplatin versus a combination of paclitaxel and cisplatin in patients with advanced non-small-cell lung cancer. *J Clin Oncol* 2000;18:3390–3399.

Giaccone G, Splinter TA, Debruyne C, et al. Randomized study of paclitaxel-cisplatin versus cisplatin-teniposide in patients with advanced non-small-cell lung cancer. The European Organization for Research and Treatment of Cancer Lung Cancer Cooperative Group. *J Clin Oncol* 1998;16:2133–2141.

Greenlee RT, Murray T, Bolden S, et al. Cancer statistics, 2000. *CA Cancer J Clin* 2000;50:7–33.

Gridelli C, Cigolari S, Gallo C, et al. Activity and toxicity of gemcitabine and gemcitabine + vinorelbine in advanced non-small-cell lung cancer elderly patients: phase II data from the Multicenter Italian Lung Cancer in the Elderly Study (MILES) randomized trial. *Lung Cancer* 2001;31:277–284.

Hensing TA, Socinski MA, Schell MJ, et al. Age does not alter toxicity or survival for patients (pts) with stage IIIB/IV non-small cell lung cancer (NSCLC) treated with carboplatin (C) and paclitaxel (P). *Proc Am Soc Clin Oncol* 2001;42. Abstract 1382.

Jiroutek M, Johnson D, Blum R, et al. Prognostic factors in advanced non-small cell lung cancer (NSCLC): analysis of Eastern Cooperative Oncology Group (ECOG) trials from 1981–1992. *Proc Am Soc Clin Oncol* 1999;40. Abstract 1774.

Johnson DR, DeVore R, Kabbinavar F, et al. Carboplatin (C) + paclitaxel (T) + RhuMab-VEGF (AVF) may prolong survival in advanced non-squamous lung cancer. *Proc Am Soc Clin Oncol* 2001. Abstract 1256.

Kelly K, Crowley J, Bunn PA Jr, et al. Randomized phase III trial of paclitaxel plus carboplatin versus vinorelbine plus cisplatin in the treatment of patients with advanced non-small-cell lung cancer: a Southwest Oncology Group trial. *J Clin Oncol* 2001a;19:3210–3218.

Kelly K, Giarritta S, Akerley W, et al. Should older patients (Pts) receive combination chemotherapy for advanced stage non-small cell lung cancer (NSCLC)? An analysis of Southwest Oncology Trials 9509 and 9308. *Proc Am Soc Clin Oncol* 2001b;42. Abstract 1313.

Komiya T, Fukuoka M, Negoro S, et al. Randomized phase III trial compared cisplatin and irinotecan (CPT-P) versus cisplatin and vindesine (VDS-P) versus irinotecan alone (CPT) in patients with advanced non-small cell lung cancer (NSCLC). The final report. Ninth World Conference on Lung Cancer 2000. Abstract 88.

Kosmidis PA, Bacoyiannis C, Mylonakis N, et al. A randomized phase III trial of paclitaxel plus carboplatin versus paclitaxel plus gemcitabine in advanced non small cell lung cancer (NSCLC). A preliminary analysis. *Proc Am Soc Clin Oncol* 2000;41. Abstract 1908.

Kunitoh H, Watanabe K, Ohashi Y, et al. Preliminary results of a randomized phase III trial of docetaxel (D) and cisplatin (P) versus vindesine (V) and P in stage IV non small cell lung cancer (NSCLC). *Proc Am Soc Clin Oncol* 2001;42. Abstract 1289.

Le Chevalier T, Brisgand D, Douillard JY, et al. Randomized study of vinorelbine and cisplatin versus vindesine and cisplatin versus vinorelbine alone in advanced non-small-cell lung cancer: results of a European multicenter trial including 612 patients. *J Clin Oncol* 1994;12:360–367.

Le Chevalier T, Brisgand D, Soria JC, et al. Long term analysis of survival in the European randomized trial comparing vinorelbine/cisplatin to vindesine/cisplatin and vinorelbine alone in advanced non-small cell lung cancer. *Oncologist* 2001;6(suppl 1):8–11.

Manegold C, Bergman B, Chemaissani A, et al. Single-agent gemcitabine versus cisplatin-etoposide: early results of a randomised phase II study in locally advanced or metastatic non-small-cell lung cancer. *Ann Oncol* 1997;8:525–529.

Martoni A, Guaraldi M, Piana E, et al. Multicenter randomized clinical trial on high-dose epirubicin plus cis-platinum versus vinorelbine plus cis-platinum in advanced non small cell lung cancer. *Lung Cancer* 1998;22:31–38.

Miller VA, Johnson D, Heelan RT, et al. A pilot trial demonstrates the safety of ZD1839 ("Iressa"), an oral epidermal growth factor receptor tyrosine kinase inhibitor (EGFR-TKI), in combination with carboplatin (C) and paclitaxel (P) in previously untreated advanced non-small cell lung cancer (NSCLC). *Proc Am Soc Clin Oncol* 2001;42. Abstract 1301.

Non-small Cell Lung Cancer Collaborative Group. Chemotherapy in non-small cell lung cancer: a meta-analysis using updated data on individual patients from 52 randomised clinical trials. *BMJ* 1995;311:899–909.

Perez-Soler R, Chachoua A, Huberman M, et al. A phase II trial of the epidermal growth factor receptor (EGFR) tyrosine kinase inhibitor OSI-774, following platinum-based chemotherapy, in patients (pts) with advanced, EGFR-expressing, non-small cell lung cancer (NSCLC). *Proc Am Soc Clin Oncol* 2001;42. Abstract 1235.

Perng RP, Chen YM, Ming-Liu J, et al. Gemcitabine versus the combination of cis-platin and etoposide in patients with inoperable non-small-cell lung cancer in a phase II randomized study. *J Clin Oncol* 1997;15:2097–2102.

Perrone F, Rossi A, Ianniello GP, et al. Vinorelbine (VNR) plus best supportive care (BSC) vs BSC in the treatment of advanced non-small cell lung cancer (NSCLC) elderly patients (pts). Results of a phase III randomized trial. *Proc Am Soc Clin Oncol* 1998;39. Abstract 1752.

Peterman AH, Socinski MA, Ribaudo J, et al. Effect of chemotherapy duration (de-fined vs. continuous) on quality of life in non-small-cell-lung cancer. *Proc Am Soc Clin Oncol* 2001;42. Abstract 1334.

Ranson M, Davidson N, Nicolson M, et al. Randomized trial of paclitaxel plus sup-portive care versus supportive care for patients with advanced non-small-cell lung cancer. *J Natl Cancer Inst* 2000;92:1074–1080.

Rapp E, Pater JL, Willan A, et al. Chemotherapy can prolong survival in patients with advanced non-small-cell lung cancer—report of a Canadian multicenter randomized trial. *J Clin Oncol* 1988;6:633–641.

Rodriguez J, Pawel J, Pluzanska A, et al. A multicenter, randomized phase III study of docetaxel + cisplatin (DC) and docetaxel + carboplatin (DCB) vs. vinorelbine + cisplatin (VC) in chemotherapy-naive patients with advanced and metastatic non-small cell lung cancer. *Proc Am Soc Clin Oncol* 2001;42. Abstract 1252.

Rosvold W, Langer CJ, McAleer C, et al. Advancing age does not exacerbate toxic-ity or compromise outcome in non-small cell lung cancer (NSCLC) patients (pts) receiving paclitaxel-carboplatin (P-C). *Proc Am Soc Clin Oncol* 1999;40. Ab-stract 1846.

Roszkowski K, Pluzanska A, Krzakowski M, et al. A multicenter, randomized, phase III study of docetaxel plus best supportive care versus best supportive care in chemotherapy-naive patients with metastatic or non-resectable local-ized non-small cell lung cancer (NSCLC). *Lung Cancer* 2000;27:145–157.

Sandler AB, Nemunaitis J, Denham C, et al. Phase III trial of gemcitabine plus cis-platin versus cisplatin alone in patients with locally advanced or metastatic non-small-cell lung cancer. *J Clin Oncol* 2000;18:122–130.

Scagliotti GV, De Marinis F, Rinaldi M, et al. Phase III randomized trial comparing three platinum-based doublets in advanced non-small cell lung cancer. *Proc Am Soc Clin Oncol* 2001;42. Abstract 1227.

Schiller JH, Harrington D, Sandler A, et al. A randomized phase III trial of four chemotherapy regimens in advanced non-small cell lung cancer. *Proc Am Soc Clin Oncol* 2000;41. Abstract 2.

Shepherd FA, Dancey J, Ramlau R, et al. Prospective randomized trial of docetaxel versus best supportive care in patients with non-small-cell lung cancer previously treated with platinum-based chemotherapy. *J Clin Oncol* 2000; 18:2095–2103.

Smith IE, O'Brien MER, Talbot DC, et al. Duration of chemotherapy in advanced non-small-cell lung cancer: a randomized trial of three versus six courses of mitomycin, vinblastine, and cisplatin. *J Clin Oncol* 2001;19:336–1343.

Socinski MA, Kies M, Schell MJ, et al. Duration of therapy in stage IIIB/IV non-small cell lung cancer (NSCLC): a multi-institutional phase III trial. *Proc Am Soc Clin Oncol* 2001;42. Abstract 1232.

Souquet PJ, Chauvin F, Boissel JP, et al. Polychemotherapy in advanced non small cell lung cancer: a meta-analysis. *Lancet* 1993;342:19–21.

Takiguchi Y, Nagao K, Nishiwaki YK, et al. The final results of a randomized phase III trial comparing irinotecan (CPT-11) and cisplatin (CDDP) with vindesine (VDS) and CDDP in advanced non-small-cell lung cancer (NSCLC). Ninth World Conference on Lung Cancer 2000. Abstract 89.

Van Meerbeeck JP, Smit EF, Lianes P, et al. A EORTC randomized phase III trial of three chemotherapy regimens in advanced non-small cell lung cancer (NSCLC). *Proc Am Soc Clin Oncol* 2001;42. Abstract 1228.

von Pawel J, von Roemeling R, Gatzemeier U, et al. Tirapazamine plus cisplatin versus cisplatin in advanced non-small-cell lung cancer: a report of the international CATAPULT I study group. Cisplatin and tirapazamine subjects with advanced previously untreated non-small-cell lung tumors. *J Clin Oncol* 2000;18:1351–1359.

Wozniak AJ, Crowley JJ, Balcerzak SP, et al. Randomized trial comparing cisplatin with cisplatin plus vinorelbine in the treatment of advanced non-small-cell lung cancer: a Southwest Oncology Group study. *J Clin Oncol* 1998;16:2459–2465.

Yuen A, Halsey J, Fisher G, et al. A Phase I/II trial of ISIS 3521, an antisense inhibitor of pkc-alpha, with carboplatin and paclitaxel in non-small cell lung cancer. *Proc Am Soc Clin Oncol* 2001. Abstract 1234.

10   TREATMENT OF LIMITED-STAGE SMALL CELL LUNG CANCER

Ritsuko Komaki

CHAPTER OVERVIEW

During the past decade, there have been major advances in the treatment of limited-stage small cell lung cancer (SCLC). Trials comparing the combination of chemotherapy and thoracic radiation therapy (TRT) with chemotherapy alone have shown that combination therapy improves survival rates.

Trials have also shown that concurrent chemotherapy and TRT is superior to sequential or alternating chemotherapy and TRT with regard to local-regional control and survival in patients with limited-stage SCLC. Today, at M. D. Anderson Cancer Center, standard treatment for this disease consists of concurrent chemotherapy and TRT, with TRT started on day 1 or after 1 cycle of chemotherapy. Accelerated TRT, prophylactic cranial irradiation for patients with a complete response to concurrent chemotherapy and TRT, and the use of supportive care—such as the use of granulocyte colony-stimulating factor, erythropoietin, and adequate antibiotics—are also standard. The role of surgery is limited in SCLC because of the nature of the disease, which often spreads to regional lymph nodes or spreads distantly.

INTRODUCTION

In the United States, approximately 20% to 25% of all lung cancer patients diagnosed each year have small cell lung cancer (SCLC). Approximately 25% of these patients have limited-stage disease—disease confined to a single hemithorax, the regional lymph nodes, the ipsilateral mediastinal lymph nodes, and the ipsilateral supraclavicular lymph nodes. Whether the presence of a malignant pleural effusion affects the outcome adversely in patients with SCLC is controversial, but patients with malignant pleural effusions are generally treated as having extensive-stage SCLC.

The outlook for patients with limited-stage SCLC has improved over the past decade, thanks to improvements in treatment. Studies have shown that the combination of chemotherapy and thoracic radiation therapy (TRT) is more effective than chemotherapy in terms of survival. Studies have also shown that concurrent chemotherapy and TRT is more effective than sequential or alternating therapy. Two-year survival rates for patients with limited-stage SCLC treated with this approach are around 4%. This represents a significant improvement over the 2-year survival rates reported in the late 1980s. This chapter will describe the development of the current treatment approach, describe details of treatment delivery at M. D. Anderson Cancer Center, and outline the various patient assessments done before, during, and after therapy.

PROGNOSTIC FACTORS

Patients with limited-stage SCLC fare better than their counterparts with extensive-stage disease (disease beyond the hemithorax, such as disease in bilateral lungs or extension beyond the chest, often to the brain, bone, bone marrow, or upper abdomen). Other patient factors influencing outcome are performance status (worse performance status correlates with worse outcome) and gender (females generally have better outcomes than males).

Age is not a significant prognostic factor in patients with limited-stage SCLC (Siu et al, 1996). Smokers who continue to smoke after the diagnosis of SCLC have worse outcomes than those who quit. Other prognostic factors associated with worse outcomes in patients with SCLC are elevated lactate dehydrogenase level, elevated alkaline phosphatase level, low sodium level, and possibly paraneoplastic syndrome. The biology of SCLC is also an important prognostic factor. Excellent reviews of the biology of SCLC have been published by Carney (1995) and Stahel and Weber (1995).

INITIAL WORKUP

The workup to define limited-stage SCLC includes a history, physical examination, pathology review, computed tomography (CT) of the chest and upper abdomen, magnetic resonance imaging of the brain, chest radiography, laboratory tests, electrocardiography, pulmonary function tests, and, in patients with a history of a myocardial infarction or other cardiovascular event or disease, adequate cardiac evaluation.

At M. D. Anderson, the first element of the workup is the pathology review since reevaluation of the pathology specimens often reveals neuroendocrine tumor, mixed adenocarcinoma, or undifferentiated large cell carcinoma with SCLC rather than pure SCLC. Pure SCLC is more sensitive to chemotherapy and radiation therapy than is the variant cell type, although there is some controversy about whether the variant cell type significantly affects patient outcome. Aisner and colleagues (1990) reviewed a series of 577 patients with limited-stage SCLC treated with chemotherapy and radiation therapy in an Eastern Cooperative Oncology Group (ECOG) protocol. Twenty-four patients (4%) had SCLC of the variant cell type. Complete response rates were 27% for patients with variant cell type and 19% for patients with classic cell type ($P = .45$). The variant cell type should be treated as non–small cell lung cancer rather than SCLC since the sensitivity of the variant cell type to chemotherapy and radiation therapy is similar to that of non–small cell lung cancer.

In patients who have good prognostic factors and negative findings on CT or magnetic resonance imaging of the brain, it is also important to evaluate for cognitive deficiency before aggressive treatment is begun (Komaki et al, 1995a). These patients are the most likely to respond to chemotherapy and TRT, and patients with a complete response would be candidates for prophylactic cranial irradiation (PCI) (see the section Prophylactic Cranial Irradiation later in this chapter). Patients in whom neurocognitive tests show severe abnormality are not candidates for PCI.

In patients with limited-stage SCLC, bone scanning and bone marrow aspiration or biopsy are indicated if the lactate dehydrogenase level is elevated, and thoracentesis is indicated if a pleural effusion is present. Follow-up imaging studies and other elements of the initial workup can be performed according to the National Comprehensive Cancer Network's clinical practice guidelines for SCLC, which outline a reasonably cost-effective strategy for the workup (NCCN, 1996).

Positron emission tomography (PET) to evaluate the extent of lung cancer, including mediastinal nodal involvement, has become fairly accurate, especially when PET is used in conjunction with CT (Pieterman et al, 2000). However, because the cost of PET for SCLC is not reimbursed by most insurers, PET is not routinely used as part of the staging workup for SCLC at M. D. Anderson.

TREATMENT

The standard treatment for patients with limited-stage SCLC consists of concurrent chemotherapy, with TRT started on day 1 or after 1 cycle of systemic chemotherapy, followed by PCI for patients who have a complete response to chemotherapy and TRT. This section will review the rationale for the current treatment approach and then describe the details of treatment as it is currently administered at M. D. Anderson.

Rationale for the Current Treatment Approach

Thoracic Radiation Therapy

The superiority of TRT to surgery in terms of survival was demonstrated in the landmark Medical Research Council trial (Fox and Scadding, 1973). In this study, patients with limited-stage SCLC were randomly assigned to surgery (71 patients) or radical radiation therapy (73 patients). Only 1% of patients treated with surgery were alive at 5 years, and these patients had eventually received palliative radiation therapy. Four percent of the patients treated with radiation therapy were alive at 5 years. Median survival times were 199 days in patients treated with surgery versus 300 days in patients treated with radiation therapy. These poor survival times might be related to the inadequate staging system in use at the time of the trial. In any case, this trial established that surgery is not the best treatment modality for patients with SCLC.

Chemotherapy

In the 1970s, recognition of the exquisite sensitivity of SCLC to chemotherapy led to replacement of radiation therapy with chemotherapy as the treatment of choice for this disease. Randomized trials of radiation therapy and chemotherapy revealed an improvement in median and 2-year survival in patients treated with chemotherapy as opposed to radiation therapy (Bunn and Ihde, 1981). Single-agent chemotherapy was soon followed by multiagent chemotherapy, which was used throughout the 1970s and early 1980s. Feld and colleagues (1993) reviewed 8 series published between 1979 and 1987 that investigated chemotherapy with and without TRT in patients with limited-stage SCLC. The authors reported an increase in 2-year survival rates from a range of 10% to 15% to a range of 25% to 30%. Most, if not all, of the improvement in outcome was attributed to more effective combination chemotherapy regimens.

Today, chemotherapy regimens commonly used to treat patients with limited-stage SCLC include etoposide, cisplatin, and paclitaxel and carboplatin and irinotecan. Paclitaxel, cisplatin, and etoposide plus concurrent radiation therapy (Ettinger et al, 2000) and ifosfamide, cisplatin, and etoposide plus concurrent radiation therapy (Glisson et al, 2000) have not been shown to have long-term benefits compared to treatment with cisplatin, etoposide, and concurrent radiation therapy for patients with limited-stage SCLC. Irinotecan has been reported to be more effective than etoposide and cisplatin for extensive-stage SCLC (Noda et al, 2002). Chemotherapy for SCLC is discussed in more detail in chapter 11.

Chemotherapy and Thoracic Radiation Therapy in Combination

Although early development of distant metastases is a critical problem in patients with SCLC, making chemotherapy an important element in the treatment regimen, intrathoracic failure becomes more important once distant metastasis is controlled. Two meta-analyses, using different methods, confirmed the value of adding TRT to chemotherapy in decreasing the rate of local recurrence and improving survival in patients with SCLC. Warde and Payne (1992) analyzed results from 11 prospective randomized trials of chemotherapy with or without TRT for patients with limited-stage disease and found an absolute increase in overall survival at 2 years from 15% to 20.4% and an absolute increase in local control at 2 years from 15% to 40% with the addition of TRT. Pignon and colleagues (1992) collected data on 2,140 patients from 16 randomized trials comparing chemotherapy alone versus chemotherapy plus TRT and found an improvement in absolute survival of 5.4% at 3 years.

Concurrent Chemotherapy and Thoracic Radiation Therapy

The very poor survival outcomes even in patients treated with combination therapy indicated that the effectiveness of both TRT and systemic chemotherapy needed to be improved. One idea for improving local and distant control in patients with SCLC was to deliver chemotherapy concurrently with radiation therapy so that chemotherapy would work as a radiosensitizer. The potential advantages of concurrent chemotherapy and radiation therapy are early use of both modalities, to provide synergistic effects; the ability to plan radiation therapy more accurately since there is no induction chemotherapy, which can obscure the original tumor volume; and short overall treatment time (high dose intensity), which prevents proliferation of clonogens. The disadvantages are enhanced normal tissue toxicity, which could necessitate dose modification or treatment breaks; inability to assess response to either modality; and, possibly, sensitization of normal tissue.

In the 1970s, concurrent chemotherapy (cyclophosphamide, doxorubicin, and vincristine) and TRT was tried at the National Cancer Institute. Patients with limited-stage SCLC who were treated with this regimen had a high response rate (90%), although the treatment-related mortality rate was 20% (Johnson et al, 1976). Because of this high mortality rate, concurrent TRT and doxorubicin has been abandoned.

Other strategies of concurrent radiation therapy and chemotherapy have been pilot-tested. McCracken and colleagues (1990) reported results from a phase II trial of the Southwest Oncology Group in which 2 courses of cisplatin, etoposide, and vincristine were given with concurrent radiation therapy 1.8 Gy per day given as a single fraction 5 days per week to a total dose of 45 Gy. Additional chemotherapy with vincristine, methotrexate, and etoposide alternating with doxorubicin and cyclophosphamide for 12 weeks was administered after the concurrent therapy. The investigators evaluated 154 patients. With a minimum period of observation of 3 years, the 2-year survival rate was 42%, and the 4-year survival rate was 30%. An updated analysis after a longer period of observation found a 5-year survival rate of 26% (Janaki et al, 1994).

Johnson and colleagues (1976, 1993) and Turrisi and colleagues (1992) reported small series of patients treated with concurrent cisplatin and etoposide with accelerated fractionation: 1.5 Gy twice daily 5 days per week for 3 weeks, for a total dose of 45 Gy. Two-year survival rates were 57% and 65%, respectively, for the Turrisi and Johnson studies. An updated analysis of the Turrisi study found a 4-year survival rate of 36% (Turrisi et al, 1999) (Table 10–1).

In the Radiation Therapy Oncology Group (RTOG) and ECOG trial 0096 (Turrisi et al, 1999), a nationwide randomized study, patients with limited-stage SCLC treated with concurrent chemotherapy (etoposide and cisplatin) and TRT (45 Gy; 1.5 Gy twice daily or 1.8 Gy daily) started on day 1 had a 2-year survival rate of 40% to 44%. The 5-year survival rates were 16% in patients treated with once-daily TRT and 26% in patients treated with twice-daily TRT—a remarkable improvement over previously reported 5-year survival rates.

The Japanese Clinical Oncology Group (Goto et al, 1999) reported a prospective randomized study in which 231 patients with limited-stage SCLC, good performance status, and age less than 76 years were treated with concurrent or sequential chemotherapy between May 1991 and January 1995. Chemotherapy consisted of paclitaxel 80 mg/m^2 on day 1 and etoposide 100 mg/m^2 on days 1 through 3 every 3 weeks for 4 cycles. Radiation therapy consisted of 45 Gy delivered in twice-daily fractions of 1.5 Gy over 3 weeks. In the concurrent-therapy group, chemotherapy and TRT were started together on day 1. In the sequential-therapy group, TRT was started after 2 cycles of chemotherapy. With a median follow-up time of

Table 10–1. Complete Response Rates and Overall Survival Rates among Complete Responders in Patients with SCLC Treated with Chemotherapy and Thoracic Radiation Therapy

Study and Type of Therapy	No. of Patients	Complete Response Rate (%)	Survival Rate (%) among Complete Responders			
			2-Year	3-Year	4-Year	5-Year
Arriagada et al (1991)						
Interdigitated	72	87	45	—	35	26
Turrisi et al (1999)						
Concurrent	36	91	54	—	36	
Komaki et al (1995b)						
Interdigitated	18	64	44	33	27	
Concurrent	29	96	70	57		

Reprinted with permission from Komaki R. Management of limited small-cell lung cancer. *Int J Clin Oncol* 2000;5:205–216.

more than 50 months, median survival time was 27.2 months in the concurrent-therapy arm and 19.5 months in the sequential-therapy arm. Survival rates in the concurrent-therapy and sequential-therapy arms, respectively, were 55.3% and 35.4% at 2 years and 30.9% and 20.7% at 3 years. Although there was no significant difference in the response rate, overall survival was superior in the concurrent-therapy arm (P = .057). The incidence of grade 3–4 leukopenia was significantly higher in the concurrent-therapy group (86.8% vs 51.3%). The incidence of nonhematologic side effects was not significantly different between the 2 groups (Goto et al, 1999).

There is both radiobiological and clinical evidence suggesting that alternating chemotherapy and TRT may improve local control and survival (Looney, 1992).

Arriagada and colleagues (1991) reported the results of 2 protocols including 72 consecutive patients with limited-stage SCLC. Patients received 2 cycles of induction chemotherapy followed by 3 cycles of TRT lasting 2 weeks each with interdigitated chemotherapy (the same regimen as that used for induction chemotherapy). Cisplatin and etoposide were used in the first trial, and cisplatin, etoposide, cyclophosphamide, and doxorubicin were used in the second trial. The results of this trial are among the most favorable reported in terms of long-term survival: the 2-year overall survival rate was 40%, and the 5-year survival rate was 26% (Table 10–1).

Investigators at M.D. Anderson retrospectively compared 2 consecutive studies investigating the sequencing and timing of chemotherapy and radiation therapy for limited-stage SCLC (Table 10–1) (Komaki et al, 1995b). The first study was called the COPE trial because of the chemotherapy regimen involved—cyclophosphamide 750 mg/m^2 intravenously (IV) day 1, vincristine 2 mg IV day 8, cisplatin 20 mg/m^2 days 1 through 3, and etoposide 100 mg/m^2 IV days 1 through 3. This trial, based on the Goldie-Coldman hypothesis, was designed to overcome drug resistance of malignant cells using interdigitated chemotherapy and TRT. After 3 cycles of induction chemotherapy (COPE), patients received 3 cycles of TRT. Each TRT cycle consisted of 1.5 Gy twice daily 5 days per week for 1 week (15 Gy per week) followed by a 2-week break. The total dose was 45 Gy in 9 weeks. COPE was given during the interval between courses of TRT, and 2 more cycles of COPE were given after TRT was completed. The goal of the 2-week breaks between periods of radiation treatments was to reduce the incidence of severe esophagitis while systemic chemotherapy was given to reduce distant metastasis and suppress clonogenic proliferation of primary cancer cells.

The second study reviewed by M.D. Anderson investigators (Wagner et al, 1994) was part of a national cooperative study in which patients received chemotherapy (cisplatin 60 mg/m^2 IV day 1 and etoposide 120 mg/m^2 IV over days 1–3 every 3 weeks for 4 cycles) with concurrent radiation therapy (1.8 Gy daily to a total dose of 45 Gy in 5 weeks or 1.4 Gy twice daily to a total dose of 45 Gy in 3 weeks) starting on day 1 of chemotherapy.

The COPE study enrolled 28 patients with limited-stage SCLC between 1987 and 1989. Eighteen of these patients had a complete response, and 8 patients had a partial response; survival rates for the complete responders at 1, 2, 3, and 4 years, respectively, were 79%, 44%, 33%, and 27%. The intergroup study of concurrent chemotherapy and TRT enrolled 33 patients from M. D. Anderson between 1990 and 1992. Follow-up time ranged from 1 to 39 months, with a median of 21 months. Twenty-nine patients had a complete response, and 4 patients had a partial response; survival rates at 1, 2, and 3 years, respectively, were 93%, 70%, and 57%. These data suggest that concurrent chemotherapy and TRT is more effective than 3 cycles of induction chemotherapy followed by interdigitated TRT and chemotherapy with regard to local and distant control as well as 2- and 3-year overall survival (Table 10–2) (Figure 10–1).

Delivery of Thoracic Radiation Therapy Early in the Course of Treatment

The timing of concurrent chemotherapy and TRT is still controversial. The National Cancer Institute of Canada Clinical Trials Group studied early versus late TRT in a randomized trial (Murray et al, 1993). A total of 308 patients were enrolled. All patients received 6 cycles of chemotherapy (cyclophosphamide, doxorubicin, and vincristine alternated with etoposide and cisplatin). Patients were randomly assigned to receive early TRT (40 Gy to the primary tumor site in 15 fractions over 3 weeks given concurrently with etoposide and cisplatin and started at week 3) or late TRT (the same radiation dose given concurrently with etoposide and cisplatin and started at week 15). After completion of all chemotherapy and TRT, complete responders received PCI, 25 Gy in 10 fractions over 2 weeks. Although complete response rates were not significantly different between the early and late TRT groups, progression-free survival ($P = .036$) and overall survival ($P = .008$) were significantly better in the early TRT group. Patients in the late TRT group had a significantly higher rate of brain

Table 10–2. **Patterns of First Site of Failure in Patients with SCLC Treated with Interdigitated or Concurrent Chemotherapy**

	Percentage of Patients with Metastases at Time of Initial Recurrence		
	Local-Regional	*Distant*	*Brain*
Interdigitated (28)	44	48	30
Concurrent (33)	30	30	0

$P < .01$.

Reprinted with permission from Komaki R. Management of limited small-cell lung cancer. *Int J Clin Oncol* 2000;5:205–216.

metastasis ($P = .006$). This study indicated that the early administration of TRT with concurrent chemotherapy improved survival, possibly by reducing the last clonogens in the primary tumor.

Chemotherapy Dose

The dose of chemotherapy is as important as the choice of chemotherapy agent in achieving a better response and survival in patients with limited-stage SCLC.

In a randomized phase III trial reported in 1993, Arriagada and colleagues randomly assigned patients to a higher-dose regimen (cisplatin 100 mg/m^2, cyclophosphamide 300 mg/m^2, doxorubicin 40 mg/m^2, and etoposide 75 mg/m^2) or a lower-dose regimen (cisplatin 80 mg/m^2, cyclophosphamide 225 mg/m^2, doxorubicin 40 mg/m^2, and etoposide 75 mg/m^2). The disease-free survival rates at 2 years were 28% for the 55 patients in the higher-dose group and 8% for the 50 patients in the lower-dose group ($P = .02$). The overall survival rates at 2 years were 43% in the higher-dose group and 26% in the lower-dose group ($P = .02$). Side effects from treatment were not increased in the higher-dose group at a median follow-up time of 33 months.

Volume Irradiated

In patients treated with chemotherapy before TRT, whether TRT should cover the prechemotherapy or postchemotherapy disease volume has been controversial. In the 1980s, significantly decreased survival rates were reported when the prechemotherapy volumes were not encompassed.

More recently, however, studies by Arriagada and colleagues (1990), Kies and colleagues (1987), and a group at the Mayo Clinic (Liengswangwong et al, 1994) have not shown any significant difference in survival between patients who receive TRT encompassing the postchemotherapy volume and those who receive TRT encompassing the prechemotherapy volume. This phenomenon might be related to better systemic chemotherapy reducing the rate of recurrence in the tumor margins. When concurrent chemotherapy and TRT are given, margins need to be tight enough (1.0–1.5 cm) not to cause severe acute toxic effects. Three-dimensional conformal treatment is one potential method for reducing the volume to critical organs while still offering an adequate dose to the gross disease.

Fractionation of Radiation Therapy

Hyperfractionated radiation therapy has been developed to improve local control and possibly survival by delivering higher doses of radiation over a shorter time. In several phase II trials of twice-daily TRT with concurrent chemotherapy, median survival times ranged from 18 months to 27 months, and 2-year survival rates ranged from 19% to 60%, with local control rates ranging from 32% to 91% (Turrisi et al, 1992; Johnson et al, 1993).

Intergroup study 0096 (Turrisi et al, 1999) was conducted through the ECOG and RTOG to investigate once-daily versus twice-daily radiation therapy with concurrent cisplatin and etoposide in patients with limited-stage SCLC. All patients received 4 cycles of chemotherapy consisting of cisplatin 60 mg/m^2 on day 1 and etoposide 120 mg/m^2 IV on days 1, 3, and 5, with treatment repeated every 21 days. The daily fractionation group received a single 1.8-Gy fraction each day, to a total tumor dose of 45 Gy in 25 fractions over 5 weeks. The twice-daily fractionation group received two 1.5-Gy fractions each day with a 4- to 6-hour interfraction interval, to a total tumor dose of 45 Gy in 30 fractions in 3 weeks. In patients who had a complete response, PCI (10 fractions of 2.5 Gy) was considered. Five-year survival was significantly better in the accelerated fractionation group (28%) than in the daily fractionation group (21%) ($P = .043$) (Turrisi et al, 1999).

Standard once-daily fractionation (1.8 Gy per fraction) versus accelerated fractionation (1.5 Gy twice daily) with a total dose of 45 Gy was investigated in a cooperative randomized trial (Arriagada et al, 1991). Radiation therapy was given with concurrent chemotherapy consisting of cisplatin 60 mg/m^2 IV day 1 and etoposide 120 mg/m^2 IV days 1 through 3 for 4 cycles. A total of 419 patients were enrolled in this randomized trial between 1988 and 1992, with 383 evaluable. Overall median survival for the entire group was 20 months, and the 2-year progression-free survival rate was 40%. The twice-daily, accelerated regimen was associated with improved survival, and there were trends towards a higher complete response rate, longer duration of response, and longer time to recurrence in the accelerated-TRT group. Side effects in the 2 arms were identical with the exception of grade 3 esophagitis, which was seen in 26% of the patients treated with twice-daily treatment and 11% of those treated with 1 fraction per day. There was no significant difference between the 2 groups in the incidence of late esophageal side effects. The treatment-related death rate was 2%. Concurrent chemotherapy and radiation therapy can be tolerated and efficacious, as shown by the 40% 2-year survival rate in a large cooperative-group trial (Turrisi et al, 1999)—twice as good as survival rates reported a decade ago (Warde and Payne, 1992).

Ariyoshi and colleagues of the Japanese Clinical Oncology Group (1994) have reported a multicenter phase II trial of concurrent cisplatin-etoposide chemotherapy and TRT for limited-stage SCLC. The chemotherapy consisted of cisplatin and etoposide repeated every 28 days for 4 to 6 cycles. TRT to the primary tumor was administered with daily fractionation according to the following schedule: 20 Gy delivered in ten 2-Gy fractions over days 2 through 12 of the first cycle of chemotherapy, and 30 Gy delivered in fifteen 2-Gy fractions delivered on days 29 through 47 of the second cycle of chemotherapy. Some patients received a 10-Gy boost. Total doses were thus 40 to 50 Gy over 7 weeks. PCI was given to complete responders after completion of treatment. Sixty-six patients were enrolled in the protocol. The median response duration was 8.7 months, the median survival time was 14.8 months, and the 2-year survival rate was 20%. The local control rate at 2 years was 40.7%. These findings indicated that the regimen used in this trial was not as effective as the regimen used in the intergroup trial in which a similar dose of TRT was given within 3 weeks or 5 weeks (Turrisi et al, 1999).

Radiation Dose to the Thorax

The radiation dose to the thorax is another controversial area (Ariyoshi et al, 1994; Cox, 1988). The National Cancer Institute of Canada conducted an important study (Coy et al, 1988) to determine the dose-response relationship for irradiation of the thorax. The investigators showed a clear dose-response relationship, with thoracic progression-free survival better among patients treated with 37.5 Gy in 15 fractions over 3 weeks than in patients treated with 25 Gy in 10 fractions over 2 weeks as consolidation therapy after completion of cisplatin-etoposide and cyclophosphamide-doxorubicin-vincristine alternating or sequential chemotherapy.

Arriagada and colleagues (1990) at the Institut Gustave-Roussy published a report of 173 patients with limited-stage SCLC treated with different doses of TRT in 3 consecutive trials. TRT was given in split courses interdigitated with chemotherapy. The total dose of TRT increased from 45 Gy (15–15–15) to 55 Gy (20–20–15) to 65 Gy (20–20–25). The 3-year local control rates were 66%, 70%, and 70%, respectively, in patients treated with the low, medium, and high TRT doses, and 5-year survival rates were 16%, 16%, and 20%, respectively. The overall rate of lethal toxicity was 10%, and this rate did not differ significantly by TRT doses. There were no significant differences in local control and survival rates between patients treated with 45 Gy and those treated with 65 Gy when effective chemotherapy was given.

Choi and colleagues (1998) conducted a phase I study designed to determine the maximum tolerated dose of radiation in daily and twice-daily fractionation with concurrent chemotherapy. The maximum tolerated dose of hyperfractionated radiation therapy was reached at 45 Gy in 30 fractions over 19 days. However, the maximum tolerated dose of daily fractionation was not reached at 66 Gy in 33 fractions over 45 days. Therefore, patients were accrued to 70 Gy in 35 fractions over 47 days. The tumor response rates varied from 78% to 100%, with no significant difference among the different dose levels. Grade 3 or more severe esophagitis and granulocytopenia were more common among the patients treated with hyperfractionated and accelerated fractionation. Doses above 40 Gy did not significantly improve the local control rate (Figure 10–2). Local recurrence after higher TRT doses is most likely due to prolongation of the duration of TRT (Komaki et al, 2000). Therefore, it seems important to keep the duration of TRT within 5 weeks rather than just escalating the total tumor dose with a prolonged duration of TRT.

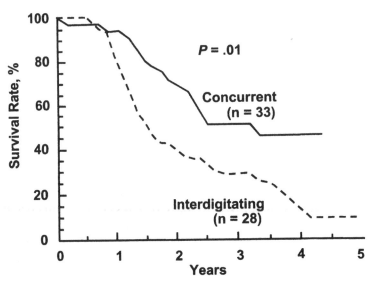

Figure 10–1. Survival in patients with limited-stage SCLC treated with concurrent (n = 33) and interdigitated (n = 28) chemotherapy. Reprinted from *International Journal of Radiation Oncology Biology and Physics,* volume 31, number 4, Komaki R, Shin DM, Glisson BS, et al. Interdigitating versus concurrent chemotherapy and radiation therapy for limited small cell lung cancer, pages 808–811, 1995, with permission from Elsevier Science.

On the basis of this theory, M. D. Anderson, together with other RTOG institutions, has initiated a study in which the dose of TRT with concurrent cisplatin and etoposide is escalated but the duration of TRT is kept within 5 weeks (RTOG 97–12) (Ritsuko Komaki, principal investigator). As of this writing, 62 patients have been enrolled, and the dose of TRT has been escalated to 64.8 Gy in 5 weeks, given in 1.5-Gy fractions during large-field TRT, followed by 1.8-Gy fractions twice daily for the boost. This approach has been better tolerated than the approach of applying large fields of TRT twice a day starting on day 1 of chemotherapy (unpublished data).

Prophylactic Cranial Irradiation

Patients who have a complete response to chemotherapy and TRT are usually treated with PCI.

The risk of brain metastasis from SCLC correlates with the length of survival, and as more effective treatment extends life, the risk of brain metastases increases (Komaki et al, 1981). An autopsy series (Nugent et al, 1979) showed that 80% of patients who died within 2 to 3 years after completion of treatment had metastases in the central nervous system (CNS),

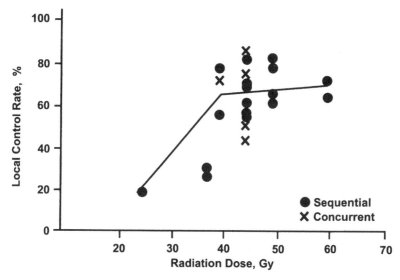

Figure 10–2.   Local control as a function of TRT dose and timing of chemotherapy and radiation therapy. Circles indicate sequential chemotherapy and TRT; "x"es indicate concurrent chemotherapy and TRT. Reprinted from Komaki R. Management of limited small-cell lung cancer. *Int J Clin Oncol* 2000;5:205–216, with permission.

including brain parenchyma, base-of-skull, leptomeningeal, and spinal cord metastases. Therapeutic irradiation of the brain in patients with clinically evident metastases has not proven effective: complete response rates range from 25% to 64%, and the median remission duration is a few months (Cox et al, 1980).

In the past, the role of PCI was controversial because of the lack of definitive evidence that it improved overall survival and because of previously reported late neurologic side effects. More efficacious and less toxic treatment was sought. Studies revealed that earlier PCI was more efficacious and that a lower total dose (24–25 Gy), smaller fraction size (2.0–2.5 Gy), delivery of PCI after completion of chemotherapy, and use of less neurotoxic chemotherapy were all important factors contributing to reduced late neurotoxicity (Komaki et al, 1985). PCI significantly reduces the incidence of brain recurrences among long-term survivors without producing obvious neurologic side effects, although the majority of studies have been done retrospectively (Shaw et al, 1993; Cull et al, 1994).

The National Cancer Institute (Johnson et al, 1996) reported excellent results in 38 patients with limited-stage SCLC treated with etoposide and cisplatin with concurrent hyperfractionated radiation therapy, 1.5 Gy twice daily to a total dose of 45 Gy over 3 weeks. The 1-year actuarial survival rate was 83%, and the 2-year actuarial survival rate was 43%. The 5-year survival rate was 19%, and the median survival time was 21.3 months. However, 34% of the patients (13 of 38) had CNS metastases as the only site of initial relapse, and all died of CNS metastases. Isolated CNS metastasis caused more than 30% of the cancer deaths in this study, which underscores the importance of PCI.

A recently reported meta-analysis of 7 randomized clinical trials has demonstrated a disease-free and overall survival advantage in those patients who underwent PCI (Auperin et al, 1999). There were several problems with the study: 4 of the 7 trials analyzed included fewer than 100 patients, which may undercut the validity of the statistical analyses; approximately 14% of all 987 patients had extensive-stage rather than limited-stage disease; and the dose fractionation in the patients who received PCI was not uniform. However, there was a trend towards a reduction in the rate of brain relapses in the subset of patients who received PCI and were treated with a total radiation dose of at least 36.0 Gy at a conventional 2 Gy per fraction. This meta-analysis did not attempt to determine the risk of long-term neurologic side effects in patients receiving and not receiving PCI.

M. D. Anderson Treatment Approach

At M. D. Anderson, radiation oncologists, medical oncologists, and thoracic surgeons discuss treatment options for each patient with limited-stage SCLC at a multidisciplinary conference and reach a consensus regarding treatment at the time of consultation in the multidisciplinary thoracic center. We always individualize our treatment recommendations. Eligible patients are offered participation in experimental protocols. For patients who are not candidates for experimental protocols, we follow institutional guidelines for treatment of SCLC.

At M. D. Anderson, patients with very large tumors in the lung, pleural effusions, or poor pulmonary function without obvious distant metastases are usually treated with a course of induction chemotherapy followed by concurrent chemotherapy and TRT. The rationale for this approach is that SCLC is sensitive to chemotherapy and thus induction chemotherapy will usually reduce the size of the tumor, reducing the volume to be treated with TRT.

The standard volume treated with TRT is the gross target volume plus a 15-mm margin around it. The clinical target volume is set as the gross target volume plus a 10-mm margin around it, and the planning target volume is set as the clinical target volume plus a 15-mm margin around it. We include the ipsilateral supraclavicular nodes if the lesion is located in the upper lobe and the bilateral supraclavicular nodes if supraclavicular or upper mediastinal nodes are grossly involved.

For lesions with hilar or mediastinal nodal involvement, the subcarinal nodes are electively irradiated with borders described in the preceding paragraph or 3 cm below the carina electively. We do not electively irradiate the contralateral hilar nodes or the lower mediastinal nodes. We use a higher-energy (6 or 18 MV) linear accelerator to avoid unnecessary scatter to the surrounding normal tissue and to give a uniform dose distribution to the target volume. TRT is done using 3-dimensional conformal radiation therapy treatment planning with inhomogeneity correction.

At M. D. Anderson, we give intravenous etoposide (120 mg/m^2) and intravenous cisplatin (60 mg/m^2) for 4 cycles starting on day 1 of TRT. Each cycle of chemotherapy lasts 21 days. TRT is given in twice-daily 1.5-Gy fractions with a 6-hour interfraction interval 5 days per week for 3 weeks, for a total tumor dose of 45 Gy. Sometimes we treat patients with a combination of irinotecan and cisplatin as induction or maintenance chemotherapy since irinotecan has been shown to be an active agent against SCLC (Noda et al, 2002). Occasionally a combination of paclitaxel and carboplatin is used, especially in patients with renal dysfunction.

For PCI at M. D. Anderson, we usually give 25 Gy in 10 fractions or 30 Gy in 15 fractions by linear accelerator with 6-MV photons to the whole brain. PCI is given to patients who have a complete response to chemotherapy and TRT and have no severe cognitive abnormality identified on neuropsychological tests. In a study of the impact of PCI on cognitive function, baseline and follow-up neuropsychological tests revealed that 83% (25/30) of patients with limited-stage SCLC had evidence of cognitive dysfunction prior to PCI, and no significant differences were found between results on pretreatment and posttreatment cognitive function tests (Komaki et al, 1995a).

ASSESSMENTS DURING TREATMENT

During treatment, patients are assessed for esophagitis, pneumonitis, neutropenic fever, anemia, and electrolyte imbalances. For severe esophagitis, local analgesics, along with oral analgesics or fentanyl citrate (Duragesic) or both, are given. Nutritional status is assessed before treatment and weekly throughout treatment. Nutritional supplements and correction of electrolyte imbalances is done promptly. Appropriate antibiotics are started immediately if patients develop neutropenic fever or bacterial infection. Granulocyte colony-stimulating factor and erythropoietin are given as indicated, usually on Friday after TRT if patients are receiving TRT. Occasionally, steroids are required for treatment of pneumonitis. Limiting the volume irradiated with TRT is the most important way to prevent pneumonitis. Concurrent doxorubicin or bleomycin with TRT is contraindicated because of the potential for damage to normal lung, heart, and skin.

KEY PRACTICE POINTS

- Concurrent chemotherapy and TRT, with TRT given early during the course of chemotherapy, is the standard treatment in patients with limited-stage SCLC.

- Patients who have very large tumors in the lung, a pleural effusion, or poor pulmonary function might need a maximum of 2 cycles of induction chemotherapy before concurrent chemotherapy and TRT.

- In patients treated with concurrent chemotherapy and twice-daily (acceler-ated) TRT, conformal radiation therapy must be used to reduce the harmful effects of treatment on the esophagus and lung.

- In patients with a complete response to concurrent chemotherapy and TRT, PCI is recommended to decrease the risk of brain metastasis and to improve survival.

- Because of the high incidence of second malignancies and local-regional and distant recurrence, patients need to have frequent check-ups after completion of the recommended treatment.

RESPONSE ASSESSMENT

Response to treatment is usually assessed 1 to 2 months after completion of the fourth cycle of chemotherapy. If clinical assessment indicates progression of disease, patients are evaluated earlier with imaging or laboratory tests or both. Assessment of response is done by repeated CT of the chest and upper abdomen, magnetic resonance imaging of the brain, bone scanning, and laboratory tests, including measurement of lactate dehydrogenase, other hepatic enzyme, and electrolyte levels; a complete blood cell count; and renal function tests. PET is not used routinely for assessment of response in patients with SCLC.

FOLLOW-UP AFTER TREATMENT

After completion of treatment, patients have check-ups every 4 to 6 weeks for the first year, then every 3 months for 2 years, then every 6 months for 3 years, and then yearly. It is very important to detect second malignancies among patients with limited-stage SCLC treated successfully and to detect locally recurrent and distant metastatic disease.

FUTURE DIRECTIONS

In the future, smoking cessation, detection of early-stage SCLC with the use of better imaging techniques or tumor markers, and better selection of patients for particular treatments should be pursued. Efficacious systemic treatment with early application of TRT, delivery of PCI with a normal tissue protector (e.g., ethyol), conformal radiation therapy with respiratory gating, appropriate supportive care to address pain, nutrition, respiratory rehabilitation, and bone marrow suppression, and development of treatments based on the biology of SCLC should all be pursued.

SUGGESTED READINGS

Aisner SC, Finkelstein DM, Ettinger DS, et al. The clinical significance of variant-morphology small-cell carcinoma of the lung. *J Clin Oncol* 1990;8:402–408.

Ariyoshi Y, Fukuoka M, Furuse K, et al. Concurrent cisplatin-etoposide chemotherapy plus thoracic radiotherapy for limited-stage small cell lung cancer. Japanese Lung Cancer Chemotherapy Group in Japanese Clinical Oncology Group. *Jpn J Clin Oncol* 1994;24:275–281.

Arriagada R, Le Chevalier T, Pignon JP, et al. Initial chemotherapeutic doses and survival in patients with limited small-cell lung cancer. *N Engl J Med* 1993;329:1848–1852.

Arriagada R, Le Chevalier T, Ruffie P, et al. Alternating radiotherapy and chemotherapy in 173 consecutive patients with limited small cell lung carcinoma. GROP and the French Cancer Center's Lung Group. *Int J Radiat Oncol Biol Phys* 1990;19:1135–1138.

Arriagada R, Pellae-Cosset B, Cueto Ladron de Guevara JC, et al. Alternating radiotherapy and chemotherapy schedules in limited small cell lung cancer: analysis of local chest recurrences. *Radiother Oncol* 1991;20:91–98.

Auperin A, Arriagada R, Pignon JP, et al. Prophylactic cranial irradiation for patients with small-cell lung cancer in complete remission. Prophylactic Cranial Irradiation Overview Collaborative Group. *N Engl J Med* 1999;341:476–484.

Bunn PA, Ihde DC. Small cell bronchogenic carcinoma: a review of therapeutic results. In: Livingston RB, ed. *Lung Cancer.* Vol 1. Boston, Mass: Nijhoff; 1981:169–208.

Carney DN. Lung cancer biology. *Semin Radiat Oncol* 1995;5:4–10.

Choi NC, Herndon JE II, Rosenman J, et al. Phase I study to determine the maximum-tolerated dose of radiation in standard daily and hyperfractionated-accelerated twice-daily radiation schedules with concurrent chemotherapy for limited-stage small-cell lung cancer. *J Clin Oncol* 1998;6:3528–3536.

Cox JD. Dose-response in small cell carcinoma [editorial]. *Int J Radiat Oncol Biol Phys* 1988;14:393–394.

Cox JD, Komaki R, Byhardt RW, et al. Results of whole-brain irradiation for metastases from small cell carcinoma of the lung. *Cancer Treatment Reports* 1980;64:957–961.

Coy P, Hodson I, Payne DG, et al. The effect of dose of thoracic irradiation on recurrence in patients with limited stage small cell lung cancer. Initial results of a Canadian Multicenter randomized trial. *Int J Radiat Oncol Biol Phys* 1988;14:219–226.

Cull A, Gregor A, Hopwood P, et al. Neurological and cognitive impairment in long-term survivors of small cell lung cancer [abstract]. *Eur J Cancer* 1994;30A(8):1067–1074.

Ettinger DS, Seiferheld WF, Abrams RA, et al. Cisplatin (P), etoposide (E), paclitaxel (T), and concurrent hyperfractionated thoracic radiotherapy (TRT) for patients (Pts) with limited disease (LD) small cell lung cancer (SCLC): preliminary results of RTOG 96–09 [abstract]. *Proc Am Soc Clin Oncol* 2000;19:490a.

Feld R, Ginsberg RJ, Payne DG. Treatment of small cell lung cancer. In: Roth JA, Ruckdeschel JC, Weisenburger TH, eds. *Thoracic Oncology.* Philadelphia, PA: Saunders; 1993:229–262.

Fox W, Scadding JG. Medical Research Council comparative trial of surgery and radiotherapy for primary treatment of small-celled or oat-celled carcinoma of bronchus. Ten-year follow-up. *Lancet* 1973;2(7820):63–65.

Glisson B, Scott C, Komaki R, et al. Cisplatin, ifosfamide, oral etoposide, and concurrent accelerated hyperfractionated thoracic radiation for patients with limited small-cell lung carcinoma: results of Radiation Therapy Oncology Group trial 93–12. *J Clin Oncol* 2000;18:2990–2995.

Goto K, Nishiwaki Y, Takada M, et al. Final results of a phase III study of concurrent versus sequential thoracic radiotherapy (TRT) in combination with cisplatin (P) and etoposide (E) for limited-stage small cell lung cancer (LD-SCLC): the Japan Clinical Oncology Group (JCOG) study [abstract]. *Proc Am Soc Clin Oncol* 1999;18:A1805. Abstract 468a.

Greenlee RT, Hill-Harmon MB, Murray T, et al. Cancer statistics, 2001. *CA Cancer J Clin* 2001;51:15–36.

Hainsworth JD, Gray JR, Stroup SL, et al. Paclitaxel, carboplatin, and extended-schedule etoposide in the treatment of small-cell lung cancer: comparison of sequential phase II trials using different dose-intensities. *J Clin Oncol* 1997;15:3464–3470.

Janaki L, Rector D, Turrisi A, et al. Patterns of failure and second malignancies from SWOG-8629: concurrent cisplatin, etoposide, vincristine, and once daily radiotherapy for the treatment of limited small cell lung cancer [abstract]. *Proc Am Soc Clin Oncol* 1994;13:331.

Johnson RE, Brereton HD, Kent CH. Small-cell carcinoma of the lung: attempt to remedy causes of past therapeutic failure. *Lancet* 1976;2(7980):289–291.

Johnson BE, Bridges JD, Sobczeck M, et al. Patients with limited-stage small-cell lung cancer treated with concurrent twice-daily chest radiotherapy and etoposide/cisplatin followed by cyclophosphamide, doxorubicin, and vincristine. *J Clin Oncol* 1996;14:806–813.

Johnson BE, Salem C, Nesbitt J, et al. Limited stage small cell lung cancer treated with concurrent hyperfractionated chest radiotherapy and etoposide/cisplatin. *Lung Cancer* 1993;9(suppl 1):S21–S26.

Kies MS, Mira JG, Crowley JJ, et al. Multimodal therapy for limited small-cell lung cancer: a randomized study of induction combination chemotherapy with or without thoracic radiation in complete responders; and with wide-field versus reduced-field radiation in partial responders: a Southwest Oncology Group study. *J Clin Oncol* 1987;5:592–600.

Komaki R, Byhardt RW, Anderson T, et al. What is the lowest effective biologic dose for prophylactic cranial irradiation? *Am J Clin Oncol* 1985;8:523–527.

Komaki R, Cox JD, Whitson W. Risk of brain metastasis from small cell carcinoma of the lung related to length of survival and prophylactic irradiation. *Cancer Treatment Reports* 1981;65:811–814.

Komaki R, Meyers CA, Shin DM, et al. Evaluation of cognitive function in patients with limited small cell lung cancer prior to and shortly following prophylactic cranial irradiation. *Int J Radiat Oncol Biol Phys* 1995a;33:179–182.

Komaki R, Milas L, Glisson B, et al. Effect of duration of thoracic radiation therapy (TRT) on the outcome of patients with limited small cell lung cancer (LSCLC) treated with chemotherapy and radiation therapy [abstract]. Radiother Oncol 2000;56:S57.

Komaki R, Shin DM, Glisson BS, et al. Interdigitating versus concurrent chemotherapy and radiotherapy for limited small cell lung cancer. Int J Radiat Oncol Biol Phys 1995b;31:807–811.

Liengswangwong V, Bonner JA, Shaw EG, et al. Limited-stage small-cell lung cancer: patterns of intrathoracic recurrence and the implications for thoracic radiotherapy. J Clin Oncol 1994;12:496–502.

Looney WB. The experimental basis of new strategies in combining chemotherapy and radiotherapy. In: Horwich A, ed. Combined Radiotherapy and Chemotherapy in Clinical Oncology. London: Edward Arnold; 1992:23–33.

McCracken JD, Janaki LM, Crowley JJ, et al. Concurrent chemotherapy/radiotherapy for limited small-cell lung carcinoma: a Southwest Oncology Group study. J Clin Oncol 1990;8:892–898.

Murray N, Coy P, Pater JL, et al. Importance of timing for thoracic irradiation in the combined modality treatment of limited-stage small-cell lung cancer. The National Cancer Institute of Canada Clinical Trials Group. J Clin Oncol 1993;11:336–344.

National Comprehensive Cancer Network. Oncology Practice Guidelines. Small cell lung cancer. Oncology (suppl) 1996;10:179–194.

Noda K, Nishiwaki Y, Kawahara M, et al. Irinotecan plus cisplatin compared with etoposide plus cisplatin for extensive small-cell lung cancer. N Engl J Med 2002;346:85–91.

Nugent JL, Bunn PA Jr, Matthews MJ, et al. CNS metastases in small cell bronchogenic carcinoma: increasing frequency and changing pattern with lengthening survival. Cancer 1979;44:1885–1893.

Pieterman RM, van Putten JW, Meuzelaar JJ, et al. Preoperative staging of non–small-cell lung cancer with positron-emission tomography. N Engl J Med 2000;343:254–261.

Pignon JP, Arriagada R, Ihde DC, et al. A meta-analysis of thoracic radiotherapy for small-cell lung cancer. N Engl J Med 1992;327:1618–1624.

Shaw E, Su J, Eagan R, et al. Analysis of long-term survival and impact of prophylactic cranial irradiation in complete responders with small cell lung cancer: analysis of the Mayo Clinic and North Central Cancer Treatment Group data bases. Proc Am Soc Clin Oncol 1993;12:328.

Siu LL, Shepherd FA, Murray N, et al. Influence of age on the treatment of limited-stage small-cell lung cancer. J Clin Oncol 1996;14:821–828.

Stahel RA, Weber E. Small cell lung cancer: the new biology. Semin Radiat Oncol 1995;5:11–18.

Turrisi AT, Glover DJ, Mason B, et al. Long-term results of platinum, etoposide and twice daily thoracic radiotherapy for limited small cell lung cancer: results on 32 patients with 48 month minimum follow-up [abstract]. Proc Am Soc Clin Oncol 1992;11:292.

Turrisi AT III, Kim K, Blum R, et al. Twice-daily compared with once-daily thoracic radiotherapy in limited small-cell lung cancer treated concurrently with cisplatin and etoposide. N Engl J Med 1999;340:265–271.

Wagner H, Kim K, Johnson DH, et al. Daily vs. twice-daily thoracic irradiation with concurrent cisplatin/etoposide chemotherapy as initial therapy for patients with limited small cell lung cancer: preliminary results of a phase III prospective intergroup trial. *Int J Radiat Oncol Biol Phys* 1994;30(suppl 1):178.

Warde P, Payne D. Does thoracic irradiation improve survival and local control in limited-stage small-cell carcinoma of the lung? A meta-analysis. *J Clin Oncol* 1992;10:890–895.

11 CHEMOTHERAPY IN THE TREATMENT OF EXTENSIVE-STAGE SMALL CELL LUNG CANCER

George R. Blumenschein, Jr.

CHAPTER OVERVIEW

Chemotherapy is the primary treatment modality for patients with extensive-stage small cell lung cancer. In this group, chemotherapy has been shown to not only improve quality of life through palliation of symptoms but also improve median survival compared with the median survival of patients who are treated with best supportive care. Eligible patients should be offered treatment in clinical trials with chemotherapy-based regimens. Patients who are not eligible for a clinical trial should be offered etoposide and cisplatin given in 3-week cycles. Patients with extensive-stage small cell lung cancer that is refractory to first-line chemotherapy or recurs after an initial response to first-line chemotherapy have a poor prognosis. Treatment options for relapsed or progressive disease include re-induction therapy with first-line chemotherapy, clinical trials, and second-line chemotherapy agents. Maintenance therapy, alternating chemotherapy, and dose intensification of chemotherapy agents have not been proven to offer any survival benefit over standard chemotherapy regimens for patients with extensive-stage small cell lung cancer. Future studies in this patient population should focus on determining the optimum combinations of new chemotherapy drugs and identifying agents with novel mechanisms of action.

INTRODUCTION

Small cell lung cancer (SCLC) is the most aggressive of the lung cancer variants. It represents approximately 20% of all lung cancer cases. SCLC is the sixth most commonly diagnosed cancer in the United States and is the most rapidly increasing type of lung cancer diagnosis. Tobacco exposure, the primary risk factor for lung cancer, is more closely associated with SCLC than with any of the other histopathologic variants of lung cancer. It has been estimated that more than 98% of patients diagnosed with SCLC have a history of cigarette smoking.

STAGING AND INITIAL WORKUP

Because SCLC is such an aggressive, rapidly spreading cancer, the staging system for this disease has only 2 categories: limited-stage disease and extensive-stage disease. Limited-stage SCLC is defined as disease that can be encompassed within a tolerable radiation field. To be considered limited stage, SCLC must be contained within 1 hemithorax, the regional lymph nodes, the contralateral mediastinal lymph nodes, and the ipsilateral supraclavicular lymph nodes. Disease outside these borders is considered extensive-stage disease. Patients with pleural effusion are generally treated as having extensive-stage SCLC. Because of its aggressive nature, SCLC disseminates early; consequently, the majority of patients with SCLC present with extensive-stage disease. Of the 34,000 patients diagnosed with SCLC each year, 60% to 70% have extensive-stage disease at the time of diagnosis.

A complete initial staging evaluation for patients with SCLC should include a history and physical examination, chest radiography, computed tomography of the chest and upper abdomen, including the adrenal glands, a bone scan, magnetic resonance imaging of the brain, complete blood cell counts, and serum chemistry studies with liver function tests (Table 11–1).

Table 11–1. Recommended Staging Workup for Patients with SCLC

History and physical examination
Pathology review
Complete blood cell count, differential leukocyte count, and platelet count
Measurement of serum concentrations of sodium, potassium, glucose,
    creatinine, total bilirubin, alkaline phosphatase, lactate dehydrogenase,
    alanine aminotransferase, and calcium
Computed tomography of the chest and upper abdomen
Chest radiography
Electrocardiography if history of heart disease
Bone scan
Magnetic resonance imaging of the brain
Bone marrow biopsy
Echocardiography if patient scheduled to receive chemotherapy with doxorubicin

Prognostic Factors

The most important prognostic factor in patients with SCLC is the stage of disease at diagnosis. Without treatment, the median survival after diagnosis of extensive-stage SCLC is 6 to 8 weeks. The next most important prognostic factors are performance status and recent weight loss. Patients who are not ambulatory and patients who have lost at least 5% of body weight in the preceding 3 to 6 months have a worse prognosis than ambulatory patients and patients with less—or no—weight loss. Other indicators of prognosis include gender, findings on serum chemistry studies, and degree of dissemination of disease. Overall, female patients fare better than their male counterparts in terms of survival. Abnormalities in serum tests—the most common of which are elevated alkaline phosphatase and lactate dehydrogenase levels and low sodium levels—portend a poor outcome. Disease involvement of more than 1 organ site also has a negative impact on prognosis. This is especially true in the case of central nervous system or liver metastasis.

Common Presenting Symptoms

In patients with extensive-stage SCLC, the primary tumor is typically centrally located. This can lead to endobronchial obstruction with related symptoms, including cough, chest pain, postobstructive pneumonia, hemoptysis, and dyspnea. Superior vena cava syndrome can also be a presenting symptom. SCLC is also associated with a number of paraneoplastic syndromes caused by overproduction of polypeptide hormones. Approximately 10% of patients will have the syndrome of inappropriate secretion of antidiuretic hormone, and 2% will have ectopic Cushing's syndrome. Neurological paraneoplastic syndromes, such as Eaton-Lambert syndrome, can also occur.

CHEMOTHERAPY FOR PREVIOUSLY UNTREATED DISEASE

In patients with previously untreated extensive-stage SCLC, combination chemotherapy is the cornerstone of treatment because of the aggressive clinical course of this disease.

Development of the Current Approach to Treatment

Numerous chemotherapy agents have been shown to be effective in the treatment of SCLC. The chemosensitive nature of this disease was demonstrated in the late 1960s in a Veterans Administration Lung Cancer Study Group trial (Green et al, 1969). In this study, patients with extensive-stage SCLC were randomly assigned to receive 3 cycles of intravenous cyclophosphamide or best supportive care. The median survival time in the chemotherapy arm was approximately double that in the control arm. These results were in noticeable contrast to the responses seen with chemotherapy for non–small cell lung cancer and led to the hope that the response of SCLC to chemotherapy would mirror that of hematologic malignancies rather than solid tumors.

This initial success with cyclophosphamide has since been duplicated with many other single agents, including the platinum analogues (e.g., cisplatin and carboplatin), alkylating agents (e.g., ifosfamide and cyclophosphamide), anthracycline analogues (e.g., doxorubicin), vinca alkaloids (e.g., vinorelbine and vincristine), and epipodophyllotoxins (e.g., etoposide and teniposide). When administered as single-agent chemotherapy in patients with previously untreated SCLC, these drugs produce overall response rates greater than 30%. Etoposide and teniposide have demonstrated the best results, with response rates in excess of 80%. Over the last several years, a number of other promising agents have been evaluated in SCLC, including the taxanes (i.e., paclitaxel and docetaxel), topoisomerase I inhibitors (e.g., topotecan and irinotecan), and gemcitabine, an antimetabolite. In chemonaive patients with SCLC, these drugs have demonstrated response rates ranging from approximately 25% to 50%.

Following the discovery that SCLC is chemosensitive and the identification of several single agents that were effective against this disease, investigators began studying combination chemotherapy regimens in patients with SCLC. By the early 1980s, the combination of cyclophosphamide, doxorubicin, and vincristine (CAV) had been established as an effective regimen in patients with SCLC and had become a standard regimen in this patient group. Later, etoposide given as a single agent was found to have efficacy against SCLC, and etoposide was then evaluated in various multiagent regimens. The most effective regimen identified was the combination of etoposide with cisplatin (EP). EP was initially evaluated in SCLC because of preclinical evidence of synergy between the 2 drugs and was subsequently discovered to have efficacy in patients with refractory SCLC previously treated with CAV.

In the 1990s, 2 studies compared single-agent chemotherapy with combination chemotherapy in patients with untreated extensive-stage SCLC. In one trial, the Medical Research Council Working Party randomly assigned 339 patients with extensive-stage SCLC and poor performance status to 4 cycles of oral etoposide (171 patients) or a standard multiagent chemotherapy regimen—either intravenous CAV or intravenous etoposide with vincristine (168 patients) (Girling, 1996). This study was stopped early as an interim analysis revealed that response rates and median survival were better in the combination-chemotherapy arm. In the second study, patients with untreated extensive-stage SCLC and either poor performance status or age 75 years or older were randomly assigned to receive either six 3-week cycles of oral etoposide 100 mg twice daily for 5 days (75 patients) or a total of 6 cycles of oral EP alternating with CAV (80 patients) (Souhami et al, 1997). This trial was also stopped early, after an interim analysis confirmed that single-agent chemotherapy was inferior to combination chemotherapy as a first-line treatment. Significantly, both studies demonstrated that even in patients with poor performance status, combination chemotherapy was superior to single-agent chemotherapy.

Combination chemotherapy is now the primary treatment modality for previously untreated extensive-stage SCLC. This is due to both the shorter remission durations seen with single-agent therapy and the lack of complete responses achieved with single-agent therapy. In addition, the concurrent administration of multiple agents has proven to have greater efficacy than the sequential administration of the same drugs.

EP and CAV produce similar response rates and median survival times in patients with chemotherapy-naive extensive-stage SCLC, but EP has emerged as the favored treatment regimen because it has less cardiac, hematologic, and neurological toxicity. The use of EP as the preferred choice for first-line chemotherapy for extensive-stage SCLC has been further bolstered by the results of a recent meta-analysis of phase III trials (Chute et al, 1999). In a review of the past 20 years of phase III trials in extensive-stage SCLC, the authors found a median survival benefit for patients treated with platinum-based regimens versus non-platinum-based regimens. Patients treated with cisplatin-based regimens had a median survival of 9.5 months, versus 7.1 months for patients treated with non-platinum-based regimens ($P = .04$).

For patients with either poor performance status or renal, neurological, or auditory impairment, carboplatin can be substituted for cisplatin in the EP regimen. The use of carboplatin in place of cisplatin is associated with decreased mucosal, neurological, and renal toxicity but increased hematologic toxicity. Cisplatin and carboplatin have been compared in various randomized trials, and the results support the equivalent efficacy of these 2 drugs.

No single first-line chemotherapy regimen has been found to be best for all patients with previously untreated extensive-stage SCLC. CAV and EP are the 2 most commonly used regimens; as noted in the preceding paragraph, the combination of etoposide and carboplatin is also used, usually in patients with contraindications to the use of EP. The choice of regimen should be dictated by the patient's concomitant medical conditions. Recommended doses and schedules for these regimens are shown in Table 11–2.

Follow-up during Therapy

Patients with extensive-stage SCLC treated with chemotherapy should have chest radiography and serum chemistry studies prior to each cycle of chemotherapy. Every 6 weeks, patients should also have restaging scans with computed tomography of the chest. A suggested treatment pathway for extensive-stage SCLC is shown in Figure 11–1.

Outcomes

With combination chemotherapy, overall response rates in patients with previously untreated extensive-stage SCLC are approximately 80%. However, complete responses are observed in only 20% to 30% of patients, and the median survival time after the initiation of chemotherapy is 7 to 10 months. Ultimately, given the poor outcomes seen with current chemotherapy regimens, all eligible patients should be encouraged to participate in clinical trials of new chemotherapy regimens.

Duration of Therapy

Because SCLC is chemosensitive, it was common practice until the 1980s to treat patients with extensive-stage SCLC with repeated courses of chemotherapy until there was evidence of tumor progression or the patient developed severe side effects. This approach to therapy evolved over

Table 11–2. First-Line Chemotherapy Regimens for Extensive-Stage SCLC

Regimen	Component Drugs and Dosages*	Cycle Length
EP	Etoposide 100 mg/m² days 1–3 Cisplatin 60 mg/m² day 1	3 weeks
CAV	Cyclophosphamide 1 g/m² day 1 Doxorubicin (Adriamycin) 50 mg/m² day 1 Vincristine 1.4 mg/m² day 1	3 weeks
EC	Etoposide 100 mg/m² days 1–3 Carboplatin AUC 6 mg/mL/min day 1	3 weeks

AUC indicates area under the curve.
*All agents given intravenously.

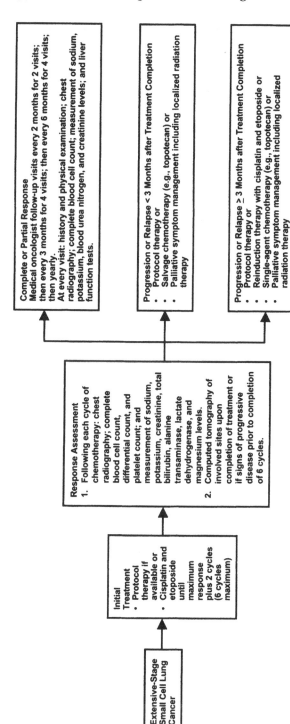

Figure 11–1.   Treatment guidelines for extensive-stage SCLC.

the years as further evaluation determined the optimum number of chemotherapy cycles. A number of randomized trials have been conducted to evaluate the benefit of either prolonged induction chemotherapy or maintenance therapy. These trials have produced conflicting results, with a modest increase in survival seen in some trials. However, a large European Organization for Research and Treatment of Cancer trial with 577 evaluable patients demonstrated no benefit. Prolonging the duration of first-line chemotherapy beyond 6 cycles has not been shown to improve survival and is not considered beneficial in the treatment of extensive-stage SCLC. Maintenance therapy (the utilization of an alternative chemotherapy regimen after achieving maximum benefit from first-line chemotherapy) has not been proven to prolong remission or survival. In addition, in the randomized trials, patients who were treated with either prolonged induction chemotherapy or maintenance chemotherapy had increased chemotherapy-related morbidity. In chemonaive extensive-stage SCLC, maximum responses to chemotherapy generally occur within the first 3 cycles of treatment. At this time, treatment beyond 6 cycles of chemotherapy is not recommended in patients with previously untreated extensive-stage SCLC.

Alternating Chemotherapy Regimens

Inspired by the Goldie-Coldman hypothesis, investigators have studied the use of alternating non-cross-resistant chemotherapy regimens in patients with chemotherapy-naive extensive-stage SCLC. In the 1980s, Goldie and Coldman theorized that the rapid alternation of non-cross-resistant chemotherapy regimens could improve the tumor cell kill rate. Various alternating-chemotherapy regimens have been studied over the years, with mixed results.

Several phase III trials investigated alternation of the 2 primary regimens used to treat extensive-stage SCLC, CAV and EP. A Canadian study done in the late 1980s had a positive outcome, with survival data favoring CAV alternated with EP over the CAV-alone arm (Evans et al, 1987). This study included 289 patients with extensive-stage SCLC who received either CAV every 3 weeks for 6 cycles or CAV alternated with EP every 3 weeks for a total of 6 cycles. The median survival times were 8 months for CAV alone and 9.6 months for the alternating regimen ($P = .03$). The Southeastern Cancer Study Group then randomly assigned patients with extensive-stage SCLC to one of 3 regimens: 6 cycles of CAV, 4 cycles of EP, or alternating CAV with EP (3 cycles each) (Roth et al, 1992). This was a large study with 437 evaluable patients. No significant differences were found between the treatment arms in terms of median survival (range, 8.1–8.6 months), response rate, or complete response rate. A similar result was obtained in a randomized study in which 288 patients with either extensive-stage SCLC or limited-stage SCLC were also treated with CAV, EP, or alternating CAV and EP (Fukuoka et al, 1991). Although a survival benefit for alternating chemotherapy was seen in patients with limited-stage SCLC, no survival benefit was seen in patients with extensive-stage SCLC, with the median survival ranging from 8 to 9 months (Fukuoka et al, 1991).

A review of the published phase III trials that have explored alternating chemotherapy regimens in extensive-stage SCLC does not clearly demonstrate a benefit in terms of survival or response for alternating chemotherapy versus a single combination-chemotherapy regimen. In addition, when patients are treated with more than a single chemotherapy regimen at a time, there is a risk of increased side effects due to overlapping drug toxicity. Increased side effects can not only result in increased morbidity but also necessitate dose reductions, which can lead to the delivery of subtherapeutic doses of chemotherapy.

Dose Intensification of Chemotherapy

Because of the responsiveness of extensive-stage SCLC to chemotherapy, the strategy of increasing the dose intensity of chemotherapy in an effort to improve patient outcomes has been studied. Multiple agents and regimens have been evaluated at length, but whether dose intensification is beneficial remains unresolved. A meta-analysis of 60 published studies that examined the question of dose intensity in SCLC failed to show an obvious benefit with respect to survival and response rates (Klasa et al, 1991). A more recent study investigated the benefit of dose intensification of the EP regimen. In this study, 90 patients with extensive-stage SCLC were randomly assigned to treatment with either standard-dose EP or high-dose EP for 2 cycles; all patients then received 2 cycles of standard-dose EP. Standard-dose EP consisted of a 3-week cycle of 80 mg/m^2 etoposide on days 1 through 3 and 80 mg/m^2 cisplatin on day 1. High-dose EP consisted of 80 mg/m^2 etoposide on days 1 through 5 and 27 mg/m^2 cisplatin on days 1 through 5. No survival benefit was observed for high-dose treatment (median survival, 11.4 months and 10.7 months, respectively, for the high-dose and standard-dose arms), but high-dose treatment was associated with an increase in overall side effects (Ihde et al, 1994).

High-dose chemotherapy combined with autologous bone marrow transplantation also has not been shown to confer a survival benefit in patients with extensive-stage SCLC. Identification of new agents that are effective against extensive-stage SCLC and the resulting new regimens may offer more promising results. However, at this time, dose intensification of chemotherapy for previously untreated extensive-stage SCLC remains investigational.

CHEMOTHERAPY FOR REFRACTORY OR RECURRENT DISEASE

Patients with SCLC that fails to respond to first-line chemotherapy or recurs after first-line chemotherapy have a poor prognosis. Recurrent SCLC is characteristically aggressive and can disseminate quickly. The median survival in this patient population is 2 to 3 months.

The results achieved with second-line therapy correlate with the length of the relapse-free interval. The most important predictors of response to second-line therapy are the degree of response to prior chemotherapy and the duration of that response. Patients can be categorized as having disease that is refractory or sensitive to chemotherapy on the basis of the duration of their relapse-free interval. Patients whose tumor never responds to first-line chemotherapy and patients who have a relapse-free interval of 3 months or less after completion of initial chemotherapy are considered to have refractory disease. Patients who have a relapse-free interval of greater than 3 months after first-line chemotherapy are considered to have sensitive disease. Patients with refractory disease have lower response rates to second-line chemotherapy than do patients with sensitive disease.

There is no established second-line chemotherapy regimen for SCLC. Patients can be treated with an alternative first-line therapy, but the results with this approach vary. CAV is somewhat active in patients who have a relapse after first-line EP, producing response rates of approximately 18%. EP, on the other hand, has generated much better results in patients whose tumor was refractory to or relapsed after first-line CAV, producing response rates of greater than 50% (Evans et al, 1985). Generally, for patients who have not yet received a platinum-based regimen, EP should be considered as a salvage regimen for relapsed SCLC. Otherwise, the choice of chemotherapy regimen should be based on the duration of the patient's relapse-free interval. Patients with a relapse occurring more than 3 months after completion of first-line chemotherapy should be considered for re-induction therapy with EP. Alternatively, these patients can be treated with a single agent, such as topotecan, if their comorbid conditions preclude the use of EP. A recent phase III study comparing topotecan with CAV in patients with recurrent SCLC (von Pawel et al, 1999) demonstrated that topotecan was equivalent to CAV in terms of efficacy and resulted in better palliation of symptoms. Patients whose disease never responds to first-line chemotherapy or recurs 3 months or less after completion of first-line chemotherapy should be treated with a single agent—for example, topotecan, irinotecan, or a taxane (see Table 11–3 for suggested doses and schedules). Given the

Table 11–3. Second-Line Chemotherapy Agents for SCLC Refractory to or Recurrent after First-Line Chemotherapy

Agent	Dosage	Cycle Length
Topotecan	1.25 mg/m^2 days 1–5	3 weeks
Paclitaxel	175 mg/m^2 day 1	3 weeks
Docetaxel	75 mg/m^2 day 1	3 weeks
Irinotecan	90 mg/m^2 weekly x 2	3 weeks

KEY PRACTICE POINTS

- In patients with previously untreated extensive-stage SCLC, first-line therapy should consist of combination chemotherapy. The use of etoposide with either cisplatin or carboplatin appears to offer the best toxicity profile and produces response rates and median survival durations similar to those achieved with other regimens.
- Combination chemotherapy is superior to single-agent chemotherapy in previously untreated patients.
- Patients should be treated until best response is seen and then given an additional 2 cycles to a maximum of 6 total cycles of chemotherapy.
- Maintenance chemotherapy, alternating chemotherapy, and dose-intense and high-dose chemotherapy have no role in the treatment of extensive-stage SCLC.
- There is no established regimen for patients with SCLC refractory to or recurrent after first-line chemotherapy. Depending on the length of the relapse-free interval, these patients should be offered therapy with either a topoisomerase I inhibitor, a taxane, an investigational agent in a clinical trial, or a combination of etoposide with a platinum analogue.
- Radiation therapy can be used for palliation of localized symptoms.

---

poor outcomes achieved with second-line chemotherapy, all eligible patients with refractory or recurrent SCLC should be offered the option of treatment within clinical trials.

PALLIATION OF SYMPTOMS

Palliation of symptoms is an important aspect of care in patients with extensive-stage SCLC. Oxygen, pain medication, and other supportive care measures can help to improve patients' quality of life. One of the most useful tools in palliative care is radiation therapy. In appropriate patients, radiation therapy can be utilized to ameliorate localized complaints, including symptomatic central nervous system metastases, bony metastases, and thoracic lesions. Palliation of symptoms is covered in detail in chapter 12.

FUTURE DIRECTIONS

There has been a marginal improvement in the survival of patients with extensive-stage SCLC over the past decade, but current results with established regimens remain unsatisfactory. New systemic therapies—not only new cytotoxic compounds but also biological agents—are needed. With improvement in the understanding of the biology of SCLC, better systemic therapy may become a reality.

SUGGESTED READINGS

Chute JP, Chen T, Feigal E, et al. Twenty years of phase III trials for patients with extensive-stage small-cell lung cancer: perceptible progress. *J Clin Oncol* 1999;17:1794–1801.

Clark R, Ihde DC. Small-cell lung cancer: treatment progress and prospects. *Oncology (Huntingt)* 1998;12:647–658; discussion 661–663.

De Vore RFI, Johnson DH. Chemotherapy for small cell lung cancer. In: Pass HI, Mitchell JB, Johnson DH, Turrisi AT, et al, eds. *Lung Cancer: Principles and Practice.* 2nd ed. Philadelphia, Pa: Lippincott Williams & Wilkins; 2000:923–939.

Elias A. Hematopoietic stem cell transplantation for small cell lung cancer. *Chest* 1999;116(suppl 6):531S–538S.

Evans WK, Feld R, Murray N, et al. Superiority of alternating non-cross-resistant chemotherapy in extensive small cell lung cancer. A multicenter, randomized clinical trial by the National Cancer Institute of Canada. *Ann Intern Med* 1987;107:451–458.

Evans WK, Osaba D, Feld R, et al. Etoposide (VP-16) and cisplatin: an effective treatment for relapse in small-cell lung cancer. *J Clin Oncol* 1985;3:65–71.

Fukuoka M, Furuse K, Saijo N, et al. Randomized trial of cyclophosphamide, doxorubicin, and vincristine versus cisplatin and etoposide versus alternation of these regimens in small-cell lung cancer. *J Natl Cancer Inst* 1991;83:855–861.

Girling DJ. Comparison of oral etoposide and standard intravenous multidrug chemotherapy for small-cell lung cancer: a stopped multicentre randomised trial. Medical Research Council Lung Cancer Working Party. *Lancet* 1996;348:563–566.

Green RA, Humphrey E, Close H, et al. Alkylating agents in bronchogenic carcinoma. *Am J Med* 1969;46:516–525.

Huisman C, Postmus PE, Giaccone G, et al. Second-line chemotherapy and its evaluation in small cell lung cancer. *Cancer Treat Rev* 1999;25:199–206.

Ihde DC. Chemotherapy of lung cancer. *N Engl J Med* 1992;327:1434–1441.

Ihde DC, Mulshine JL, Kramer BS, et al. Prospective randomized comparison of high-dose and standard-dose etoposide and cisplatin chemotherapy in patients with extensive-stage small-cell lung cancer. *J Clin Oncol* 1994;12:2022–2034.

Johnson DH. Management of small cell lung cancer: current state of the art. *Chest* 1999;116(suppl 6):525S–530S.

Kelly K. New chemotherapy agents for small cell lung cancer. *Chest* 2000;117(4 suppl 1):156S–162S.

Klasa RJ, Murray N, Coldman AJ. Dose-intensity meta-analysis of chemotherapy regimens in small-cell carcinoma of the lung. *J Clin Oncol* 1991;9:499–508.

Murren J, Glatstein E, Pass HI. Small cell lung cancer. In: De Vita VT Jr, Hellman S, Rosenberg SA, eds. *Cancer: Principles and Practice of Oncology.* 6th ed. Philadelphia, Pa: Lippincott Williams & Wilkins; 2001:983–1018.

Roth BJ, Johnson DH, Einhorn LH, et al. Randomized study of cyclophosphamide, doxorubicin, and vincristine versus etoposide and cisplatin versus alternation of these two regimens in extensive small-cell lung cancer: a phase III trial of the Southeastern Cancer Study Group. *J Clin Oncol* 1992;10:282–291.

Sandler AB. Current management of small cell lung cancer. *Semin Oncol* 1997;24:463–476.

Schiller JH, Adak S, Cella D, et al. Topotecan versus observation after cisplatin plus etoposide in extensive-stage small-cell lung cancer: E7593—a phase III trial of the Eastern Cooperative Oncology Group. *J Clin Oncol* 2001;19:2114–2122.

Souhami RL, Spiro SG, Rudd RM, et al. Five-day oral etoposide treatment for advanced small-cell lung cancer: randomized comparison with intravenous chemotherapy. *J Natl Cancer Inst* 1997;89:577–580.

von Pawel J, Schiller JH, Shepherd FA, et al. Topotecan versus cyclophosphamide, doxorubicin, and vincristine for the treatment of recurrent small-cell lung cancer. *J Clin Oncol* 1999;17:658–667.

12 PALLIATIVE CARE IN PATIENTS WITH LUNG CANCER

Joe B. Putnam, Jr.

CHAPTER OVERVIEW

Palliation of symptoms may be required at any point in a lung cancer patient's care. Moving from "therapy-oriented care" to "comfort-oriented care" poses special challenges to the physician and the health care team: they must attempt to optimize the function of each individual patient and to communicate the care plan to the patient's family and friends. Relief of dyspnea and pain are of critical importance to the patient's welfare. Appropriate nutrition and relief of other symptoms are also important components of the patient's care. The challenge to the individual physician is to consider all the options available for the patient's comfort and then to select the best options with the patient and the family.

INTRODUCTION

Lung cancer will affect an estimated 169,500 men and women in the United States in 2001 and will be the cause of death of 157,400. Only about 15% of patients with lung cancer can be treated with curative intent with local modalities (surgery and radiation therapy) alone. Approximately 25% to 35% of patients are diagnosed with metastatic disease, for which primary therapy includes combinations of chemotherapy, radiation therapy, and other therapies in an attempt to treat and palliate the systemic manifestations of the disease and to improve survival. A third group of patients have advanced-stage lung cancer localized to the hemithorax, for which combinations of chemotherapy, surgery, and radiation therapy may be considered.

The optimal treatment of lung cancer is an area of intense investigation among numerous physicians from many specialties. However, despite the best efforts of physicians, nurses, family members, and patients, few patients diagnosed with lung cancer experience long-term survival. In patients with advanced-stage or metastatic disease, initial strategies include therapy that aims to enhance local and systemic control and improve survival. When therapy directed at improving control and prolonging survival no longer represents an optimal treatment plan for an individual patient, alternatives must be considered. These alternatives may be described as comfort-oriented care, or palliative care. In patients treated with palliative intent, therapeutic interventions are directed toward palliation of symptoms. Physicians and nurses continue to provide medical care, and the patient is not abandoned.

The purpose of this chapter is to describe the evaluation and treatment of patients with lung cancer receiving comfort-oriented care. Using a patient-centered approach, the chapter will describe methods of palliation of specific symptoms.

PATIENT EVALUATION

At M. D. Anderson Cancer Center, patients with lung cancer have their performance status assessed at initial evaluation. Performance status is evaluated to assist in determining the patient's individual fitness for therapy. Patients with poor performance status may be more likely to be offered palliative therapy. Changes in performance status may suggest a transition from therapy-oriented care to comfort-oriented care. Several performance scales are available for grading the overall physical status of patients with lung cancer. Performance scales are useful because they define in a broad but reproducible manner the patient's activities and functional limitations and provide an indirect measure of general health status at a specific point in time. Commonly used performance scales include the modified Zubrod performance scale (Zubrod et al, 1960), which is used by the Eastern Cooperative Oncology Group to measure the performance of patients enrolled in its clinical trials (Oken et al, 1982), the Karnofsky performance scale (Karnofsky, 1961), the European Organization for Research and Treatment of Cancer Quality of Life Questionnaire (EORTC QLQ-C30) (Hollen and Gralla, 1996) and its lung cancer module (EORTC QLQ-LC13) (Langendijk et al, 2000), the Functional Assessment of Cancer Therapy—Lung quality of life instrument, and the Lung Cancer Symptom Scale (Cella et al, 1995; Hollen and Gralla, 1996). The Zubrod and Karnofsky scales are shown in Table 12–1. Other performance scales, such as the Medical Outcomes Study Short Form Survey (SF-36), may be used as measures of general health. In the M. D. Anderson Thoracic Center, physicians most often use the Zubrod and Karnofsky performance scales.

Patients treated in the context of clinical trials may have specific performance measures assessed at every outpatient visit. At M. D. Anderson, the Zubrod or Karnofsky performance status and pain status are measured at each visit.

After primary (or additional) therapy has been completed, patients are screened for symptoms. In the M. D. Anderson Thoracic Center, we screen all patients for symptoms before treatment and at each postoperative visit. The symptoms screened for are listed in Tables 12–2 and 12–3. Special attention is paid to weight loss, pain, and dyspnea.

Table 12–1.   Performance Status Scales/Scores

ECOG or Zubrod Scale		Karnofsky Score
0	Asymptomatic and fully active	100%
1	Symptomatic; fully ambulatory; restricted in physically strenuous activity	80%–90%
2	Symptomatic; ambulatory; capable of self-care; more than 50% of waking hours are spent out of bed	60%–70%
3	Symptomatic; limited self-care; spends more than 50% of time in bed, but not bedridden	40%–50%
4	Completely disabled; no self-care; bedridden	20%–30%

ECOG indicates Eastern Cooperative Oncology Group.

Table 12–2.   Preoperative Symptoms Measured in the Thoracic Center

Zubrod performance score	Pain
Anorexia	Degree of pain
Bone pain or symptoms	Mild / moderate / severe
Cough	Pneumonia
Diarrhea	Pneumothorax
Degree of diarrhea	Gastroesophageal reflux
Mild / moderate / severe	Degree of reflux
Dysphagia	Mild / moderate / severe
Degree of dysphagia	Shortness of breath / dyspnea
Mild / moderate / severe	Degree of dyspnea
Fatigue	Mild / moderate / severe
Fever	Other
Hemoptysis	Symptom duration (of longest-lasting
Hoarseness	symptom)
Horner's syndrome	
Myasthenia	
Neurological symptoms	

Table 12–3.   Postoperative Symptoms Measured in the Thoracic Center

Zubrod performance score	Incisional pain
Bone pain or symptoms	Degree of incisional pain
Cough	Mild / moderate / severe
Diarrhea	Neurological symptoms
Degree of diarrhea	Gastroesophageal reflux
Mild / moderate / severe	Degree of reflux
Dysphagia	Mild / moderate / severe
Degree of dysphagia	Shortness of breath / dyspnea
Mild / moderate / severe	Degree of dyspnea
Fatigue	Mild / moderate / severe
Fever	Other
Hemoptysis	
Hoarseness	

Symptoms and Palliative Treatment Approaches

Constitutional Symptoms

The majority of patients with lung cancer develop fatigue, general malaise, anorexia, and weight loss during or after therapy. In many cases, these symptoms are not specific indicators of a particular systemic or organ-specific problem but rather constitutional symptoms due to a combination of the patient's individual health, the tumor burden, sequelae of therapy, and the patient's nutritional status.

Modification of social habits (such as alcohol use) and addictions (such as tobacco addiction) and efforts to ensure proper hydration and nutrition—including calorie counts and use of nutritional supplements and vitamins—may ameliorate constitutional symptoms and improve the patient's sense of well-being. In patients treated with chemotherapy or radiation therapy, special efforts should be made to attenuate treatment-specific side effects (see chapter 13) to enhance the patient's sense of well-being.

Symptoms Due to Brain Metastases

The majority of patients with lung cancer have locally advanced disease or metastases at diagnosis. Brain metastases may present with seizures, and bone metastases may present with pain.

Brain metastases—even metastases involving the dura—can be successfully resected, and resection of brain metastases can result in significantly improved quality of life (Rumana et al, 1998) and survival. Survival in patients with brain metastases as the only site of distant spread may be better than survival in patients with unresectable or more diffuse metastatic disease.

In patients with lung cancer who have brain metastases at the time of diagnosis of their disease, the brain metastases are frequently resected before the primary lung tumor is treated. In this situation, recommended treatment for the primary tumor would be resection in patients with clinical stage I or II disease or concurrent chemotherapy and radiation therapy in patients with clinical stage III or IV disease (Bonnette et al, 2001).

In patients with lung cancer who develop brain metastases after the completion of definitive therapy for their primary tumor, resection of the brain metastases is recommended whenever possible in physiologically fit individuals.

Radiation therapy for brain metastases can also produce excellent results. Good symptom relief and improved function can be expected with this approach.

Depression

More insidious than physical symptoms of lung cancer, but perhaps more devastating for patients with lung cancer, is depression. Depression during end-of-life care may be variable and can be difficult to treat to the patient's or family's satisfaction. Pharmacologic and psychiatric therapy may be of great value in patients with depression and their families.

Pain

A complete discussion of the numerous options available for pain relief in patients with lung cancer is beyond the scope of this chapter. Good sources of detailed information on this topic include the National Comprehensive Cancer Network Practice Guidelines for Cancer Pain (Benedetti et al, 2000), which offer a detailed algorithm for treatment of cancer-related pain, and the Web site of M. D. Anderson's Pain Research Group, which lists several excellent resources (Pain Research Group, 2002).

Oral medications with short-acting and long-acting opioids can produce excellent results in patients with lung cancer–related pain. Although some individual practitioners have concerns about patients becoming addicted to or overusing medications, patients rarely develop addiction problems related to narcotics. More commonly, physicians fail to prescribe sufficient pain medication for patients during end-of-life care.

At M.D. Anderson, an acute pain management service and a chronic pain management service, both under the direction of the Department of Anesthesiology, provide excellent pain management services for patients who have undergone pulmonary resection, for patients undergoing pain evaluation, and for patients with bony metastases or other metastatic disease that causes pain.

Patients' pain is evaluated frequently (every time vital signs are measured), and patients and families are advised to bring any pain problems to the attention of physicians and nurses. The pain management services work closely with the patient, the physicians and nurses on the primary service treating the patient, and the patient's family to develop an effective pain-management plan. The plan is monitored and modified as needed to enhance pain control. Because depression often exacerbates pain, the pain management services often prescribe a combination of narcotics and antidepressants.

In patients with painful bone or vertebral metastases, external-beam radiation therapy, systemic radiopharmaceuticals, chemotherapy, or hormonal therapy can bring about good attenuation of pain (Janjan, 2001). Current external-beam techniques and conformal radiation therapy techniques allow for high doses to be delivered to the tumor or the symptomatic metastasis with minimal injury to adjacent normal structures (e.g., the heart, esophagus, normal lung, or spinal cord) (Stevens et al, 2000). Radiation therapy is not required in every case of an observed primary tumor or metastasis; rather, radiation therapy should be reserved for cases in which it is expected to improve tumor- or metastasis-related symptoms.

Symptoms of Advanced-Stage Lung Cancer

Symptoms of Superior Sulcus Tumors

Superior sulcus tumors (lung cancers arising from the apex of the lung) account for approximately 3% of non–small cell lung cancers. In patients with superior sulcus tumors, surgery to improve function and relieve pain should always be considered. Growth of superior sulcus tumors leads to progression of symptoms, and if the tumor is inadequately or incompletely treated, it may encase the brachial plexus, resulting in a "flail" extremity without function. A forequarter amputation may be required for control of the tumor and relief of pain.

In a retrospective review of 143 patients with superior sulcus tumors treated at M.D. Anderson (Komaki et al, 2000), overall 5-year survival rates were 47% for patients with stage IIB disease, 14% for patients with stage IIIA disease, and 16% for patients with stage IIIB disease. Patients with R2 resections (incomplete resection) who received 55 to 64 Gy as postoperative radiation therapy had a 5-year survival rate of 82%, compared to 56% in patients who received 50 to 54 Gy.

Tumors involving the superior sulcus are frequently treated inadequately and inconsistently with 30 Gy of external-beam radiation to the primary tumor prior to resection. No prospective trial has proven the benefit of this approach over surgery alone, and the use of radiation therapy before surgery has several theoretical disadvantages. First, if primary radiation therapy is inadequate, accelerated repopulation may occur. Second, if negative margins are not achieved, the chance for optimal local control is lost. Third, resection of tumors abutting or invading the brachial plexus after radiation therapy can be challenging. Finally, definitive postresection radiation therapy can be performed in a more consistent and complete manner than can preoperative radiation therapy.

The treatment of patients with superior sulcus tumors should involve a multidisciplinary approach, with patients evaluated by a medical oncologist, a radiation oncologist, and a thoracic surgeon. This approach optimizes the definition of the extent and stage of the tumor and optimizes decisions regarding whether preoperative or postoperative therapy or alternatives to surgery (e.g., definitive chemotherapy and radiation therapy) should be considered.

At M.D. Anderson, patients with superior sulcus tumors are treated initially with surgery. After pathological evaluation and final staging, postoperative radiation therapy is used for any microscopic residual disease. The dose of radiation therapy may exceed 60 Gy. The benefits of radiation therapy given in this manner are improved local control of the tumor and the use of each therapeutic modality (surgery and radiation therapy) in an optimal fashion.

In 1999, investigators at M.D. Anderson published results of a study showing that superior sulcus tumors with vertebral invasion can be treated successfully with surgery (Gandhi et al, 1999). Most of the 17 patients in the study received postoperative external-beam radiation therapy. No perioperative deaths occurred, and the 2-year actuarial survival rate was 54%. Patients with a superior sulcus tumor that invades the vertebral column (stage IIIB disease) can undergo resection with a combined approach including posterior-lateral thoracotomy, lobectomy with en bloc chest wall resection, laminectomy, vertebrectomy, anterior spinal column reconstruction with methylmethacrylate, and spinal instrumentation (York et al, 1999). An additional study examined the outcomes of preoperative chemotherapy and radiation therapy followed by resection for clinical T3 and T4 superior sulcus tumors (Rusch et al, 2000). Five-year survival rates were 46% for stage IIB disease, 0% for stage IIIA disease, and 13% for stage IIIB disease. Treatment of disease that has metastasized to the spine has also been accomplished with resection and reconstruction with good results (Gokaslan et al, 1998).

Lung-Sparing Surgery to Prevent Dyspnea

In patients with advanced lung cancer, complex operations designed to spare uninvolved lung parenchyma and thereby prevent dyspnea may be considered. These techniques include bronchial sleeve resection, bronchoplasty, pulmonary artery sleeve resection, pulmonary arterioplasty, and tracheal resection. These techniques are infrequently required; however, they may be critical in patients predicted to have marginal pulmonary reserve after surgery.

Bronchial sleeve resection with or without pulmonary artery resection and reconstruction can be accomplished with excellent results and good long-term survival. Morbidity, mortality, and functional data suggest that such reconstructions are comparable to lobectomy in terms of pulmonary function (Rendina et al, 1999, 2000). The 5-year survival rate in studies of this approach was 18.6% for patients with disease designated stage IIIA or IIIB.

Tracheal resection and reconstruction for airway obstruction is also infrequently performed. More commonly, for tracheal or bronchial tumors causing obstruction, surgeons use palliative techniques of external-beam radiation therapy and internal radiation therapy (brachytherapy) supplemented with laser ablation—or even mechanical fulguration—or placement of expandable metal stents (covered or noncovered) (see the section Intraluminal Tumor later in this chapter). Patients with isolated primary tracheal tumors, such as adenoid cystic carcinomas or squamous cell carcinomas, have good results after complete resection. Postoperative radiation therapy is generally considered in these cases (Mathisen, 1999; Mitchell et al, 1999). Consistent success requires excellent surgical technique and meticulous attention to detail. Gentle handling of tissue, avoidance of disruption of the tracheal blood supply, anastomosis under no tension, and complete resection of the neoplasm with negative margins are necessary.

Pulmonary or Respiratory Insufficiency

Problems related to pulmonary or respiratory insufficiency predominate at all stages of the care of lung cancer patients. Cigarette smoking, a terrible addiction, is the most prevalent cause of lung cancer and associated pulmonary diseases. Patients with lung cancer frequently present with impaired pulmonary function due to smoking. In addition, lung cancer treatment can cause pulmonary or respiratory insufficiency: surgical removal of lung tissue and radiation-induced damage of lung tissue can impair ventilation, perfusion, or both. Finally, the tumor itself can cause pulmonary or respiratory problems.

Dyspnea

The management of dyspnea must be directed toward its source. Causes of dyspnea include chronic obstructive pulmonary disease, recurrent pleural effusion, and airway obstruction secondary to intrinsic or extrinsic compression. Primary treatment directed toward local control of these entities may include surgery, chemotherapy, radiation therapy, or combinations of these therapies.

Dyspnea due to chronic obstructive pulmonary disease can be palliated with careful medical management; specific attention to lung resection techniques, including lung-sparing surgery; or the use of 3-dimensional conformal radiation therapy in lieu of standard external-beam radiation therapy. These approaches increase the likelihood of local control at the same time as they relieve dyspnea. Limitations of lung-sparing surgery (wedge resection, or segmentectomy), or lung-sparing radiation therapy (3-dimensional conformal therapy) may include a greater likelihood of recurrence and the need for additional therapy in the future.

The preoperative or pretreatment evaluation of patients with impaired pulmonary function can include (in addition to the routine history and physical examination) radiographic studies and pulmonary function testing, such as complete spirometry, measurement of the diffusing capacity of the lung for carbon monoxide, xenon ventilation perfusion lung scanning, and oxygen consumption testing. These studies can be considered in patients who have undergone resection or treatment for metastatic disease.

Malignant Pleural Effusions

Malignant pleural effusions frequently cause dyspnea and loss of function. Pleural fluid accumulated in the chest may be treated symptomatically with simple drainage by thoracentesis. However, many patients have recurrent effusions. In these patients, treatment options are much more varied.

Treatment for patients with initial or recurrent malignant pleural effusions should focus on relief of symptoms of dyspnea and restoration of normal activity (Antony et al, 2000). The traditional practice of arbitrarily requiring pleurodesis (obliteration of the pleural space), achieved by in-hospital drainage with chemical or other agents, may subject the patient to a prolonged hospitalization or other interventions that may significantly reduce quality of life and remaining survival time outside the hospital. At M.D. Anderson, our standard approach is to manage malignant pleural effusions on an outpatient basis.

Etiology. Numerous benign, infectious, and malignant causes can lead to recurrent pleural effusions (Light, 1999, 2000). Patients with cancer frequently develop recurrent malignant pleural effusions secondary to their disease. The cancers most often associated with malignant pleural effusions are non–small cell lung cancer, breast cancer, lymphoma, and ovarian cancer. Increased levels of vascular endothelial growth factor are present in malignant pleural effusions (Zebrowski et al, 1999). In 25% of patients with cancer, malignant cells in the effusion may not be identified by pathologic examination.

Prognosis. Median life expectancy in cancer patients with malignant pleural effusions ranges from 3 to 9 months depending upon the histologic subtype of the primary tumor (Sanchez-Armengol and Rodriguez-Panadero, 1993). In one prospective randomized study, the median survival time for all patients with malignant pleural effusions was 90 days (Putnam et al, 1999).

Therapy. Treatment options for malignant pleural effusion include thoracentesis or repeat thoracentesis; tube thoracostomy, drainage, and sclerotherapy using talc, bleomycin, or other material (Patz et al, 1998); placement of a chronic indwelling pleural catheter (Pleurx Pleural Catheter; Denver Biomedical, Inc., Golden, Colo); placement of a pleuroperitoneal shunt; and thoracoscopy with drainage and talc insufflation.

In the past, successful treatment of malignant pleural effusions required hospitalization for chest tube drainage, sclerosis, and, hopefully, pleurodesis, followed by removal of the drainage catheters. If pleurodesis could not be achieved, the treatment was designated as "failed," and the patient was then treated with the best available means. In contrast, today's "patient-centered" treatment focuses on relief of the patient's symptoms and restoration of normal function. Pleurodesis is not required to accomplish these goals.

Sclerotherapy. Many agents have been used with success in sclerotherapy for malignant pleural effusions. The most commonly used agent, talc (de Campos et al, 2001), may be insufflated during thoracoscopy or applied as a slurry during closed chest tube drainage. In one prospective study (Olak and Desler, 1993), 501 patients with pleural effusions were randomly assigned to treatment with 4 to 5 grams of talc delivered through a chest tube (234 patients) or video-assisted thoracic surgery (VATS) with drainage of the effusion and talc insufflation (235 patients). Multiple confounding problems occurred in each group, including death prior to 30 days after treatment (13% of patients in the chest tube group; 9.4% of patients in the VATS group), failure to administer talc, inability to re-expand the lung to more than 90% of the intrathoracic (hemithorax) volume, and lack of follow-up data. In evaluable patients who survived at least 30 days after completion of treatment, the rate of freedom from recurrent effusions at 30 days was the same in both groups (70% [82 of 117 patients] in the chest tube group and 79% [103 of 131 patients] in the VATS group).

Small-bore catheter drainage with bleomycin or talc sclerotherapy has also been performed with success (Belani et al, 1998; Marom et al, 1999; Parulekar et al, 2001).

Chronic Indwelling Pleural Catheter.   Between 1994 and 1999, a prospective randomized trial was conducted at M. D. Anderson and 10 other centers to compare the effectiveness and safety of an indwelling pleural catheter (Pleurx) (Figure 12–1) with the effectiveness and safety of a chest tube and doxycycline sclerosis for treatment of cancer patients with symptomatic recurrent malignant pleural effusions (Putnam et al, 1999). The potential benefits of catheter-based treatment were outpatient management, improved quality of life, reduced medical costs, and improved function.

A total of 144 patients were randomly assigned to either an indwelling pleural catheter or a chest tube and doxycycline sclerosis. (Talc was not available at all centers at the time of the study.) For every 2 patients treated with a pleural catheter, 1 patient was stratified to treatment with a chest tube and doxycycline sclerosis. Chest tubes were placed with a simple surgical procedure (Figure 12–2). A modified Borg scale for dyspnea, the dyspnea component of the Guyatt chronic respiratory questionnaire, and Karnofsky performance status score were used to compare the 2 groups. Outcomes measured included control of pleural effusion, length of hospitalization, morbidity, and survival.

There was no difference between the 2 groups in performance status or initial dyspnea scores. Median survival was 90 days in both the chest tube and pleural catheter groups. Patients with lung or breast cancer had a 90-day survival rate of approximately 70%; patients with other cancer types (as a group) had a 90-day survival rate of less than 40%. After treatment, both the chest tube and pleural catheter groups showed similar significant improvements in the Guyatt chronic respiratory questionnaire scores and had similar morbidity. There were no treatment-related deaths.

Initial treatment success (pleurodesis achieved in the chest tube group; drainage of effusion and relief of dyspnea in the pleural catheter group) was achieved in 64% of the patients treated with a chest tube and sclerosis, compared to 92% of those treated with a chronic indwelling catheter. Seventy percent of patients treated with a pleural catheter experienced spontaneous pleurodesis. Seventy-one percent of patients with a chest tube had pleurodesis, although 28% of these patients developed a recurrence of their pleural effusion after treatment. The mean time of hospitalization was shorter in the pleural catheter patients: 1 day versus 6.5 days.

The Pleurx catheter is ideal for patients with "trapped lung" and for patients with a chronically recurring pleural effusion without a diagnosis of malignancy (Figure 12–3). Use of the catheter allows the patient and/or his or her family to relieve the dyspnea while draining the pleural fluid at

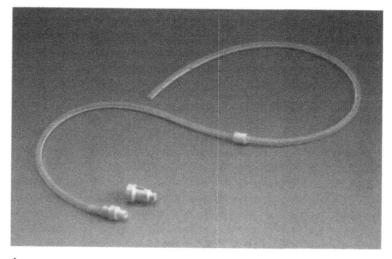

A

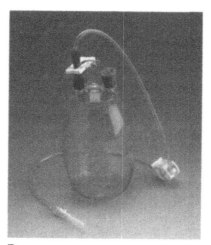

B

Figure 12–1. Pleurx catheter. The Pleurx catheter (A) is a soft silastic catheter fenestrated on the end that goes into the pleural cavity. A Teflon sheath provides a foundation for fibroblast ingrowth to minimize the risk of infection. The external arm ends with a 1-way valve and cap. This 1-way valve can be accessed using the "obturator," which appears much like a stiff 16-gauge Angiocath intravenous catheter (Becton-Dickinson, Franklin Lakes, NJ). (B) A prepackaged vacuum bottle is used to drain the pleural fluid (to a maximum of 600 mL). No more than 1,200 mL of fluid (2 bottles) is removed at any single time. The stiff plastic obturator is used to access the pleural catheter and drain the fluid. The vacuum automatically withdraws sufficient fluid. When the catheter and vacuum source have stopped draining the pleural fluid, the catheter is removed. Typically when less than 10 mL has been drained every other day for 1 week, the catheter may be removed.

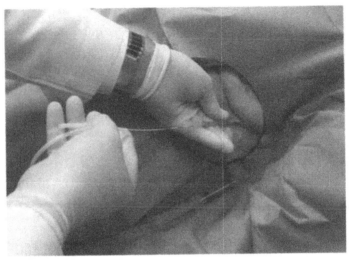

A

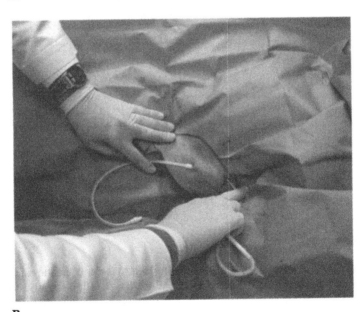

B

Figure 12–2. Techniques of inserting a Pleurx pleural catheter. Patients are typically selected on the basis of symptomatic and recurrent pleural effusion. Patients
should have a free-flowing pleural effusion that can be easily diagnosed with plain
chest roentgenograms (posterior-anterior, lateral, and bilateral decubitus films). In
patients without a history of bleeding problems and in patients with no history of
thrombocytopenia, coagulation studies and platelet studies are not generally obtained. In patients who have had chemotherapy within the previous 4 weeks, coagulation profiles are obtained. *(Legend continues on next page)*

home. In this manner, the patient and family can intervene directly against symptoms of dyspnea that the patient experiences as a result of the recurring pleural effusion. Typically drainage is performed every other day. Patients tolerate this well and are able to maintain an independent and functional life outside the hospital.

Outpatient Management of Malignant Pleural Effusions.   On the basis of the successful multi-institutional experience with indwelling pleural catheters, we hypothesized that outpatient management of patients with malignant pleural effusion could be accomplished with an indwelling pleural catheter at significant cost savings (Putnam et al, 2000). We compared hospitalization and early charges between 100 patients (40 inpatients, 60 outpatients) treated with pleural catheters and 100 patients (all inpatients) treated with chest tube drainage and sclerosis. Outcomes evaluated were control of pleural effusion, length of hospitalization, morbidity, and survival.

We found no pretreatment or posttreatment differences in Zubrod performance scores or symptoms between the 2 groups. Mean hospitalization time was 8 days for inpatients whether they were treated with a chest tube or a pleural catheter. Overall survival was 50% at 90 days. Survival did not differ by treatment for any group. In patients treated with pleural catheters, there were no catheter-related deaths, no emergency operations, and no major bleeding. Eighty-one percent of patients treated with pleural catheters experienced no side effects. The economic impact of pleural catheters was significant. For patients treated in-hospital, mean charges ranged from $7,000 to $11,000. Patients treated as outpatients (60 pleural catheter patients) had mean charges of $3,400. Outpatient pleural catheter drainage was safe, cost-efficient, and successful and was associated with minimal morbidity. No hospitalization was required for patients initially evaluated as outpatients. Outpatient management of malignant pleural effusions is now our standard of care.

Figure 12–2. *(continued)*   Typically patients have undergone at least 1 thoracentesis to prove that the symptoms can be relieved with drainage of the fluid. In patients with chronic long-standing pleural disease, shortness of breath may not be related to the pleural effusion but may instead be related to significant pleural disease or to underlying impaired lung function. Patients undergo insertion of the Pleurx catheter in a procedure room. They are provided supplemental oxygen as needed and monitored for heart rate and rhythm, blood pressure, and oxygen saturation.

(A) With the patient under local anesthesia, a suitable site in the anterior axillary line is identified and anesthetized. After localization of the pleural fluid with a 22-gauge needle, a flexible wire is placed into the pleural cavity using the Seldinger technique. (B) A counter-incision is made, and the Pleurx catheter is placed via a subcutaneous tunnel. The Teflon cuff is identified and placed subcutaneously 1 cm from the exit site. *(Figure continues on page 234)*

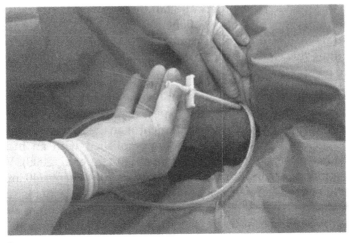

C

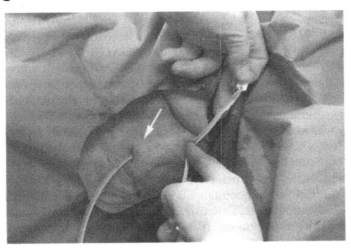

D

Figure 12–2. *(continued)*   (C) The intercostal tract into the pleural space is dilated using a dilator surrounded by a "peel-away" sheath. (D) The subcutaneous tunnel. The fenestrated end of the silastic catheter has been placed through the "peel-away" sheath. The catheter exits the skin inferior and medial to the insertion site of the catheter through a counter-incision. A Teflon cuff, which is integral to the catheter, is placed just under the skin approximately 1 cm from the exit site (arrow). The peel-away sheath is removed after the catheter is guided into the chest. Fluoroscopy is not necessary.

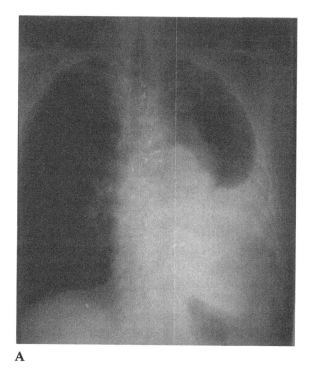

A

Figure 12–3. Patient with malignant pleural effusion and "trapped lung." In this patient, persistent shortness of breath and "pressure" in the chest were relieved with insertion of a Pleurx catheter. (A) Before pleural catheter insertion. (*Figure continues on page 236*)

Extrinsic Compression of Airway

Extrinsic compression of the trachea or bronchi may be treated when possible with surgical resection. On occasion, lung cancer may not invade directly into the compressed structure; however, this external compression may still impair ventilation. With resection of the primary tumor, the cause of the compression can be removed, and the normal ventilation mechanics can be restored. If such external compression cannot be alleviated surgically or if the risks of surgery outweigh the benefits, external-beam radiation therapy can be considered.

Computed tomography, magnetic resonance imaging, and bronchoscopy are performed by the surgeon or pulmonologist to assess the involvement of the tracheal mucosa. Biopsies, brushings of the tracheal or bronchial mucosa, and washings are performed to assist in the diagnosis of invasion of the mucosa. External compression of the trachea or mainstem bronchi may be treated with placement of indwelling expandable

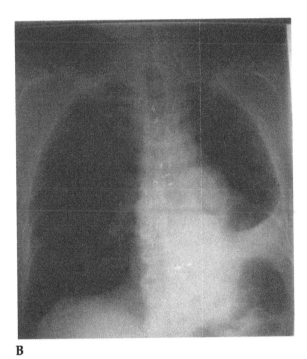

B

Figure 12–3. *(continued)* (B) After pleural catheter insertion.

stents. The stents are placed in the operating room under fluoroscopic guidance while the patient is under general anesthesia. Control of hemoptysis with flexible or rigid bronchoscopy and laser ablation may be required prior to placement of the stent.

Intraluminal Tumor

Lung tumors may obstruct portions of the main-stem bronchus and by extension obstruct the distal trachea. Growth of tumor in this area can obstruct the contralateral main-stem bronchus as well. In such situations, patients experience significant shortness of breath. Some patients with intraluminal tumor experience a true airway emergency necessitating immediate treatment.

All patients with hemoptysis and all patients with airway obstruction must be treated in the operating room with rigid bronchoscopy. Flexible bronchoscopy in the patient with airway obstruction cannot always reestablish an airway quickly enough to prevent respiratory arrest. Treatment in the operating room with a trained team consisting of an experienced thoracic anesthesiologist, a thoracic surgeon, and adept nurses is required for successful results. All equipment that may be required in the treatment of airway obstruction must be on hand in the operating room, including a flexible bronchoscope with appropriate biopsy forceps; flexible brushes; topical epinephrine; topical anesthetics; and a rigid bronchoscope for performing biopsies, mechanical fulguration, and laser treatment.

If the tumor completely occludes the distal trachea, it may be necessary to "core out" the trachea lumen to provide an airway and permit oxygenation. This procedure requires technical facility with rigid bronchoscopy and adept manipulation of biopsy and extraction forceps. Rigid bronchoscopes of various sizes are used to dilate a stricture or push through the obstructing tumor, gradually improving the airway.

With the airway established, laser ablation of the tumor can be performed. Bleeding from the cut edges of the tumor may be controlled with topical epinephrine. In patients in whom the tumor has eroded through the bronchus into the pulmonary artery, extraction of the tumor to open the airway may result in exsanguination. Emergency thoracotomy and lobectomy may be considered in such cases but is frequently futile.

Additional techniques for relieving airway obstruction include external-beam radiation therapy, mechanical fulguration via rigid bronchoscopy, stent placement, dilation, laser ablation, and brachytherapy.

Brachytherapy may be performed to enhance airway control after definitive surgery and external-beam radiation therapy. Brachytherapy is a technique in which a radiation source (such as an iridium bead) is inserted through a small catheter placed under direct bronchoscopic guidance into the involved airway. Brachytherapy permits delivery of specified doses of radiation to a very small area—generally tissues within 1 to 2 cm of the source. In this way, radiation therapy may be used to treat the intraluminal tumor without significant structural damage to surrounding thoracic structures. Brachytherapy may be done on an outpatient basis with good results.

The most frequent complication of endobronchial brachytherapy is hemoptysis. The risk of hemoptysis depends on the prior radiation dose the patient has received. Patients who have not had prior external-beam radiation therapy have a relatively low risk of significant hemoptysis. However, patients who have had prior external-beam radiation therapy have a small risk of fatal hemoptysis. Because of the risk of complications, brachytherapy should be used with caution. Endobronchial radiation therapy is only one of multiple methods—including stent placement, cryotherapy, and laser ablation—for managing recurrent endobronchial disease.

ALIMENTATION AND NUTRITION

Many patients with lung cancer have cachexia during the later stages of their disease, and cachexia may be exacerbated by treatment. Patients

---

KEY PRACTICE POINTS

- Many patients with lung cancer present with impaired pulmonary function.
- Surgery may be used to palliate symptoms in patients with lung cancer—e.g., surgery may be used for drainage of pleural effusion and for optimizing impaired airways.
- Outpatient management of malignant pleural effusions is cost-effective and is the standard of care at M.D. Anderson.
- Rigid bronchoscopy while the patient is under general anesthesia is the standard of care for patients with hemoptysis and for those with airway obstruction.
- External-beam radiation therapy and/or brachytherapy may be used for focused treatment of lung tumors aimed at improving dyspnea related to airway obstruction.
- An integrated pain management program for both inpatient and outpatient pain problems is of great value for patients.
- Proper nutrition and hydration may enhance quality of life.

---

with the later stages of disease typically have decreased appetite and thus may have difficulty maintaining adequate nutrition with an appropriately balanced diet. We have found that consultations with our nutritional service are of great help for these patients in improving their quality of life and their sense of well-being. During consultations, the dietician discusses calorie counts and ways in which the patient can achieve intake of sufficient calories, vitamins, and other supplements. In patients with significant radiation esophagitis, placement of a feeding tube (nasogastric) or a gastrostomy tube (percutaneous) or a feeding jejunostomy (via laparoscopy) may be considered. Patients are frequently dehydrated and must be encouraged to supplement their diet with sufficient liquids.

SUGGESTED READINGS

Antony VB, Lodenkemper R, Astoul P, et al, for the American Thoracic Society. Management of malignant pleural effusions. *Am J Respir Crit Care Med* 2000;162:1987–2001.

Belani CP, Pajeau TS, Bennett CL. Treating malignant pleural effusions cost consciously. *Chest* 1998;113(1 suppl):78S–85S.

Benedetti C, Brock C, Cleeland C, et al. NCCN Practice Guidelines for Cancer Pain. *Oncology (Huntingt)* 2000;14:135–150.

Bonnette P, Puyo P, Gabriel C, et al. Surgical management of non-small cell lung cancer with synchronous brain metastases. *Chest* 2001;119:1469–1475.

Cella DF, Bonomi AE, Lloyd SR, et al. Reliability and validity of the Functional Assessment of Cancer Therapy-Lung (FACT-L) quality of life instrument. *Lung Cancer* 1995;12:199–220.

de Campos JR, Vargas FS, de Campos Werebe E, et al. Thoracoscopy talc poudrage: a 15-year experience. *Chest* 2001;119:801–806.

Gandhi S, Walsh GL, Komaki R, et al. A multidisciplinary surgical approach to superior sulcus tumors with vertebral invasion. *Ann Thorac Surg* 1999; 68:1778–1784.

Gokaslan ZL, York JE, Walsh GL, et al. Transthoracic vertebrectomy for metastatic spinal tumors. *J Neurosurg* 1998;89:599–609.

Hollen PJ, Gralla RJ. Comparison of instruments for measuring quality of life in patients with lung cancer. *Semin Oncol* 1996;23(2 suppl 5):31–40.

Janjan N. Bone metastases: approaches to management. *Semin Oncol* 2001;28(4 suppl 11):28–34.

Karnofsky D. Meaningful clinical classification of therapeutic responses to anticancer drugs [editorial]. *Clin Pharmacol Ther* 1961;2:709–712.

Komaki R, Roth JA, Walsh GL, et al. Outcome predictors for 143 patients with superior sulcus tumors treated by multidisciplinary approach at the University of Texas M.D. Anderson Cancer Center. *Int J Radiat Oncol Biol Phys* 2000;48:347–354.

Langendijk JA, ten Velde GP, Aaronson NK, et al. Quality of life after palliative radiotherapy in non-small cell lung cancer: a prospective study. *Int J Radiat Oncol Biol Phys* 2000;47:149–155.

Light RW. Management of pleural effusions. *J Formos Med Assoc* 2000;99:523–531.

Light RW. Useful tests on the pleural fluid in the management of patients with pleural effusions. *Curr Opin Pulm Med* 1999;5:245–249.

Marom EM, Patz EF Jr, Erasmus JJ, et al. Malignant pleural effusions: treatment with small-bore-catheter thoracostomy and talc pleurodesis. *Radiology* 1999;210:277–281.

Mathisen DJ. Primary tracheal tumor management. *Surg Oncol Clin N Am* 1999;8:307.

Mitchell JD, Mathisen DJ, Wright CD, et al. Clinical experience with carinal resection. *J Thorac Cardiovasc Surg* 1999;117:39–52.

Oken MM, Creech RH, Tormey DC, et al. Toxicity and response criteria of the Eastern Cooperative Oncology Group. *Am J Clin Oncol* 1982;5:649–655.

Olak J, Dresler CM. Sclerosis of pleural effusions by talc thoracoscopy versus talc slurry: a phase III study. Cancer and Leukemia Group B (CALGB #9334). 1993.

Pain Research Group other sites page. The University of Texas M.D. Anderson Cancer Center Web site. Available at: http://prg.mdanderson.org/links.htm. Accessed: January 7, 2002.

Parulekar W, Di Primio G, Matzinger F, et al. Use of small-bore vs large-bore chest tubes for treatment of malignant pleural effusions. *Chest* 2001;120:19–25.

Patz EF Jr, McAdams HP, Erasmus JJ, et al. Sclerotherapy for malignant pleural effusions: a prospective randomized trial of bleomycin vs doxycycline with small-bore catheter drainage. *Chest* 1998;113:1305–1311.

Putnam JB Jr, Light RW, Rodriguez RM, et al. A randomized comparison of indwelling pleural catheter and doxycycline pleurodesis in the management of malignant pleural effusions. *Cancer* 1999;86:1992–1999.

Putnam JB Jr, Walsh GL, Swisher SG, et al. Outpatient management of malignant pleural effusion by a chronic indwelling pleural catheter. *Ann Thorac Surg* 2000;69:369–375.

Rendina EA, De Giacomo T, Venuta F, et al. Lung conservation techniques: bronchial sleeve resection and reconstruction of the pulmonary artery. *Semin Surg Oncol* 2000;18:165–172.

Rendina EA, Venuta F, De Giacomo T, et al. Sleeve resection and prosthetic reconstruction of the pulmonary artery for lung cancer. *Ann Thorac Surg* 1999;68:995–1001.

Rumana CS, Hess KR, Shi WM, et al. Metastatic brain tumors with dural extension. *J Neurosurg* 1998;89:552–558.

Rusch VW, Parekh KR, Leon L, et al. Factors determining outcome after surgical resection of T3 and T4 lung cancers of the superior sulcus. *J Thorac Cardiovasc Surg* 2000;119:1147–1153.

Sanchez-Armengol A, Rodriguez-Panadero F. Survival and talc pleurodesis in metastatic pleural carcinoma, revisited. Report of 125 cases. *Chest* 1993; 104:1482–1485.

Stevens CW, Lee JS, Cox J, et al. Novel approaches to locally advanced unresectable non-small cell lung cancer. *Radiother Oncol* 2000;55:11–18.

York JE, Walsh GL, Lang FF, et al. Combined chest wall resection with vertebrectomy and spinal reconstruction for the treatment of Pancoast tumors. *J Neurosurg* 1999;91(suppl 1):74–80.

Zebrowski BK, Yano S, Liu W, et al. Vascular endothelial growth factor levels and induction of permeability in malignant pleural effusions. *Clin Cancer Res* 1999;5:3364–3368.

Zubrod CG, Schneiderman M, Frei E III, et al. Appraisal of methods for the study of chemotherapy of cancer in man: comparative therapeutic trial of nitrogen mustard and triethylene thiophosphoramide. *J Chron Dis* 1960;11:7–33.

13 PREVENTION AND MANAGEMENT OF SEQUELAE OF MULTIMODALITY THERAPY

*Ara A. Vaporciyan, Jason F. Kelly,
and Katherine M. W. Pisters*

CHAPTER OVERVIEW

The advent of more effective chemotherapeutic agents and more effective methods of delivering radiation therapy has led to the more frequent use of multimodality therapy in the treatment of non–small cell lung cancer. Careful patient selection and close cooperation between the various members of the multidisciplinary team are requirements for successful multimodality therapy. Every member of the multidisciplinary team must be aware of the effects of each treatment modality on the delivery of subsequent treatments. Close collaboration between members of the team helps to ensure that any possible problem will be addressed early, before it can progress to cause irreversible morbidity or a delay in the delivery of planned therapy.

Multimodality regimens involving chemotherapy should only be used in patients with a Zubrod performance status score of 0 or 1 and adequate bone marrow, liver, and kidney function. The addition of chemotherapy to radiation therapy increases the frequency and severity of the most common acute radiation-induced side effects—esophagitis, skin reactions, pneumonitis, and pericarditis. In patients with unresected disease treated with chemotherapy and definitive radiation therapy, severe esophagitis occurs in approximately one third of patients treated with a sequential approach (chemotherapy followed by radiation therapy) and approximately two thirds of patients treated with a concurrent approach. Symptomatic relief with analgesics and nutritional support are the mainstays of treatment for patients with severe esophagitis. Preoperative radiation therapy and, to a lesser extent, preoperative chemotherapy increase the risk of surgery-related complications, including wound infections and dehiscence, persistent air leak, and bronchopleural fistula. The use of meticulous dissection, reinforced staple lines, and pulmonary sealants can reduce the incidence of parenchymal air leaks, while the use of rotational flaps, such as intercostal muscle flaps and pericardial fat pad flaps, can limit problems with the bronchial closure.

INTRODUCTION

In certain subsets of patients with non–small cell lung cancer (NSCLC), multimodality therapy is more effective than single-modality therapy in reducing the incidence of tumor recurrence and improving overall survival. Today, many patients with NSCLC are treated with a multimodality approach. However, the combination of several different treatment modalities, each associated with particular side effects, can lead to increased overall morbidity. To successfully implement this aggressive form of treatment, clinicians must understand the risks inherent in the treatment plan and the available methods for minimizing these risks and managing any side effects that occur. Each discipline involved in the care of patients with NSCLC (medical oncology, radiation oncology, and thoracic surgery) will have its own set of concerns depending on the order in which the treatment modalities are administered.

At M.D. Anderson Cancer Center, all possible permutations of the 3 standard modalities of therapy (chemotherapy, surgery, and radiation therapy) are currently or have been part of our armamentarium for the treatment of NSCLC. This chapter will discuss the most common side effects associated with multimodality therapy and describe our efforts to minimize side effects and treat those that do occur.

PATIENT SELECTION

Careful patient selection is critical for the success of multimodality therapy. Many important factors must be considered in selecting the optimal treatment approach for an individual patient, including disease stage, performance status, weight loss, the presence of comorbid illnesses, baseline cardiopulmonary function, and hematopoietic, hepatic, and renal function. A rigorous staging workup is essential to accurately determine the clinical stage. The elements of the staging workup are described in detail in chapter 2.

MEDICAL ONCOLOGY

At M. D. Anderson, only patients with excellent performance status (a score of 0 or 1 on the Zubrod scale) are treated with multimodality therapy that includes chemotherapy. Clinical trials of multimodality therapy involving chemotherapy have excluded patients with a Zubrod performance status of 2 or greater. Most trials have also excluded patients with significant weight loss. In addition, patients with active hemoptysis, lobar atelectasis, or postobstructive pneumonia are not considered candidates for multimodality therapy that involves chemotherapy. These patients are treated with single-modality therapy. Adequate bone marrow, liver, and kidney function is confirmed prior to the initiation of treatment in all patients scheduled to receive chemotherapy in combination with surgery or radiation therapy.

Preoperative Chemotherapy

In patients who meet the criteria outlined in the preceding paragraph, full doses of systemic chemotherapy can be given prior to surgical resection. Many different chemotherapy regimens have been evaluated in the preoperative setting, the majority based on platinum. In general, the side effects of preoperative chemotherapy in patients with stage IB to IIIA NSCLC are similar to or less severe than the side effects seen when the same chemotherapy regimens are given to patients with inoperable disease with good performance status. Radiographic response rates are generally higher with preoperative chemotherapy than with the same regimens given in the setting of metastatic disease.

In patients treated with preoperative chemotherapy, pulmonary function is measured not only before chemotherapy but also in the interval between chemotherapy and surgery to assess for pulmonary toxicity. This is especially important for patients treated with chemotherapeutic agents with known pulmonary toxicity (e.g., mitomycin and gemcitabine).

Many investigators have evaluated the use of both chemotherapy and radiation therapy prior to surgery. Some investigators have administered these modalities sequentially, while others have administered them concurrently. When both modalities are utilized prior to surgery, rates of surgery-related morbidity and mortality may be higher than rates seen with chemotherapy alone before surgery. Moreover, many chemotherapy agents require substantial dose reduction when they are given concurrently with radiation therapy, and such dose reductions may reduce the efficacy of chemotherapy. There is little evidence from the literature to support the routine use of the combination of chemotherapy and radiation therapy before surgery.

Postoperative Chemotherapy

Many investigators have evaluated the use of chemotherapy or chemotherapy and radiation therapy after surgery for lung cancer. Unfortunately, the majority of these trials have not found a survival benefit associated with the use of postoperative treatment. In most studies, only 50% to 70% of the intended 4 cycles of chemotherapy was actually administered. A variety of factors have contributed to this problem, but in general, patients with NSCLC who have undergone thoracotomy have poor tolerance of adjuvant treatment.

Chemotherapy with Definitive Irradiation

There are several factors to consider when chemotherapy and definitive thoracic irradiation is planned. If a sequential chemotherapy–radiation therapy approach is undertaken, most chemotherapeutic agents can be delivered at full dose. If treatment is delivered in a concurrent fashion, chemotherapy doses often require reduction. Specific side effects of the combination of chemotherapy and definitive thoracic irradiation are discussed in the section Radiation Oncology later in this chapter.

Oncologists should prescribe regimens as published in the peer-reviewed medical literature. There is now extensive experience with vinca alkaloid and cisplatin regimens administered concurrently with full-dose radiation therapy (Radiation Therapy Oncology Group trial 94–10) (Curran et al, 2000). In addition, there is extensive information from phase II trials on the use of weekly taxanes and carboplatin concurrently with radiation therapy. Gemcitabine is a potent radiosensitizer, and trials conducted to date have found that administration of this agent in combination with radiation therapy significantly increases treatment toxicity.

It is unclear whether additional doses of systemic chemotherapy should be administered before or after concurrent chemotherapy and definitive radiation therapy. Ongoing phase III randomized trials are addressing these issues.

Radiation Oncology

Acute Side Effects

The most common acute side effects of external-beam irradiation are skin reactions, esophagitis, anorexia, nausea, and fatigue. Other acute side effects, such as pneumonitis and pericarditis, are possible but occur infrequently.

Skin reactions after radiation therapy range from mild erythema localized within the treatment portal to moist desquamation. When the skin is intact, these changes are managed with an emollient moisturizer such as Aquaphor ointment. A thin layer of this hydrogenated petrolatum is applied to the affected skin area daily after radiation therapy. It is important for patients to understand that applying a moisturizer prior to a radiation treatment may actually intensify the reaction. In cases in which the skin has sloughed, a half-strength diluted solution of 3% hydrogen peroxide solution and water is applied with gauze to clean away dead skin and reduce the risk of superinfection. This cleansing is followed by application of 1% hydrocortisone cream to reduce inflammation and pruritus. Silvadene cream can also be used. For more severe reactions, particularly those involving a large area of desquamation, an occlusive dressing is applied to provide a moisture barrier until the new epithelial layer forms, though this requires stopping radiation therapy until the desquamation resolves or removing the dressing prior to each radiation treatment.

Esophagitis is the major dose-limiting side effect of thoracic irradiation. Even with conformal treatment planning and treatment delivery, a portion of the esophagus receives a significant radiation dose during pulmonary irradiation. After 2 to 3 weeks of conventional daily radiation treatments, patients develop mild dysphagia. Reactions earlier than this usually represent thrush or gastroesophageal reflux and should be treated with antifungals or H2 blockers, respectively. Often patients will describe not pain but rather a glomus sensation or a feeling that food is sticking in place. This discomfort usually responds to analgesic therapy. A topical agent such as viscous lidocaine alone or in a mouthwash preparation with diphenhydramine and aluminum hydroxide or magnesium hydroxide suspension can provide immediate relief, especially if the agent is applied before meals. Sucralfate (Carofate) slurries can also be used. Many patients respond well to combination analgesics, such as hydrocodone and acetaminophen, taken before meals and bedtime. As odynophagia progresses, elixir formulations are often better tolerated than tablets. For more refractory cases of odynophagia, narcotics such as morphine or oxycodone are used. Time-release formulations are given twice daily and supplemented with smaller doses of the immediate-release preparation given as needed for breakthrough pain. This approach allows rapid, effective dose titration to meet patients' analgesic needs. Transdermal fentanyl is used for patients who have difficulty managing multiple medication doses. Potential disadvantages of transdermal fentanyl include longer time to onset of pain relief and less flexibility in dose modification. Patients treated with narcotic analgesics are counseled regarding opiate-induced constipation and are instructed to take senna and docusate sodium (Senokot-S) to maintain bowel regularity. Lactulose syrup is another option for patients who tend towards obstipation.

Nutritional support plays an important role during radiation therapy for lung cancer. All patients treated with definitive radiation therapy meet with a staff dietician within the first 2 weeks after therapy is started. The dietician explains that patients who avoid losing weight during radiation therapy tolerate treatment better and have a better chance of avoiding treatment interruption or prolonged recovery after treatment is completed. The dietician reviews the patient's protein and caloric intake, identifies any areas requiring improvement, and recommends specific dietary modifications to help patients maintain good nutrition during therapy. When patients are eating less because of decreased appetite or esophagitis, the foods they do eat need to be rich in protein and calories. For the treatment and recovery period, no restrictions are placed on fat or oil intake. Patients are advised that once swallowing starts to be difficult, they should avoid eating foods that are hard or rough, heavily seasoned, or extreme in temperature. Likewise, they are advised to avoid beverages with alcohol, high acid content (e.g., citrus juice), or carbonation. Many commercial dietary supplements are available (e.g., Ensure, Boost, and Ultracal) to help patients maintain their weight during radiation therapy. Usually 6 to 8 cans per day are required if these are the sole source of calories. Patients who lose more than 10% of their baseline body weight are eligible to have a percutaneous endoscopic or fluoroscopic gastrostomy feeding tube placed. Direct infusion of liquid nutrition enables patients to continue their treatment program without needing an interval recovery time. If anorexia is a problem, megestrol acetate (Megace) can be used. Dexamethasone is not recommended during radiation therapy because of potential problems with pneumonitis.

Postoperative Radiation Therapy

In the postoperative setting, patients usually start radiation therapy after their first check-up with their surgeon, 4 to 6 weeks after surgery. To minimize the risk of radiation-related dehiscence, radiation therapy is not started less than 10 to 14 days after surgery. Whether a lobe or an entire lung is removed must be taken into account when adjuvant mediastinal irradiation is planned. The proportion of the total lung volume that receives a dose of 20 Gy or higher must be kept as low as possible to decrease the risk of acute radiation pneumonitis or late radiation fibrosis. As a general guideline, the proportion of the total lung volume receiving 20 Gy or more should be less than 40%. Since this percentage is recommended for patients with normal lung capacity, the total lung volume treated to 20 Gy should be proportionately less for patients who have undergone pulmonary resection. Patients who develop pneumonitis with symptoms of dyspnea, non-productive cough, and low-grade fever after postoperative radiation therapy are usually referred to a pulmonologist for corticosteroid and bronchodilator inhaler therapy. Symptomatic pulmonary fibrosis is uncommon, but when it occurs, it is also managed with the assistance of a pulmonologist. In patients with symptomatic pulmonary fibrosis, supplemental oxygen, steroids, and bronchodilators can help ease symptoms, but the underlying process is usually irreversible.

Radiation Therapy before Surgery or Chemotherapy

Radiation therapy delivered in the preoperative setting can produce side effects similar to those seen with postoperative radiation therapy, but the severity is usually less since the total radiation dose is usually lower than the dose used for definitive irradiation. Patient care and symptom management are also the same as in other settings. Usually patients are given at least 2 weeks to recover from their radiation therapy before additional treatment—either surgery or chemotherapy—is begun.

When surgery is planned, patients typically rest 4 to 6 weeks after the completion of radiation therapy before re-evaluation and surgery scheduling. If surgery is delayed for more than 2 months after the completion of preoperative radiation therapy, the difficulty of resection may be increased because of radiation-induced scarring. Because of the potential for treatment delay and the lower radiation doses required with preoperative radiation therapy, we favor a postoperative approach. This allows the boost volume to be better defined by the surgery–radiation oncology team and allows for full-dose chemoradiation if surgery is not possible. It is imperative that a multidisciplinary approach be used to coordinate the care of patients receiving neoadjuvant radiation therapy. At M.D. Anderson, the involved physicians and surgeons evaluate patients before therapy is begun to ensure that they are candidates for surgery and are likely to benefit from neoadjuvant treatment. This coordination helps prevent a delay in surgery for patients with resectable disease and also ensures that patients with inoperable disease do not receive an inadequate or interrupted course of radiation therapy.

Definitive Thoracic Irradiation with Chemotherapy

Definitive radiation therapy with concurrent chemotherapy has been shown to benefit selected patients who have no or minimal weight loss (<5%–10% from baseline) and have a Zubrod performance status score of 0 or 1 or the equivalent score on another performance status scale. Data from a prospective, randomized trial (Curran et al, 2000) have shown that approximately one third of patients who receive chemotherapy followed by definitive radiation therapy and up to half of patients who receive concurrent chemotherapy and definitive radiation therapy experience severe esophagitis (National Cancer Institute Common Toxicity Criteria grade 3 or 4). This severe esophagitis can necessitate dietary modification, narcotic analgesics, and, for patients who have lost more than 10% of their body weight, feeding tube placement. Another factor that can influence acute side effects in patients treated with chemoradiation is the daily radiation dose—especially when patients receive greater than 2 Gy per day, as in the case of hyperfractionated treatment delivering 1.2 to 1.5 Gy twice daily. When chemotherapy is given concurrently with hyperfractionated radiation therapy, approximately two thirds of patients experience severe esophagitis. This excess toxicity explains why concurrent chemotherapy and hyperfractionated radiation therapy is currently restricted to the protocol setting.

Late Side Effects

Late or chronic complications of radiation therapy are defined as complications occurring or persisting 90 days or later after the completion of treatment. When radiation therapy is carefully planned and delivered with respect to normal tissue tolerances, severe late complications are not routinely seen. In addition to the previously mentioned dose guidelines for the total volume of lung treated, the doses to the spinal cord, heart, and esophagus must be considered (Table 13–1). When these dose limits (based on 1.8–2.0 Gy per fraction) are respected, the risk of severe complications, such as cardiomyopathy or myelitis, is less than 5% at 5 years after therapy. In contrast to acute side effects, long-term side effects are more directly related to the dose per fraction or individual radiation treatment than to the total radiation dose. The risk of more intense late complications increases as the dose per fraction increases. In the randomized, prospective intergroup trial comparing sequential chemotherapy and radiation therapy versus concurrent chemotherapy and once-daily radiation therapy versus concurrent chemotherapy and twice-daily radiation therapy (Curran et al, 2000), the late complication rate was about 17% in all 3 arms. This finding suggests that adding concurrent chemotherapy to radiation therapy does not increase the rate of late complications. The intergroup trial also found that the different rates of acute esophagitis in the 3 arms did not translate into correspondingly different rates of late esophageal stricture, indicating that acute radiation-related complications do not predict for late complications.

THORACIC SURGERY

In general, of the 3 modalities available for the treatment of patients with lung cancer, surgery is associated with the highest incidences of treatment-related morbidity (15%–40%) and mortality (1%–12%). The occurrence of surgery-related side effects and deaths is minimized through

Table 13–1.   Suggested Maximum Doses to Critically Sensitive Normal Structures

Organ and Portion Irradiated	Maximum Dose, Gy
Normal lung	
Ipsilateral lung (entire lung)	25
40% of total lung volume (ipsilateral and contralateral lungs combined)	20
Spinal cord	
10 cm	48
$\leqslant$ 20 cm	< 48
Heart	
< 50%	50
50%–99%	45
Entire organ	40
Esophagus	
< 5 cm	70
5–9.9 cm	60
10–19.9 cm	50
$\geqslant$ 20 cm	40

careful attention to the preoperative assessment, the technical conduct of the operation, and postoperative management.

The potential complications after pulmonary resection are numerous and have been discussed extensively in many sources. The delivery of preoperative chemotherapy or radiation therapy increases the risk of certain surgery-related complications and thus must be taken into account throughout the evaluation and treatment of the patient if increased morbidity is to be avoided. Not only the surgeon but also every other member of the multidisciplinary team must be aware of the potential problems that can arise during multimodality therapy and lead to increased morbidity. Early identification and prompt correction of problems avoids delays in the delivery of planned therapy and prevents the development of irreversible morbidity.

Preoperative Assessment

In the preoperative assessment of patients with lung cancer, the first issue addressed is the timing of surgery after chemotherapy and/or radiation therapy.

After chemotherapy, the recovery interval before surgery is usually 3 to 5 weeks. For most patients, this is ample time for recovery of adequate bone marrow function and nutritional status. An overall white blood cell count below 4×10^9/L or an absolute neutrophil count below 2×10^9/L is considered a relative contraindication to surgery. In patients with persistent low white blood cell counts after chemotherapy, either the recovery interval is prolonged (if the white blood cell count is slightly diminished) or recombinant granulocyte colony-stimulating factor (e.g., Neupogen) is administered (if the white blood cell count is significantly diminished). In patients with persistent anemia after chemotherapy, recombinant erythropoietin (e.g., Procrit) is administered to restore normal hemoglobin levels and minimize the need for perioperative transfusions. Patients with prechemotherapy weight loss and those who sustain weight loss during chemotherapy benefit from aggressive nutritional support during the interval between chemotherapy and surgery. Patients with extreme weight loss may require enteral access and continuous feedings. All these maneuvers to restore adequate bone marrow function and nutritional status are performed efficiently only if the oncologist and the surgeon maintain close communication. If either functions without knowledge of the other's treatment plan, then potentially correctable problems may go uncorrected or result in delay of the planned treatment.

After radiation therapy, the recovery interval before surgery is at least 1 week for each 10 Gy delivered. Earlier attempts at surgery are associated with increased morbidity due to the still-resolving inflammation, which makes dissection more difficult, and radiation-associated edema and pneumonitis. As in patients treated with preoperative chemotherapy, the recovery period in patients treated with preoperative radiation therapy is spent maximizing the patient's condition for surgery. For example, patients with nutritional impairment due to esophagitis (see the section Radiation Oncology earlier in this chapter) are given aggressive nutritional support. Communication between the radiation oncologist and the surgeon is of paramount importance. If the delay between completion of radiation therapy and surgery is greater than 2 months, the technical difficulty of surgery is greatly magnified because of increasing fibrosis. By maintaining good communication, the radiation oncologist and the surgeon can identify and correct problems early, thus avoiding unnecessary delays in surgery and minimizing postoperative morbidity.

Surgical Technique

In patients treated with preoperative chemotherapy or radiation therapy, the technical details of pulmonary resection are adjusted to reduce the risk of specific postoperative complications.

Meticulous Dissection

The most important technique is meticulous dissection. Gentle handling of the tissue, a surgical axiom, cannot be stressed enough in patients undergoing thoracic surgery after preoperative chemotherapy or radiation therapy.

Minimal and careful dissection diminishes blood loss, parenchymal damage, and devascularization of the bronchus. Tissue integrity is lowered by preoperative therapy, and the addition of indiscriminate dissection can lead to the need for a longer period of chest tube drainage secondary to persistent air leakage or, in the most extreme case, bronchial stump dehiscence and empyema. One area that deserves special attention is dissection around the pulmonary artery. The pulmonary artery is already a delicate structure, and in patients who have undergone preoperative chemotherapy or radiation therapy, additional precautions are required. First, the pulmonary artery should be isolated at the hilum; vascular control can then be obtained with the use of a tourniquet. The pulmonary artery branches can then be dissected with minimal risk of uncontrolled bleeding.

Additional Measures for Preventing Air Leaks

Diminished tissue integrity after either radiation therapy or chemotherapy significantly increases the risk of parenchymal air leak after dissection. Persistent air leakage necessitates a longer period of chest tube drainage, which results in an increase in the severity of postoperative pain and a prolonged hospital stay. The primary method for avoiding air leaks is meticulous dissection. However, in patients with severe emphysema (common in lung cancer patients) who have undergone preoperative therapy, additional methods beyond meticulous dissection are usually required to avoid significant parenchymal air leaks. Several methods are available, and some are suited to a particular area at risk.

One common area of parenchymal damage leading to air leaks is the interlobar fissures. The use of linear automatic stapling devices to complete these fissures is commonplace. However, although this approach is adequate in patients who are chemotherapy naive and radiation therapy naive, nonreinforced staple lines often lead to parenchymal damage and air leak in patients who have undergone preoperative therapy. The staples often tear through the weakened tissue, a problem similar to that seen in severely emphysematous patients undergoing volume-reduction surgery. Reinforcement of the staple line with commercially available strips of bovine pericardium or Gore-Tex membranes can greatly diminish the risk of this problem.

An additional method available for preventing air leaks after upper lobectomy is the construction of a pleural tent. This technique involves mobilization of the apical pleura so that it drapes over the surface of the remaining lung. The resulting apposition of tissue (lung and pleura) facilitates rapid closure of parenchymal defects. The residual apical cavity is not drained but rather allowed to fill with fluid and eventually disappears because of shifting mediastinal structures and elevation of the diaphragm.

Unfortunately, the aforementioned methods of preventing air leaks (reinforcement of staple lines and creation of pulmonary tents) are not applicable in the setting of parenchymal damage sustained during exposure of the pulmonary artery at the base of the interlobar fissures. Until recently, meticulous dissection was the only method available for preventing air leaks in this area. However, a number of tissue sealants have now become available that have variable degrees of success. FocalSeal-L (Genzyme Corporation, Cambridge, MA) is an approved pulmonary sealant that is applied topically and then activated with a light source. It can be used for broad areas of parenchymal injury encountered during dissection in the interlobar fissures or during lysis of pulmonary adhesions. The resulting biodegradable expandable adherent patch has been shown in clinical trials to reduce the duration of air leaks. The hemostatic fibrin sealant Tisseel (Baxter Healthcare Corporation, Deerfield, IL), while not specifically designed as a parenchymal sealant, has also been used with some success.

Additional Methods for Preventing Bronchial Stump Dehiscence

One of the most significant areas of concern in patients undergoing pulmonary resection, especially in preoperatively irradiated patients, is the development of a bronchial stump dehiscence. The fistula that forms as a result is termed a bronchopleural fistula. This complication, and the resulting empyema, can be life-threatening and are very difficult to treat, often requiring reoperation.

The best solution is prevention. Every effort should be made to avoid devascularization of the bronchus during dissection. The use of staples rather than stitches for closure has not been shown to influence the rate of development of bronchopleural fistula, but the speed, reproducibility, and ease of use associated with current stapling devices are certainly advantageous. Even with adherence to meticulous dissection, however, additional efforts to reinforce the closure are recommended, especially after the delivery of any preoperative radiation therapy or after a bronchial anastomosis is constructed (i.e., after sleeve lobectomy or carinal pneumonectomy).

At M.D. Anderson, we usually use viable rotational flaps to buttress the bronchial stump. The most common scenarios in which we utilize pedicled flaps are listed in Table 13–2. A number of pedicled flaps are available; the most commonly utilized are the pericardial fat pad flap and the intercostal muscle flap. These flaps provide the most reliable coverage and should be utilized whenever possible. However, harvesting these flaps requires some experience. Inadvertent damage to the flap's blood supply during harvesting can lead to a nonviable flap. Application of a nonviable flap is worse than using no flap at all. An additional method of coverage is the use of broad-based rotational flaps of pericardium or diaphragm. These flaps, however, provide less reliable coverage then the pedicled flaps and require repair of a defect in the structure of origin. They are simpler to harvest and can be used when an adequate intercostal or pericardial fat pad flap is unavailable. Pleural flaps should not be used for reinforcement of the bronchial stump because their vascular supply is unreliable and because

Table 13–2.   Indications for Pedicled Flap Coverage of a Bronchial Stump or Bronchial Anastomosis

Procedure Performed	Chemotherapy	Preoperative Therapy Delivered		
		Radiation Therapy < 50 Gy	Radiation Therapy ≥ 50 Gy	Chemoradiation
Lobectomy	Flap coverage not indicated	Flap coverage not indicated	Case dependent*	Case dependent*
Sleeve lobectomy	Flap coverage indicated	Flap coverage indicated	Flap coverage indicated	Flap coverage indicated
Pneumo-nectomy	Case dependent when right lung removed; flap coverage not indicated when left lung removed	Flap coverage indicated when right lung removed; not indicated when left lung removed	Flap coverage indicated	Flap coverage indicated

* The decision whether to employ flap coverage requires examination of such factors as the lobe resected, the patient's overall health status, the presence of obstructive pneumonia, and the proximity of the pulmonary artery to the bronchial stump.

these flaps retract owing to scarring. Details on harvesting of these flaps and their applications are available in a variety of surgical textbooks.

Postoperative Management

The postoperative management of patients treated with multimodality therapy is not significantly different from that of patients treated with standard thoracic surgery alone. The application of aggressive pulmonary toilet and a prompt and determined search for any infectious source is critical. Postoperative anemia is more common in patients treated with multimodality therapy. These patients frequently have some degree of mild anemia or diminished bone marrow reserve before surgery. Hemoglobin levels are evaluated on the first, third, and fifth postoperative days. Significant anemia is treated with transfusions; milder anemia is treated with the use of erythropoietin (e.g., Procrit). Iron supplementation is administered carefully to avoid exacerbating the constipation often associated with narcotics used in the postoperative period.

Electrolyte abnormalities after surgery are also more common in patients treated with multimodality therapy. Subclinical renal toxicity from neoadjuvant chemotherapy may become apparent in the postoperative phase as a loss of electrolytes. Electrolyte levels are monitored during the

KEY PRACTICE POINTS

- The increasing use of multimodality therapy in the treatment of NSCLC mandates an understanding of the specific morbidity associated with combinations of different treatment modalities.
- Successful use of multimodality therapy requires that all physicians be aware of all aspects of the treatment plan prior to the initiation of therapy. This allows early identification and prevention of many of the potential problems that can arise during therapy.
- Although chemotherapy is often included in multimodality regimens, patients with NSCLC who have undergone thoracotomy have consistently poor tolerance of adjuvant chemotherapy.
- Administration of chemotherapy concurrently with radiation therapy necessitates drug dose reductions. Even with these reductions, however, the addition of chemotherapy to radiation therapy increases the frequency and intensity of skin reactions and esophagitis.
- After the completion of chemotherapy, a recovery interval of approximately 3 to 5 weeks is usually required prior to surgery.
- After the completion of radiation therapy, a recovery period of approximately 1 week for every 10 Gy administered is required prior to surgery.
- Aggressive nutritional support during every phase of multimodality therapy is critical.
- Meticulous surgical technique and the liberal use of vascularized pedicled tissue flaps to reinforce bronchial closure are the hallmarks of successful thoracic surgery in patients treated with preoperative chemotherapy or radiation therapy.

first 3 days after surgery or until patients resume a normal diet. Hypomagnesemia and hypophosphatemia are not uncommon, and magnesium and phosphate levels are monitored during the postoperative period and corrected as needed.

Adequate postoperative nutritional intake is unrelentingly maintained. In patients in whom poor intake is suspected, calorie counts are obtained during the postoperative period to document adequate caloric intake (at least 20–25 kcal/kg/day with 1.5 g protein/kg/day). Inadequate nutritional intake is corrected with the use of oral supplements (e.g., Ensure, Boost, and Ultracal). Continued inadequate nutritional intake may necessitate placement of enteral feeding tubes (Dobbhoff tubes or percutaneous gastrostomy tubes) to ensure adequate caloric intake.

Finally, wound care, especially in irradiated fields, is given special attention. In patients with any evidence of cellulitis, early initiation of antibiotics is standard practice. Large seromas are drained percutaneously using sterile technique. Smaller seromas are treated only if they become symptomatic.

SUGGESTED READINGS

Curran WJ Jr, Scott C, Langer C, et al. Phase III comparison of sequential vs concurrent chemoradiation for patients with unresected stage III non-small cell lung cancer (NSCLC): initial report of Radiation Therapy Oncology Group (RTOG) 9410. *Proceedings of the American Society of Clinical Oncology* 2000;19. Abstract 1891.

Harris SU, Nahai F. Intrathoracic muscle transposition. Surgical anatomy and techniques of harvest. *Chest Surg Clin N Am* 1996;6:501–518.

Putnam JB Jr. Complications of multimodality therapy. *Chest Surg Clin N Am* 1998;8:663–680.

Siegenthaler MP, Pisters KM, Merriman KW, et al. Preoperative chemotherapy for lung cancer does not increase surgical morbidity. *Ann Thorac Surg* 2001;71:1105–1111.

14 PREVENTION AND EARLY DETECTION OF LUNG CANCER

Edward S. Kim and Fadlo R. Khuri

CHAPTER OVERVIEW

Lung cancer is the leading cause of death in the United States, causing more deaths annually than breast cancer, prostate cancer, or colon cancer. The causal relationship between smoking and lung cancer is well established. From a public health standpoint, then, smoking prevention and smoking cessation campaigns are attractive tools for reducing the incidence of lung cancer and thus the number of deaths from this disease. However, such campaigns have met with only limited success: despite millions of dollars worth of spending on media campaigns highlighting the dangers of smoking, the prevalence of smoking in the United States has decreased less than 1% per year over the past 10 years. Chemoprevention—the use of natural or synthetic agents to reverse, suppress, or prevent carcinogenesis before the development of invasive cancer—has shown some promise in preventing lung cancer in patients at high risk for the disease. Among the potential chemopreventive agents under study are retinoids, α-tocopherol, selenium, lipoxygenase inhibitors, cyclooxygenase inhibitors, and green tea. However, the field of lung cancer chemoprevention is a relatively new area of investigation, and more studies will be needed before definitive lung cancer chemoprevention recommendations can be made.

INTRODUCTION

Lung cancer is the leading cause of cancer-related death worldwide. Lung cancer is also the leading cause of death in the United States, causing more deaths than breast cancer, prostate cancer, or colon cancer, and its incidence continues to rise. It is projected that more than 158,000 people in the United States will lose their lives to lung cancer in 2001.

The causal relationship between tobacco use and lung cancer is well documented on both an epidemiologic and a molecular basis. Approximately 85% of lung cancers are believed to be directly linked to smoking. Thus, strategies designed to deter people from beginning to smoke and to help smokers quit are very attractive from a public health standpoint. However, smoking prevention and smoking cessation efforts have met with only limited success. Smoking rates among US men leveled off in the late 1990s. However, despite millions of dollars in national campaigns highlighting the dangers of smoking, smoking rates are still increasing among US women and adolescents. By the mid-1980s, lung cancer had overtaken breast cancer as the leading cause of cancer-related death in US women.

A second approach to preventing lung cancer is chemoprevention—the use of natural or synthetic agents to prevent the development of cancer in individuals at high risk for the disease. Investigation of chemoprevention strategies has increased in recent years as the molecular basis of lung cancer development has become better understood.

In parallel with efforts to prevent lung cancer, efforts are under way to reduce the public-health burden of lung cancer by developing screening tests that can detect lung cancer at its earliest and most treatable stages. Potential early-detection methods examined to date include chest radiography, spiral computed tomography (CT), and positron emission tomography.

This chapter will detail lung cancer prevention and early-detection efforts, with special emphasis on the chemoprevention efforts ongoing at M. D. Anderson Cancer Center and other leading academic institutions.

MODEL OF LUNG CANCER DEVELOPMENT

Adler, in 1912, was one of the first researchers to propose that tobacco might have a role in bronchogenic carcinoma. Other scientists in the early 1900s also supported the apparent relationship between cigarette smoking and lung cancer, even suggesting that cessation of smoking could prevent lung carcinoma. In the 1930s, Ochsner and DeBakey observed that the increase in cigarette sales might be related to the simultaneous rising incidence of lung cancer (Ochsner and DeBakey, 1940).

Today, the link between smoking and lung cancer development is explained in terms of two concepts: field cancerization and the multistep model of carcinogenesis.

The concept of field cancerization, introduced during the 1950s by Auerbach and colleagues (Auerbach et al, 1957), applies to cancers of the aerodigestive tract. This concept states that carcinogen exposure results in diffuse epithelial injury throughout the aerodigestive tract and that genetic changes and premalignant and malignant lesions in one region of the field translate into an increased risk of cancer development in the entire field. For example, epidermoid carcinoma of the oral epithelium is caused by exposure to a preconditioned carcinogenic agent. If exposure to this agent is prolonged, irreversible cellular changes occur, and the carcinogenic process progresses. One consequence of field cancerization is multiple primary tumors, both synchronous and metachronous. The concept of second primary tumors was initially described by Warren and Gates in 1932 and has since been discussed by other investigators. The field cancerization hypothesis has been supported by recent studies: areas of carcinoma in situ and metaplasia have been found to occur in the bronchial epithelium after prolonged exposure to inhaled carcinogenic agents, specifically cigarette smoke, and there is increasing molecular evidence that these areas of histologic change are causally related to the development of lung cancer.

The multistep model of carcinogenesis holds that the development of cancer is a multistep process in which exposure to a carcinogen (for example, in the case of lung cancer, any of the multiple carcinogens identified in cigarette smoke) results in repeated damage and repair until the accumulated exposure triggers a transformation from normal to premalignant cells (from normal cells to metaplasia and dysplasia) and eventually to frank carcinoma.

SMOKING PREVENTION AND CESSATION INTERVENTIONS

The 2000 Surgeon General's report on tobacco, *Reducing Tobacco Use: A Report of the Surgeon General,* warns that "tobacco use will remain the leading cause of preventable illness and death in this Nation and a growing number of other countries until tobacco prevention and control efforts are commensurate with the harm caused by tobacco use" (USDHHS, 2000).

In this report, the Surgeon General pointed out that educational, clinical, regulatory, economic, and comprehensive approaches to tobacco prevention and control are all available but differ substantially in their techniques. Economic, regulatory, and comprehensive approaches are likely to have the greatest long-term, population impact. Educational and clinical approaches are of greater importance in helping individuals.

There is agreement that smoking prevention interventions (efforts to deter individuals from beginning to smoke) and smoking cessation interventions (efforts to get smokers to quit) are the most proven measures for preventing primary lung cancer and are the keys to creating a smoke-free society. For further information, the Surgeon General's report can be viewed at www.cdc.gov/tobacco.

Link between Smoking and Lung Cancer

The evidence for the relationship between smoking and lung cancer is clear. The risk of lung cancer increases with the number of cigarettes smoked and the number of years of smoking, earlier age at onset of smoking, higher degree of inhalation, higher tar and nicotine content, and use of unfiltered (as opposed to filtered) cigarettes. In addition, among ex-smokers, the risk of lung cancer decreases proportionately with the number of years after quitting.

More than 3,000 chemicals have been identified in tobacco smoke. Polynuclear aromatic hydrocarbons, such as benzopyrenes, account for a significant proportion of tobacco's tumorigenic activity. Upon activation by specific enzymes in human tissue, including lung tissue, the compounds become mutagenic. These activated carcinogens bind to DNA by inducing activating point mutations, such as K-*ras* mutations, at codons 12, 13, and 61. Nitrosamines are also present in tobacco smoke and have a propensity to induce tumors in the lungs of both animals and humans.

Smoking Prevention Interventions

Interventions have been developed to prevent people from beginning to smoke. Advertising campaigns targeting youth have been an area of focus. Advertising campaigns have also focused on young women—especially those who are or could become pregnant. In both groups—youth and women—the prevalence of smoking is increasing.

Unfortunately, despite multiple campaigns emphasizing the dangers of tobacco use, the prevalence of smoking in the United States has declined only 0.5% per year over the past 10 years. Since the Surgeon General's 1964 report on the dangers of smoking, more than 40 million Americans have quit smoking. However, there are still 50 million smokers in the United States today—thus the need for smoking cessation interventions.

Smoking Cessation Interventions

Mounting evidence indicates that the risk of lung cancer in smokers who quit decreases proportionately with the number of years since the quit date. Additional evidence for the benefits of smoking cessation comes from studies showing that lung cancer patients who continue to smoke after their diagnosis have a higher risk of developing recurrences or second primary tumors than do patients who quit when they are diagnosed.

Smoking cessation programs have evolved over time. More than 300 methods are cited in the literature. During the 1960s and 1970s, group therapy, hypnosis, self-help manuals, nicotine analogues, and conditioning-based approaches were popular. In the 1980s, nicotine gum, acupuncture, and physician counseling were the mainstays of smoking cessation programs. The 1990s saw the introduction of the transdermal nicotine patch and the drug bupropion (Zyban). In 1997, Hurt and colleagues reported that bupropion was effective in smoking cessation; this finding was verified in 1999 by Jorenby and colleagues, who found that the combination of the nicotine patch and bupropion was superior to either method alone.

Smoking cessation programs are strongly encouraged for all patients who participate in lung cancer chemoprevention trials or undergo treatment of lung cancer at M. D. Anderson. Physicians educate patients about the benefits of smoking cessation and then offer referrals to our Tobacco Cessation Clinic.

CHEMOPREVENTION

Chemoprevention is an attempt to decrease the burden of lung cancer on society by augmenting the limited success of smoking prevention and smoking cessation programs in decreasing the risk of smoking-related cancer.

In 1976, Sporn coined the term chemoprevention, which is defined as the use of natural or synthetic chemical agents to reverse, suppress, or prevent carcinogenic progression before the development of invasive cancer. Chemoprevention uses knowledge gained from basic biological research to design clinical interventions that attempt to halt the process of carcinogenesis. Chemoprevention in the aerodigestive tract is predicated on the concepts of field cancerization and the multistep model of carcinogenesis, which are discussed in the section Model of Lung Cancer Development earlier in this chapter.

Strategies targeting arrest or reversal of 1 or several of the steps in the multistep process of carcinogenesis may impede the development of cancer. This paradigm has been described particularly well in studies involving cancers of the head and neck, which have focused on oral premalignant lesions, including leukoplakia and erythroplakia, and their associated risk of progression to cancer. Most of the potential chemopreventive agents studied in lung cancer are agents that have first shown promise in the chemoprevention of head and neck cancer.

This section will discuss general strategies of chemoprevention; agents studied for their potential chemopreventive effect in aerodigestive tract malignancies, including lung cancer; major lung cancer chemoprevention trials undertaken to date; and potential new molecular targets for chemoprevention strategies.

Strategies

Chemoprevention strategies target the carcinogenic process at early and potentially reversible stages, focusing on inhibition of 1 or many steps in the progression towards cancer. As a cell's exposure to carcinogens increases, genetic mutations and other processes occur that eventually lead to excessive proliferation of genetically altered cells and, eventually, cancer. Chemoprevention strategies include primary prevention in groups at high risk, reversal of premalignant lesions, and prevention of second primary tumors.

Primary Prevention in High-Risk Groups

At present, there is no standard way to determine which patients are at high risk for the development of lung cancer. Chemoprevention trials have studied patients who are believed to be at high risk for the development of cancer. Specific factors used at present to define high risk include a smoking history of 20 to 30 pack-years; a previous tobacco-related cancer, including head and neck, lung, esophagus, or bladder cancer; and sputum atypia. In the future, it may be possible to identify high-risk patients through measurement of specific molecular markers (for more information, see the section Potential New Molecular Targets later in this chapter).

Reversal of Premalignant Lesions

Various agents have been studied in the treatment of patients with sputum atypia or bronchial squamous metaplasia. One study showed improvement of bronchial epithelial metaplasia in smokers treated with folate and vitamin B12 supplementation. However, because of problems with the consistency of the end points, positive results must be viewed with temperance. Larger trials with biological end points (see the section Potential New Molecular Targets later in this chapter) will be needed to confirm treatment efficacy. Trials targeting intermediate biological markers may well be the most promising element in control of lung cancer.

Prevention of Second Primary Tumors

In patients with resected non–small cell lung cancer (NSCLC), second primary tumors occur at the rate of 2% to 4% per year. Agents that have proven successful in the prevention of second primary malignancies in patients treated for head and neck cancer are being studied for their efficacy in patients treated for lung carcinoma.

Agents

Numerous agents have been studied for their chemopreventive effect against cancers of the aerodigestive tract, including retinoids, β-carotene, vitamin E (α-tocopherol), and selenium. Some of the newer agents to be tested—including lipoxygenase inhibitors and cyclooxygenase (COX) inhibitors—focus on modulation of specific biological markers in patients with high-risk features.

Retinoids

Retinoids have been studied extensively as potential chemopreventive agents. Retinoids have been investigated for their efficacy in primary prevention of cancer, reversal of premalignant lesions, and prevention of second primary malignancies.

Vitamin A was first noted to be an essential nutrient in 1913, and its deficiency was associated with changes in epithelial histology as early as 1925. Deficiency of vitamin A is possibly associated with bronchial metaplasia and increased incidence of lung cancer. Vitamin A exists as preformed vitamin A (retinol esters, vitamin A, and retinal) and provitamin A carotenoids (β-carotene and metabolic precursors of retinol).

Retinoids occur in both natural forms (retinyl palmitate and retinol) and synthetic forms (fenretinide, or N-[4-hydroxyphenyl]retinamide; all-*trans*-retinoic acid; 13-*cis* retinoic acid [13-cRA; isotretinoin]; and 9-*cis* retinoic acid). Retinoids play important roles in normal cell growth and differentiation as well as in regulation of apoptosis.

Landmark trials by Hong and colleagues (1986, 1990) showed that 13-cRA was effective in reversing premalignant lesions such as oral leukoplakia. Furthermore, at high doses, 13-cRA was effective in preventing second primary tumors in patients who had been definitively treated for a prior head and neck cancer. However, 13-cRA was poorly tolerated at the dose used in the studies—50 to 100 mg/m^2/day. This finding led to the use of lower 13-cRA doses in subsequent trials to reduce toxicity and improve compliance. In the trials by Hong and colleagues, after 54.5 months of follow-up, there was still no difference in the rates of recurrence between the 13-cRA-treated group and the placebo group (Benner et al, 1994). However, there continued to be a statistically significant lower incidence of second primary tumors in the 13-cRA-treated group compared with the placebo group (14% vs 31%). These results suggested that other aerodigestive malignancies, including lung cancer, might be similarly preventable with 13-cRA.

An ongoing randomized chemoprevention trial in head and neck squamous cell cancer (HNSCC) using low-dose 13-cRA to prevent second primary tumors in patients definitively treated for stage I or II disease was launched in 1991. An interim analysis of this study (Khuri et al, 2001a) reported recurrence and second primary tumor incidence according to prior tumor stage as well as smoking status (current, former, or never). Among 1,081 patients for whom adequate follow-up was available, primary tumors recurred in 2.8% and second primary tumors occurred in 4.3% annually. The rate of second primary tumor development was higher among patients with stage II HNSCC than among patients with stage I HNSCC. In addition, active smokers had a significantly higher recurrence rate compared with former smokers and never smokers (3.7% vs 2.2% vs 2.4%). This prospective study demonstrated for the first time the impact of active smoking status on recurrence of second primary tumors.

An intergroup trial utilizing low-dose 13-cRA (30 mg/day) to prevent second primary tumors in patients who underwent successful resection of stage I NSCLC found that 13-cRA was associated with no improvement in rates of second primary tumors, recurrence, or mortality and was possibly harmful in current smokers and beneficial in never smokers.

An ongoing randomized, placebo-controlled trial at M. D. Anderson is studying the toxicity and efficacy of treatment with 13-cRA plus α-tocopherol and 9-*cis*-retinoic acid in former smokers. All patients undergo a standard bronchoscopy with endobronchial biopsies done at 6 predetermined sites. The patients are treated for 3 months and then have another biopsy.

In a trial involving patients with a previously resected stage I NSCLC, retinyl palmitate was shown to decrease the incidence of second primary tumors (Pastorino et al, 1993) (for details on this trial, see the section Prevention with Retinoids later in this chapter). However, trials of retinyl palmitate that have evaluated the reversal of intermediate end points, such as sputum atypia, have failed to show any improvement. In addition, randomized trials of retinoids in subjects with squamous metaplasia have yet to demonstrate that treatment with these agents produces a significant response.

β-Carotene

β-Carotene has been clinically evaluated more extensively than any other carotenoid. β-Carotene is present as a nutrient in many fruits and vegetables. It has antioxidant activity and can stimulate immune function. Original epidemiologic data showed a deficiency of or low levels of β-carotene in patients with lung cancer, and animal models clearly document that β-carotene protects against tumorigenesis. However, clinical trials involving supplementation with pharmacologic doses of β-carotene have produced counterintuitive results.

Surprisingly, in 2 large randomized studies, active smokers who received supplemental β-carotene demonstrated an increased incidence of lung cancer and a higher likelihood of dying of lung cancer compared with active smokers who did not receive this carotenoid (ATBC Cancer Prevention Study Group, 1994; Omenn et al, 1996). (Details of these studies are given in the section Primary Prevention in High-Risk Groups later in this chapter.) Several theories exist to explain this phenomenon, but the cause is still uncertain. One theory proposes that under conditions of highly oxidative stress, such as exist in the lungs of active smokers, β-carotene may display pro-oxidant capacities.

As a result of the increased incidence of lung cancer (and of lung cancer–related death) seen in these randomized trials, all clinical trials of β-carotene in active smokers have been halted.

α-Tocopherol

α-Tocopherol is also a putative antioxidant and has been shown to have an inhibitory effect on the growth of normal smooth muscle cells as well as an antiproliferative effect on malignant cell lines in vitro. Recent epidemiologic data, however, failed to show a significant association between α-tocopherol and lung cancer. The efficacy of α-tocopherol in the chemoprevention of lung cancer has not been demonstrated in clinical studies performed to date, but more adequately powered studies are needed. In limited studies, α-tocopherol has been shown to have a possible preventive effect on other cancers.

Selenium

Selenium is a component of glutathione peroxidase, an oxidative enzyme that was first recognized as an essential trace element more than 40 years ago. Epidemiologic data suggest an inverse relationship between selenium intake and lung cancer. A 1991 U.S. study comparing the relationship between cancer mortality rates and environmental selenium levels in forage crops by county showed that mortality rates for all cancers were significantly lower in counties with intermediate or high selenium levels. Shamberger and Frost first proposed selenium's role in cancer prevention in 1969. Since then, further research in animal studies has shown that selenium compounds can inhibit and retard carcinogenesis at higher dose levels.

While studies have shown that high levels of natural selenium are associated with significant hepatotoxic effects—a finding that has limited research efforts—synthetic organoselenium compounds have been reported to be effective and less toxic chemopreventive agents in laboratory animals. The synthetic compound 1,4-phenylenebis(methylene)selenocyanate is one of several synthetic compounds that have shown efficacy in inhibiting lung tumors in laboratory animals.

A major clinical trial by Clark and colleagues attempted to determine whether a nutritional supplement of selenium would decrease the incidence of basal cell and squamous cell carcinomas of the skin (Clark et al, 1996). This multicenter, double-blind, randomized trial evaluated 1,312 patients aged 18 to 80 years who had a history of skin cancer. Patients were given 200 μg of selenium (in the form of a 0.5-g high-selenium brewer's dried yeast tablet) or placebo daily. Although selenium had no effect on skin cancer incidence, secondary end point analyses revealed that selenium supplementation was associated with a significantly lower incidence of nonskin cancer and with lower nonskin and overall cancer mortality rates. In addition, rates of lung cancer, prostate cancer, and colon cancer were all significantly reduced in patients in the selenium arm.

Other studies, however, have produced conflicting evidence regarding the benefit of selenium supplementation in preventing cancer. From the epidemiologic data, it is unclear whether selenium acts alone or as part of a combination of antioxidants.

These observations have led to an intergroup trial to study selenium in lung cancer. This randomized trial was launched in 2000 and is studying the effects of supplemental selenium in preventing second primary tumors in patients with stage I NSCLC (T1N0M0 and T2N0M0). The target accrual is more than 2,000 patients. It is hoped that this study will define a possible role for selenium in lung cancer chemoprevention.

Further drug development and large prospective clinical trials are necessary to confirm selenium's role in the chemoprevention of lung cancer. Only then can public health recommendations regarding selenium supplementation be made.

Lipoxygenase Inhibitors

Eicosanoids, which are formed when lipoxygenases combine with arachidonic acid, are thought to play a role in tumor promotion, tumor progression, and metastatic disease. The eicosanoids include prostaglandins, leukotrienes, thromboxanes, and hydroxyeicosatetraenoic acids (HETEs).

Studies of cancer cells show that lipoxygenase inhibitors, which combine with lipoxygenase and thereby prevent its substrate-enzyme combination with arachidonic acid and the formation of eicosanoids, have a chemopreventive effect in animal models of lung cancer.

Lipoxygenase metabolites such as leukotrienes and HETEs have been shown to be associated with lung cancer growth, and 5-lipoxygenase mRNA has been found to be overexpressed in lung cancer tissue. Studies in human lung cancer cell lines found that 5-lipoxygenase is stimulated by the autocrine growth factors gastrin-releasing peptide and insulin-like growth factor, which have also been found to stimulate production of 5-HETE. 5-HETE stimulated proliferation in cancer cells, but treatment of these same cells with lipoxygenase inhibitors decreased proliferation. Furthermore, studies in animals showed that lipoxygenase inhibitors significantly reduced the multiplicity of NNK-induced tumors in strains of A/J mice.

Clinical trials have shown a chemopreventive effect of lipoxygenase inhibitors in other tumor types, but at this writing, no clinical data exist regarding the utility of lipoxygenase inhibitors in the prevention of aerodigestive-tract malignancies.

Cyclooxygenase Inhibitors

COX-1 and COX-2 are enzymes involved in the conversion of arachidonic acid to prostaglandins. Physiologic functions of COX-1 include platelet thromboxane production, cytoprotection of the stomach, and renal vasodilation. COX-2 has a role in inflammation that has been linked to carcinogenesis.

Studies of COX inhibitors in lung cancer have been limited, but the National Health and Nutrition Examination Survey found that aspirin was associated with a statistically lower risk of lung cancer (Schreinemachers and Everson, 1994). Two COX genes have been cloned—COX-1 and COX-2. These genes have similar enzymatic activities as well as more than 60% amino acid homology. A recent study demonstrated expression of COX-2 in normal bronchial epithelial cells, type I and II pneumocytes, smooth muscle cells, vascular endothelial cells, and inflammatory mononuclear cells (Hida et al, 1998). Substantially increased expression of COX-2 was seen in 70% of adenocarcinomas of the lung, with only a fraction of small cell lung cancers and squamous cell carcinomas expressing COX-2. COX-2 expression was upregulated in a proportion of premalignant lung lesions as well. Further, COX-2 protein expression was detected in precursors of lung carcinomas (Hida et al, 1998). Interestingly, in a separate study (Mestre et al, 1997), retinoid treatment of human oral squamous carcinoma cells suppressed basal levels of COX-2 and epidermal growth factor–mediated and phorbol ester–mediated induction of COX-2 protein.

With the advent of selective COX-2 inhibitors, clinical trials exploring the role of these agents in the chemoprevention of aerodigestive-tract cancers may soon be at hand. At M.D. Anderson, we are planning to perform a randomized, placebo-controlled phase II clinical trial in current and former smokers, examining the effect of COX-2 inhibition on biomarkers of lung cancer risk and COX-2–dependent signaling pathways. After bronchoscopy, patients will be treated with celecoxib or placebo for 3 months and observed for an additional 3 months. We will study the effect of celecoxib treatment on lung tissue and arachidonic acid metabolites in the bronchial epithelium of current and former smokers. Trials such as these will help define the role of COX-2 inhibition in the prevention of lung cancer in high-risk patients.

Green Tea

Green tea has generated significant interest as a potential chemopreventive agent. Around the world, tea is the most widely consumed beverage after water. Tea is derived from the plant *Camilla sinensis* and is processed as black tea (78%), green tea (20%), or oolong tea (2%). Western countries consume more black tea, whereas Asian countries consume more green tea. Unlike green tea, black tea is fermented. It has been hypothesized that the low lung cancer incidence in Japan, where the prevalence of smoking is high, can be attributed to the consumption of green tea.

Green tea contains antioxidants called polyphenols. One third to one half of green tea is made up of a combination of catechins and flavonols. The major catechins include epicatechin, (-)-epicatechin-3-gallate, (-)-epigallocatechin, and (-)-epigallocatechin-3-gallate, the primary component. There is about 300 to 400 mg of polyphenols in one cup (8 ounces) of green tea.

Lung cancer chemoprevention trials with green tea have been limited by problems with patient recall. In 2 studies, evaluations were based on patient interviews and questionnaires, and the precise amounts of green tea ingested could not be quantified. One trial showed an inverse relationship and the other showed a positive relationship between green tea consumption and lung cancer incidence. A third study measured frequencies of sister-chromatid exchange in mitogen-stimulated peripheral lymphocytes of smokers, nonsmokers, smokers who consumed green tea, and smokers who consumed coffee. Results showed high rates of sister-chromatid exchange in smokers but similarly lower rates of sister-chromatid exchange in both smokers who consumed green tea and nonsmokers, implying a benefit of green tea for smokers.

In a recently completed phase I trial conducted at M. D. Anderson, the effect of green tea extract was studied in 49 patients with solid tumors (Pisters et al, 2001). Side effects were mild, and no responses were seen. Ten patients with stable disease completed 6 months of treatment with green tea extract. Further investigations are needed to clarify the efficacy of green tea in lung cancer chemoprevention.

Major Chemoprevention Trials in Lung Cancer

Several major lung cancer chemoprevention trials have been conducted. These trials have focused on β-carotene, α-tocopherol, selenium, and vitamin A because epidemiologic studies have indicated lower rates of lung cancer in individuals with high serum levels of these agents.

Methodologic Issues

When lung cancer incidence is used as the end point in lung cancer chemoprevention trials, these trials take years to complete. Conducting trials in populations with a high risk of lung cancer can help shorten the time needed before any effect is seen. One such population would be patients cured of small cell lung cancer, in whom the rate of second primary tumors is twice as high as the rate in patients treated for early-stage head and neck cancer or lung cancer.

Primary Prevention in High-Risk Groups

The α-tocopherol, β-carotene (ATBC) cancer prevention study (ATBC Cancer Prevention Study Group, 1994) was a randomized, double-blind, placebo-controlled primary-prevention trial in which 29,133 Finnish male smokers received either α-tocopherol (50 mg/day) alone, β-carotene (20 mg/day) alone, both α-tocopherol and β-carotene, or a placebo. The men were between 50 and 69 years of age, and all smoked 5 or more cigarettes per day. Patients were followed up for 5 to 8 years. Lung cancer incidence, the primary end point, did not change with the addition of α-tocopherol alone, nor did the overall mortality rate. However, both groups that received β-carotene supplementation (alone or with α-tocopherol) had an 18% increase in the incidence of lung cancer. There appeared to be a stronger adverse effect from β-carotene in the men who smoked more than 20 cigarettes a day. This trial raised the serious issue that pharmacologic doses of β-carotene could be harmful in active smokers.

The β-carotene and retinol efficacy trial (CARET) (Omenn et al, 1996) confirmed the results of the ATBC trial. CARET was a randomized, double-blind, placebo-controlled trial that tested the combination of 30 mg of β-carotene and 25,000 IU of retinyl palmitate against placebo in 18,314 men and women aged 50 to 69 years who were at high risk for lung cancer. The majority of the participants (14,254) had a smoking history of at least 20 pack-years and were either current smokers or recent ex-smokers. The remaining participants (4,060 men) were deemed to be at high risk for lung cancer because of extensive occupational exposure to asbestos. Lung cancer incidence was the primary end point. This trial was stopped after 21 months because there was no evidence of benefit from chemopreventive therapy but there was a 28% increase in lung cancer incidence in the active-intervention group. The overall lung cancer mortality rate increased 17% in this group.

Subgroup analysis of the ATBC study and CARET has provided few explanations for the increase in lung cancer incidence in participants receiving β-carotene. It seems that β-carotene has a harmful effect only in heavy smokers or those with previous exposure to asbestos. Current recommendations call for these people to avoid large doses of supplemental β-carotene.

The Physicians Health Study, a randomized, double-blind, placebo-controlled trial, studied 22,071 healthy male physicians (Hennekans et al, 1996). About half of them (11,036) received 50 mg of β-carotene on alternate days, and the other 11,035 men received placebos. The use of supplemental β-carotene had virtually no effect on lung cancer incidence or lung cancer–related mortality during a 12-year follow-up period.

In China, a study evaluating β-carotene, α-tocopherol, and selenium in the prevention of gastric and esophageal cancer showed a nonsignificant decrease in the risk of lung cancer in a small group of patients (Li et al, 1993).

Prevention of Second Primary Tumors

Prevention with Retinoids.   Several studies have investigated the chemo-preventive effect of retinoids in patients with resected NSCLC. No firm conclusions can be made regarding retinoids in lung cancer on the basis of the trials completed to date.

In one trial (Pastorini et al, 1993), 307 patients with completely resected stage I NSCLC were randomly assigned to receive 12 months of treatment with retinyl palmitate (300,000 IU per day) or no treatment. At a median follow-up time of 46 months, patients who received retinyl palmitate had a 35% lower incidence of second primary tumors (3.1% vs 4.8%, $P = .045$). As in studies in patients with head and neck cancer, retinoid treatment had no effect on survival duration or the rate of recurrence of initial primary tumors.

In the EUROSCAN study, 2,592 patients—60% with a history of head and neck cancer and 40% with a history of lung cancer—were randomly assigned to receive supplementation with retinyl palmitate, N-acetylcys-teine, both drugs in combination, or placebo for 2 years (van Zandwijk et al, 2000). Patients were divided into 2 groups: current and former smokers (93.5%) and never smokers (6.5%). The study found no benefit of chemo-preventive agents in terms of survival, event-free survival, or second primary tumors. However, the authors did not verify smoking status through measurement of urine cotinine levels, and the authors did not present information about the impact of smoking status on second primary tumors and recurrence.

US-Intergroup trial NCI 91–0001, a randomized, double-blind study of low-dose 13-cRA after complete resection of stage I NSCLC, completed accrual in April 1997 with 1,486 participants (Lippman et al, 2001). The study objectives included evaluating the efficacy of 13-cRA in reducing the incidence of second primary tumors, determining the qualitative and quantitative toxicity of daily low-dose 13-cRA treatment, and comparing the overall survival rates of patients receiving 13-cRA and those receiving a placebo. Patients were required to have complete resection of primary stage I NSCLC (postoperative disease stage of T1 or T2N0) 6 weeks to 3 years prior to registering. At this writing, a total of 1,166 randomized, eligible patients have been followed for a median of 3.5 years. There were no significant differences between the arms with respect to mortality, recurrences, or second primary tumors. However, subset analyses suggested that 13-cRA was harmful in current smokers and beneficial in never smokers.

The effects of various retinoids in patients with resected NSCLC need to be further investigated.

Prevention with Selenium.   Selenium is also being studied for prevention of second primary tumors. An ongoing Eastern Cooperative Oncology Group trial is studying the effect of daily selenium supplementation in patients with stage I lung cancer.

Potential New Molecular Targets

Understanding of lung tumorigenesis at the molecular level opens the way for new natural or synthetic agents to be developed that can interrupt this process and prevent tumor recurrence. Understanding of lung tumorigenesis at the molecular level also provides investigators with biomarkers that can be used as markers of high risk for the development of lung cancer and as intermediate markers of response to treatment. This section will discuss some of the genes and proteins known or believed to play a role in lung tumorigenesis and describe how knowledge of these genes and proteins has been translated—or may be translated in the future—into new chemopreventive therapies.

Retinoic Acid Receptor-β

Evidence is increasing that retinoids and their nuclear receptors are important in modulating differentiation of malignant cells and suppressing progression of premalignant lesions to malignant ones by redirecting differentiation. Retinoic acid receptor-β (RAR-β) expression may serve as a useful intermediate marker in lung carcinogenesis.

Multiple researchers have demonstrated abnormal expression of RAR-β in head and neck cancer and lung cancer. Further studies, by Lotan and colleagues, showed that RAR-β mRNA expression increased in 18 of 22 patients with oral premalignant lesions that responded clinically to 13-cRA compared with 8 of 17 patients with oral premalignant lesions that did not respond to 13-cRA as assayed by in situ hybridization ($P = .04$) (Lotan et al, 1995b).

Analysis of lung tissue specimens—including specimens of normal, metaplastic, dysplastic, and neoplastic tissue and tissue from the margins of resected lung cancer specimens—showed that RAR-β was not detected in 50% of dysplastic tissues and in more than 50% of lung adenocarcinomas and squamous cell carcinomas (Lotan et al, 1995a). In addition, RAR-γ and retinoic X receptor-β have been found to be underexpressed in NSCLC in vivo. Decreased RAR-β expression is observed in histologically normal bronchial epithelium at the margins of resection of lung tumors.

A randomized study testing 4-hydroxyphenylretinamide in chronic smokers with bronchial metaplasia or dysplasia showed no effect on RAR-β expression (Kurie et al, 2000). In another trial testing 13-cRA versus placebo in active smokers with bronchial metaplasia, 13-cRA did not increase reversal of metaplasia or dysplasia as compared with results in the placebo arm (Khuri et al, 2001b). However, among volunteers who quit smoking, treatment with 13-cRA induced expression of RAR-β in patients with bronchial metaplasia and dysplasia.

Another study (Xu et al, 1999) tested the effect of 13-cRA on RAR-β expression in the bronchial epithelium of 68 chronic smokers. In this study, 6 months of treatment with 13-cRA (1 mg/kg/day) resulted in increased RAR-β expression independent of current smoking status or reversal of squamous metaplasia, indicating that RAR-β may indeed serve as an intermediate biomarker in aerodigestive cancers. Ayoub and colleagues verified these findings by sampling bronchial brushings and measuring RAR-β activity in 188 patients who were chronic smokers (Ayoub et al, 1999). Patients with low RAR-β expression were randomly assigned to receive 13-cRA (30 mg/day) or a placebo. RAR-β was again demonstrated to be upregulated with retinoid treatment, confirming the findings of the earlier study. Interestingly, in a subgroup of 40 patients in whom palatal brushings were obtained in addition to bronchial brushings, 27 patients had similar RAR-β expression in palatal and bronchial brushings.

Although most of the available evidence regarding RAR-β is consistent with the notion that low RAR-β expression is associated with poor prognosis, not all the studies to date support this conclusion. Khuri and colleagues conducted a retrospective analysis in which the relationship between RAR-β mRNA expression and prognosis was examined in 158 cases of pathologic stage I NSCLC (Khuri et al, 2000). Surprisingly, strongly positive RAR-β expression, compared with lack of RAR-β expression, denoted poorer prognosis with respect to overall and 5-year survival rates. Thus, strong intratumoral expression of RAR-β may indicate a poor prognosis for patients with stage I NSCLC.

Further research is needed to clarify the relationship between RAR-β expression and prognosis and the role of RAR-β expression as an intermediate biomarker in patients with lung cancer.

p53

The *p53* tumor suppressor gene has been mapped to the short arm of chromosome 17 (17p13). Point mutations that inactivate this tumor suppressor gene remove important cell-cycle regulatory constraints and regulation of apoptosis, contributing to accelerated cancer growth. *p53* mutations are the most frequent genetic alteration in lung cancer. *p53* mutations may serve as early indicators of lung cancer development. Gene therapy to restore normal *p53* gene function and cytotoxic therapy designed to specifically target cells with mutant *p53*—approaches currently being studied in the treatment of existing malignancy—may one day prove to be useful chemoprevention approaches.

Immunohistochemical studies of the aerodigestive tract have detected overexpression of *p53* in regions of premalignant dysplasia and carcinoma in situ but no overexpression of *p53* in normal bronchial mucosa. Of note, *p53* mutations have been found adjacent to primary tumors as well as in distant locations in the aerodigestive tract, which supports the field cancerization concept. This suggests that genetic damage resulting in p53 protein accumulation and possibly *p53* gene mutation may be an early event in lung carcinogenesis, preceding lung cancer invasion. Thus, mutant p53 protein may be a good target marker for early cancer detection.

In some patients with cancer, mutated *p53* can mount a humoral response to abnormal levels of the protein. Screening patients at high risk for lung cancer for the presence of anti-p53 antibodies in the serum may serve as a biomarker for early lung cancer detection.

Studies of p53 and retinoids have been performed in oral premalignant lesions. The level of p53 protein detected correlated with increased histologic progression of the lesions. However, *p53* expression was not affected by treatment with 13-cRA, and there was no correlation between p53 protein accumulation and retinoid resistance, making the mechanism of resistance unclear. Future gene therapy strategies in combination with other treatment modalities may hold answers to these puzzles.

Restoration of normal *p53* gene function using gene therapy is being studied in clinical trials as a potential treatment for lung cancer. Direct injection of a retroviral vector with wild-type *p53* has proved to be successful in a limited number of patients; in these patients, induction of apoptosis was more frequent in posttherapy than in pretherapy tissue samples. Future treatment approaches may include intrabronchial aerosol delivery of *p53* and T cell–mediated immunotherapy against mutant *p53*.

Several methods have been developed targeting the *p53* gene and p53 protein to halt or reverse the process of tumorigenesis and metastasis. ONYX-015 is an adenovirus with the 55-kD *E1B* gene deleted, which replicates and causes certain cancer cells to die. Although preclinical in vitro results have varied, clinical data with ONYX-015 have been definitive. Selective intratumoral replication and tumor-selective tissue destruction have been documented in phase I and II clinical trials of ONYX-015 in patients with recurrent, refractory HNSCC. However, durable responses and clinical benefit were seen in fewer than 15% of these patients. A multicenter phase II trial undertaken in 1997 showed that ONYX-015 in combination with chemotherapy resulted in more durable responses than those seen with chemotherapy alone in patients with recurrent HNSCC. The efficacy of ONYX-015 in combination with chemotherapy has led to the launching of a phase III trial comparing the combination of cisplatin and fluorouracil with ONYX-015 versus the same chemotherapy alone.

These studies of various treatment approaches in patients with *p53* mutations may lead one day to the creation of chemoprevention strategies for patients with similar molecular defects.

RAS

RAS genes are mutated in approximately 30% of lung adenocarcinomas, and mutated *RAS* genes can be found in premalignant lesions in smokers. Activation is due to a point mutation. Mutations in k-*ras* predict a poorer prognosis in both early-stage and late-stage NSCLC. Eventually, the signal cascade activates nuclear proto-oncogene products such as those generated by the *MYC* genes.

Farnesyl transferase inhibitors (FTIs) are a novel class of compounds that inhibit a critical enzymatic step in the constitutive expression of mutated *RAS* genes. In preclinical studies utilizing HNSCC cell lines and NSCLC cell lines, SCH66336, a novel tricyclic peptidomimetic compound designed by Schering-Plough, appears to have extensive activity. Other FTIs have been developed and are being tested in the clinical setting (e.g., R115777, Janssen Pharmaceutica, Inc.)

Preclinical data from Moasser and colleagues had indicated that the addition of FTIs to either paclitaxel or epothilones was able to overcome acquired resistance to these tubulin toxins in a variety of different cancer cell lines (Moasser et al, 1998). We reported results of a phase I trial of SCH66336 in combination with paclitaxel in adults with solid tumors (Kim et al, 2001). Patients received paclitaxel at doses ranging from 135 mg/m^2 to 175 mg/m^2 in combination with oral SCH66336, which was started 7 days prior to the paclitaxel, at doses ranging from 100 mg twice daily to 150 mg twice daily. The maximum tolerated dose was found to be 175 mg/m^2 of paclitaxel every 3 weeks with SCH66336 at 100 mg twice daily. Of 24 patients, 21 were evaluable for assessment for response and toxicity. Side effects were acceptable, with the dose-limiting side effects being neutropenic fever and, occasionally, grade 3 diarrhea. Responses were quite striking: 8 (38%) of 21 evaluable patients had a major confirmed response, and only 5 of 21 patients had disease progression by cycle 3 of combination therapy. Responses were seen in NSCLC, HNSCC, and various salivary gland tumors, with 1 individual having stable disease for a total of 24 cycles of therapy encompassing 19 months.

Given the promising results with FTIs in lung cancer treatment and their mild toxicity profile, we are planning a multi-institutional, randomized, double-blind, placebo-controlled chemoprevention trial utilizing the FTI R115777 in patients at high risk for the development of lung cancer. To be eligible for the trial, patients must have undergone definitive treatment for a tobacco-related cancer, must have a smoking history of at least 30 pack-years, and must have evidence of sputum atypia. After a baseline bronchoscopy, patients will take study medication for 6 months and will then be observed for 6 months. We will evaluate bronchial histologic changes in precancerous areas and changes in Ki-67 expression in response to treatment. This trial is planned to begin accrual in late 2001.

Epidermal Growth Factor Receptor

Epidermal growth factor receptor (EGFR/erbB-1) is part of the erbB family of receptor tyrosine kinases, which also includes erbB-2, erbB-3, and erbB-4. The erbB family members can form either homodimers or heterodimers upon ligand binding to the cytoplasmic domain of the receptors, which can lead to phosphorylation of the tyrosine residues and further activation of the downstream signal transduction pathways, including *ras*/mitogen-activated protein kinase, phosphatidylinositol-3 kinase, and STAT-3. The signal transduction pathway can lead to tumor cell proliferation as well as invasion and metastasis.

Overexpression of EGFR has been observed in a variety of human cancers, including breast, ovarian, prostate, bladder, lung, brain, and pancreas. In HNSCC, EGFR expression is reported in approximately 90% of specimens and is associated with a poor prognosis. Therefore, a number of strategies to block or downregulate EGFR have been developed in an effort to inhibit tumor proliferation and improve overall clinical outcome.

Kurie and colleagues reported that increased EGFR expression in bronchial metaplasia, although it was a potential biomarker for lung carcinogenesis, did not significantly contribute to histologic evaluation of response to retinoids (Kurie et al, 1996). erbB-2 is highly expressed in 10% to 15% of NSCLCs and appears to correlate with shorter survival time in lung cancer. These receptor tyrosine kinases send signals to the guanosine triphosphate–binding RAS protein, which in turn transmits information to effectors downstream.

Strategies targeting lung cancer include the use of tyrosine kinase inhibitors and monoclonal antibodies to EGFR. C225 (cetuximab), a monoclonal antibody to EGFR, has been shown to be highly specific for the receptor in inhibiting the growth of human tumor xenografts in nude mice. Furthermore, the anti-EGFR monoclonal antibodies appear to enhance the antitumor efficacy of chemotherapy agents, such as cisplatin and doxorubicin, as well as the in vitro radiosensitivity of HNSCC cells. Phase I/II studies of anti-EGFR monoclonal antibodies in various solid tumors—including HNSCC, NSCLC, and colorectal cancer—have shown encouraging results.

ZD1839 (Iressa), a selective EGFR tyrosine kinase inhibitor aimed at inhibiting signal transduction, is currently under clinical investigation. Phase I clinical trials have confirmed that ZD1839 given as a single agent has predictable, reversible mechanism-based, significant antitumor activity with only mild toxicity. Preclinically, ZD1839 also appears to potentiate the antitumor and apoptotic effects of several cytotoxic agents, including the platinums and taxanes, against a number of human tumor xenografts, including NSCLC, vulvar cancer, and prostate cancer. Because of the efficacy and acceptable toxicity profile observed in phase I trials, particularly in NSCLC, ZD1839 is currently being studied in phase III clinical trials for the treatment of advanced NSCLC.

At M.D. Anderson, we are currently planning a multi-institutional, randomized, double-blind, placebo-controlled chemoprevention trial utilizing ZD1839 in patients at high risk for the development of lung cancer. To be eligible for the trial, patients must have undergone definitive treatment for a tobacco-related cancer, must have a smoking history of at least 30 pack-years, and must have evidence of sputum atypia. After a baseline bronchoscopy, patients will take study medication for 6 months and will then be observed for 6 months. We will evaluate bronchial histologic changes in precancerous areas and changes in Ki-67 expression in response to treatment. This trial is planned to begin accrual in late 2001.

Future Directions in Lung Cancer Chemoprevention

The future of lung cancer chemoprevention remains open to innovation. The mechanisms underlying lung tumorigenesis are becoming better understood. Thus, novel chemopreventive agents will continue to be investigated in an ongoing attempt to prevent the development of lung cancer and thus reduce mortality from this disease. Basic translational research combining molecular markers and novel chemical agents in the clinical setting is truly the future direction of chemoprevention. Efforts are ongoing to find molecular markers that can be used to identify patients at high risk and thus permit more specific targeting of chemoprevention efforts. With targeting of high-risk patients and with improvements in side effect profiles that lead to better compliance, chemoprevention may have a profound impact on the prevention of lung cancer.

Large prevention trials are necessary to provide definitive evidence that will spur enactment of new antitobacco health policies. However, such large trials are expensive, and problems with compliance among the participants are frequent. In addition, such studies take years to complete. The identification of biomarkers that can be used as intermediate end points of efficacy may help allay costs and allow easier and earlier assessment of treatment effectiveness.

Because tobacco use remains the single most prevalent cause of lung cancer, smoking prevention and cessation campaigns need to continue.

SCREENING FOR EARLY DETECTION OF LUNG CANCER

Given the disappointing results to date of clinical trials of NSCLC prevention strategies, early detection of NSCLC, when the disease is most likely to be curable, is now of great interest. Methods of early detection studied to date include chest radiography and, more recently, spiral CT and positron emission tomography.

KEY PRACTICE POINTS

- Smoking prevention and smoking cessation interventions remain essential in the prevention of lung cancer.
- Patients with a history of heavy smoking (> than 30 pack-years) may be at increased risk for developing lung cancer.
- Patients with a history of a definitively treated early-stage lung or head and neck cancer are at increased risk for the development of second primary tumors.
- Patients with a history of heavy smoking or prior tobacco-related cancers should seek clinical trials of potential chemopreventive agents.
- Active smokers and people with a history of exposure to asbestos should avoid large doses of supplemental β-carotene.
- Plans are under way to test novel biological agents, including inhibitors of ras, EGFR, and COX, in chemoprevention trials.
- Preliminary studies indicate that spiral CT may have utility in the early detection of lung cancer; however, further investigation is needed.

Spiral Computed Tomography

Recent studies have tested the efficacy of screening individuals at high risk for lung cancer with spiral CT. The results, while provocative, are not yet definitive, and debate continues as to whether they are sufficient to mandate broad lung cancer screening programs.

The Early Lung Cancer Action Project is a US study that uses chest radiography and low-dose spiral CT to screen individuals at high risk for lung cancer. In 1999, investigators reported the results of baseline screening in 1,000 asymptomatic smokers or former smokers who had smoked at least 1 pack of cigarettes per day for 10 years or 2 packs per day for 5 years (Henschke et al, 1999). All participants were 60 years of age or older. All participants underwent chest radiography and low-dose spiral CT. CT detected 1 to 6 noncalcified pulmonary nodules in 233 patients (23%), while chest radiography detected 1 to 6 calcified nodules in 68 patients (7%). Twenty-seven (11%) of the 233 CT-detected lesions were malignant, compared with 7 (10%) of the 68 lesions detected with chest radiography. Twenty-three of the 27 CT-detected tumors and 4 of the 7 radiography-detected tumors were early-stage.

The Anti-Lung Cancer Association is a Japanese program that has screened 1,669 patients at high risk for lung cancer with annual spiral CT scans (Kaneko et al, 2000). This program found that CT was superior to chest radiography in the detection of smaller, peripheral lung cancers.

In 1,000 patients, 27 lung cancers were detected with CT, 23 of which were early stage, and 7 lung cancers were detected with chest radiography, 4 of which were early stage.

Although these studies show the potential promise of spiral CT in screening patients at high risk for lung cancer, additional trials will be needed before routine CT scanning in patients at risk can be deemed effective.

Positron Emission Tomography

Positron emission tomography scanning is increasingly being used in the staging of various cancers. Its role in screening for early detection of lung cancer, however, has not been defined.

SUGGESTED READINGS

Adler I. Primary Malignant Growths of the Lung and Bronchi: A Pathological and Clinical Study. London, England: Longmans, Green; 1912.

Alpha-Tocopherol, Beta Carotene Cancer Prevention Study Group. The effect of vitamin E and beta carotene on the incidence of lung cancer and other cancers in male smokers. *N Engl J Med* 1994;330:1029–1035.

Auerbach O, Gere JB, Forman JB, et al. Changes in the bronchial epithelium in relation to smoking and cancer of the lung. *N Engl J Med* 1957;256:98–104.

Ayoub J, Jean-Francois R, Cormier Y, et al. Placebo-controlled trial of 13-cis-retinoic acid activity on retinoic acid receptor-beta expression in a population at high risk: implications for chemoprevention of lung cancer. *J Clin Oncol* 1999;17:3546–3552.

Benner SE, Pajak TF, Lippman SM, et al. Prevention of second primary tumors with isotretinoin in patients with squamous cell carcinoma of the head and neck: long-term follow-up. *J Natl Cancer Inst* 1994;86:140–141.

Clark LC, Combs GF Jr, Turnbull BW, et al. Effects of selenium supplementation for cancer prevention in patients with carcinoma of the skin. A randomized controlled trial. Nutritional Prevention of Cancer Study Group. *JAMA* 1996;276:1957–1963.

Hennekans CH, Buring JE, Manson JE, et al. Lack of effect of long-term supplementation with beta-carotene on the incidence of malignant neoplasms and cardiovascular disease. *N Engl J Med* 1996;334:1145–1149.

Henschke CI, McCauley DI, Yankelevitz DF, et al. Early Lung Cancer Action Project: overall design and findings from baseline screening. *Lancet* 1999; 354:99–105.

Hida T, Yatabe Y, Achiwa H, et al. Increased expression of cyclooxygenase 2 occurs frequently in human lung cancers, specifically in adenocarcinomas. *Cancer Res* 1998;58:3761–3764.

Hong WK, Endicott J, Itri LM, et al. 13-cis-retinoic acid in the treatment of oral leukoplakia. *N Engl J Med* 1986;315:1501–1505.

Hong WK, Lippman SM, Itri LM, et al. Prevention of second primary tumors with isotretinoin in squamous-cell carcinoma of the head and neck. *N Engl J Med* 1990;323:795–801.

Hong WK, Spitz MR, Lippman SM. Cancer chemoprevention in the 21st century: genetics, risk modeling, and molecular targets. *J Clin Oncol* 2000;18(suppl 21):9s-18s.

Hong WK, Sporn MB. Recent advances in chemoprevention of cancer. *Science* 1997;278:1073–1077.

Hurt RD, Sachs DP, Glover ED, et al. A comparison of sustained-release bupropion and placebo for smoking cessation. *N Engl J Med* 1997;337:1195–1202.

Jorenby DE, Leischow SJ, Nides MA, et al. A controlled trial of sustained-release bupropion, a nicotine patch, or both for smoking cessation. *N Engl J Med* 1999;340:685–691.

Kaneko M, Kusumoto M, Kobayashi T, et al. Computed tomography screening for lung carcinoma in Japan. *Cancer* 2000;89(11 suppl):2485–2488.

Khuri FR, Kim ES, Lee JJ, et al. The impact of smoking status, disease stage, and index tumor site on second primary tumor incidence and tumor recurrence in the head and neck retinoid chemoprevention trial. *Cancer Epidemiol Biomarkers Prev* 2001a;10:823–829.

Khuri FR, Lee JS, Lippman SM, et al. Modulation of proliferating cell nuclear antigen in the bronchial epithelium of smokers. *Cancer Epidemiol Biomarkers Prev* 2001b;10:311–318.

Khuri FR, Lotan R, Kemp BL, et al. Retinoic acid receptor-beta as a prognostic indicator in stage I non-small-cell lung cancer. *J Clin Oncol* 2000;18:2798–2804.

Kim ES, Glisson BS, Meyers ML, et al. A phase I/II study of the farnesyl transferase inhibitor (FTI) SCH66336 with paclitaxel in patients with solid tumors [abstract]. *Proc Am Assoc Cancer Res* 2001;42. Abstract 2629.

Kim ES, Hong WK, Khuri FR. Prevention of lung cancer. The new millennium. *Chest Surg Clin N Am* 2000;10:663–690.

Kurie JM, Lee JS, Khuri FR, et al. N-(4-hydroxyphenyl)retinamide in the chemoprevention of squamous metaplasia and dysplasia of the bronchial epithelium. *Clin Cancer Res* 2000;6:2973–2979.

Kurie JM, Shin HJ, Lee JS, et al. Increased epidermal growth factor receptor expression in metaplastic bronchial epithelium. *Clin Cancer Res* 1996;2:1787–1793.

Li JY, Taylor PR, Li B, et al. Nutrition intervention trials in Linxian, China: multiple vitamin/mineral supplementation, cancer incidence, and disease-specific mortality among adults with esophageal dysplasia. *J Natl Cancer Inst* 1993;85:1492–1498.

Lippman SM, Lee JJ, Karp DD, et al. Randomized phase III intergroup trial of isotretinoin to prevent second primary tumors in stage I non-small-cell lung cancer. *J Natl Cancer Inst* 2001;93:605–618.

Lotan R, Sozzi G, Ro J, et al. Selective suppression of retinoic acid receptor beta (RAR beta) expression in squamous metaplasia, and in non-small cell lung cancers (NSCLC) compared to normal bronchial epithelium. *Proc Am Soc Clin Oncol* 1995a;14:165. Abstract 345.

Lotan R, Xu XC, Lippman SM, et al. Suppression of retinoic acid receptor-beta in premalignant oral lesions and its up-regulation by isotretinoin. *N Engl J Med* 1995b;332:1405–1410.

Mestre JR, Subbaramaiah K, Sacks PG, et al. Retinoids suppress epidermal growth factor-induced transcription of cyclooxygenase-2 in human oral squamous carcinoma cells. *Cancer Res* 1997;57:2890–2895.

Moasser MM, Sepp-Lorenzino L, Kohl NE, et al. Farnesyl transferase inhibitors cause enhanced mitotic sensitivity to Taxol and epothilones. *Proc Natl Acad Sci U S A* 1998;95:1369–1374.

Ochsner A, DeBakey M. Carcinoma of the lung. *Arch Surg* 1940;Dec:209–258.

Omenn GS, Goodman GE, Thornquist MD, et al. Effects of a combination of beta carotene and vitamin A on lung cancer and cardiovascular disease. *N Engl J Med* 1996;334:1150–1155.

Pastorino U, Infante M, Maioli M, et al. Adjuvant treatment of stage I lung cancer with high-dose vitamin A. *J Clin Oncol* 1993;11:1216–1222.

Patz EF Jr, Goodman PC, Bepler G. Screening for lung cancer. *N Engl J Med* 2000; 343:1627–1633.

Pisters KM, Newman RA, Coldman B, et al. Phase I trial of oral green tea extract in adult patients with solid tumors. *J Clin Oncol* 2001;19:1830–1838.

Schreinemachers DM, Everson RB. Aspirin use and lung, colon and breast cancer incidence in a prospective study. *Epidemiology* 1994;5:138–146.

Shamberger RJ, Frost DV. Possible protective effect of selenium against human cancer. *Can Med Assoc J* 1969;100:682.

Slebos RJ, Kibbelaar RE, Dalesio O, et al. K-ras oncogene activation as a prognostic marker in adenocarcinoma of the lung. *N Engl J Med* 1990;323:561–565.

Sporn MB. Approaches to prevention of epithelial cancer during the preneoplastic period. *Cancer Res* 1976;36:2699–2702.

US Department of Health and Human Services. *Reducing the Use of Tobacco: A Report of the Surgeon General*. Atlanta, Ga: US Department of Health and Human Services, Centers for Disease Control and Prevention, National Center for Chronic Disease Prevention and Health Promotion, Office on Smoking and Health; 2000.

van Zandwijk N, Dalesio O, Pastorino U, et al. EUROSCAN, a randomized trial of vitamin A and N-acetylcysteine in patients with head and neck cancer or lung cancer. For the European Organization for Research and Treatment of Cancer Head and Neck and Lung Cancer Cooperative Groups. *J Natl Cancer Inst* 2000;92:977–986.

Warren S, Gates O. Multiple primary malignant tumors: a survey of the literature and statistical study. *Am J Cancer* 1932;51:1358.

Xu XC, Lee JS, Lee JJ, et al. Nuclear retinoid acid receptor beta in bronchial epithelium of smokers before and during chemoprevention. *J Natl Cancer Inst* 1999;91:1317–1321.

15 MOLECULAR EVENTS IN LUNG CANCER AND IMPLICATIONS FOR PREVENTION AND THERAPY

Walter N. Hittelman, Jonathan M. Kurie,
and Stephen G. Swisher

Chapter Overview

Lung cancer development is thought to involve a multistep tumorigenesis process occurring in a field of carcinogenic exposure. The molecular events associated with lung cancer development involve genetic and epigenetic changes involving oncogenes, tumor suppressor genes, and regulatory genes that affect basic cellular processes, including growth, immortalization (escape from senescence), evasion from cell death, sustained angiogenesis, and the ability to take over the epithelium, invade, and metastasize. The process of lung cancer development is augmented by molecular changes that enhance genomic instability, especially in the setting of chronic exposure of the lung to carcinogens. Knowledge of the lung tumorigenesis pathway and direct measurement of these changes in lung tissue provide the opportunity to assess the risk of cancer in individuals exposed to carcinogens such as tobacco smoke, to directly examine the impact of chemopreventive treatments on the lungs, to aid in early detection, to assess prognosis in patients with established lung cancer, and potentially to identify the most appropriate treatment approach for an individual's tumor. Knowledge of the molecular attributes of lung tumors also provides the opportunity to develop therapies directly targeted to correcting defective cellular pathways, either through inhibition of dysregulated signaling or through replacement of defective genes. Molecular therapeutic approaches are now being used in the preventive setting as well as in the therapeutic setting in combination with surgery, radiation therapy, and chemotherapy.

Introduction

Lung cancer remains a major challenge in the world. Despite improvements in staging and the application and integration of surgery, radiation therapy, and chemotherapy, the 5-year survival rate for individuals with lung cancer remains around 15%. One reason for this low survival rate is that many lung cancers are detected at an advanced stage and thus are difficult to manage. Another reason for the low survival rate is the high frequency of second primary tumors in individuals definitively treated for a first primary lung tumor (i.e., about 2% per year in patients with non–small cell lung cancer and 4% to 6% per year in patients with small cell lung cancer). Progress toward decreasing the morbidity of lung cancer will depend on the development of new strategies for prevention, early detection, and treatment that are tailored specifically for this disease. The development of new strategies in turn will depend on a better understanding of the etiology and biology of lung cancer development and its response to intervention. Once this understanding is achieved, new strategies can be developed that specifically target basic processes important for lung cancer development and progression. The purpose of this chapter is to provide insight into the molecular etiology and biology of lung cancer development and to discuss how this information can be translated into targeted strategies for prevention and therapy.

MOLECULAR EPIDEMIOLOGY OF LUNG CANCER

Tobacco exposure, air pollution, and exposure to organic chemicals, metals, fibers, and radon are thought to be major etiologic factors for lung cancer. Chronic exposure to cigarette smoke is believed to be responsible for 90% of lung cancer cases, and lung cancer risk increases with smoking intensity and duration. For example, individuals with a 20-pack-year smoking history have an approximately 10% lifetime risk of developing lung cancer. While smoking cessation is thought to reduce lung cancer risk, the impact of cessation is not detectable until a few years after an individual stops smoking. Moreover, smoking cessation may ultimately reduce the relative cancer risk by only half. For this reason, more than 50% of new lung cancer cases arise in former smokers.

Cigarette smoke includes a complex mixture of more than 4,000 chemical compounds that are delivered to the lungs in both gas and tar phases. Of these, more than 40 have been identified as carcinogens. In some cases, the chemicals are procarcinogens (e.g., benzo(a)pyrene and nitrosamines) that need to be activated to induce DNA damage. In other cases, the compounds are directly reactive unless detoxified by the host. Molecular epidemiologic studies are beginning to identify intrinsic host factors that place some individuals, especially those with a history of chronic smoking, at increased lung cancer risk compared to others. Most intrinsic factors identified thus far reflect levels of carcinogen metabolism, DNA repair capabilities, and other measures of intrinsic cellular sensitivity to mutagens. In case-control studies that take tobacco exposure into account, these factors can provide statistically significant risk ratios—that is, their presence is found at higher frequencies in individuals with lung cancer than in matched controls. However, the detected risk ratios usually fall in the range of 1.5 to 10. In some cases, combinations of these risk factors are associated with risk ratios on the order of 30 to 40. While this is not sufficient for individualized clinical management decisions, it may be useful for identifying subgroups of individuals who might benefit from more intense and interventive strategies for risk determination.

The identification of intrinsic pathways that may influence carcinogen metabolism has led to preventive strategies geared to interfere with carcinogen activation and enhance detoxification of reactive intermediates. While preclinical models have suggested a number of potentially useful chemopreventive agents, some of which are found in the normal diet (e.g., fruit, cruciferous vegetables, nuts, garlic, and onion), none of these agents have so far shown an impact on lung cancer incidence in prospective prevention studies. Of concern, 2 studies suggested a potential increase in lung cancer incidence in individuals who continued to smoke while receiving beta-carotene. Thus, the balance of reactions that influence carcinogen metabolism may differ between current and former smokers, and this may need to be considered in the design of chemoprevention trials. Lung chemoprevention trials now ongoing at M. D. Anderson Cancer Center are aimed at identifying differences between current and former smokers in their response to different forms of chemopreventive intervention.

FIELD CANCERIZATION AND MULTISTEP LUNG TUMORIGENESIS

Lung tumor development has been proposed to reflect a "field cancerization" process whereby the whole tissue is exposed to carcinogenic insult (e.g., from tobacco smoke) and is at increased risk for multistep tumor development. Several types of clinical and laboratory data support this notion. First, from a clinical perspective, the field cancerization notion is supported by findings of synchronous primary lung tumors (frequently exhibiting dissimilar histologic features and distinct genetic signatures) and by the finding of an increased risk of second primary tumors in the same carcinogen-exposed field in individuals surviving a first aerodigestive tract cancer. Second, individuals with an increased risk for developing lung cancer (e.g., heavy smokers) often exhibit lesions in the lungs such as bronchial metaplasia or dysplasia or sputum cell abnormalities, and these lesions often arise at multiple sites within the carcinogen-exposed lung. Third, autopsy studies have demonstrated that 90% to 100% of tissue sections derived from the lungs of most light smokers, from all heavy smokers, and from individuals with lung cancer show evidence of epithelial change throughout the lung field, including loss of cilia, basal cell hyperplasia, and carcinoma in situ. The degree of histologic change correlates strongly with the extent of tobacco exposure. Fourth, biochemical, molecular, and cellular examination of lung tissue from current and former smokers with or without cancer demonstrates various types of genetic and epigenetic changes associated with carcinogen exposure, including the presence of DNA adducts, chromosome changes, gene mutations, gene amplification, gene deletions, and gene methylation. These changes can be detected throughout the exposed lung even though lung cancer typically develops at only one or several sites.

Lung cancer development is also thought to reflect a multistep tumorigenesis process whereby genetic changes accumulate over time and lead to the outgrowth of clonal cell populations within the lung exhibiting increasing hallmarks of tumorigenesis. Like field cancerization, the notion of multistep lung tumorigenesis is supported by a variety of clinical, histologic, and molecular studies. For example, in a classic study, Saccomano and colleagues evaluated serial sputum specimens from individuals at risk for lung cancer and found evidence for increasing degrees of histologic abnormalities over time (Saccomano et al, 1974). However, the rate of progression from premalignancy to cancer was highly variable from individual to individual.

Molecular Changes Associated with Lung Cancer Development

Molecular characterizations of lung tumors over the years have led to the identification of a number of types of genetic changes that occur frequently.

Oncogenes

The earliest genetic abnormalities discovered were genes that appeared to be associated with a gain of function and were termed oncogenes. When oncogenes are transfected into normal cells, they induce these cells to exhibit a tumor phenotype, such as the ability to grow in an anchorage-independent setting or to form tumors in nude mice. It was later discovered that oncogenes arise from changes in normal genes, which were termed proto-oncogenes. In some cases, the genetic change involves a mutation in the gene sequence such that the gene product becomes constitutively active. An example of this type of mutation is k-*ras* mutation, which is found in nearly 30% to 50% of lung adenocarcinomas and 15% to 20% of all non–small cell lung cancers but occurs rarely in small cell lung cancer. In other cases, the genetic changes are associated with gene amplification or gene translocation and enhanced expression of the gene product. An example of this type of change is *myc* gene amplification, which occurs in 15% to 30% of small cell lung carcinomas but in only 5% to 10% of non–small cell lung carcinomas. Other oncogenes frequently found to be altered in lung cancer include tyrosine kinase receptor genes, such as HER-2/*neu*; genes for growth signaling molecules, such as *raf*; phosphoinositide 3-kinase (PI3K); and growth-promoting genes, such as cyclin D1 and cyclin E.

Tumor Suppressor Genes

A second type of genetic change associated with lung cancer development involves changes in genes that are associated with loss of function and thus are called tumor suppressors. When tumor suppressor genes are transfected into tumor cells, they can reverse the tumor phenotype. These genes have been discovered through loss of heterozygosity (LOH) studies in which one chromosome allele is deleted from the genome and the remaining allele is deleted or inactivated through other mechanisms.

A prime example of a tumor suppressor is the *p53* gene, thought to be important in controlling cell growth and cell death in response to stress. The *p53* gene is mutated in more than 50% of lung cancers, and this is frequently accompanied by deletion of the wild-type allele. Importantly, it has been reported that the nature of the *p53* mutation reflects the type of carcinogen associated with lung cancer development. For example, the types of *p53* mutations found in individuals exposed to cigarette smoke are different from those found in individuals exposed to carcinogens such as radon or metals.

Another tumor suppressor gene frequently altered in lung cancer is the retinoblastoma *(Rb)* gene, which is an important regulator of cell growth. Inactivation of both *Rb* alleles is common in lung cancer, and loss of protein expression is seen in about 90% of small cell lung carcinomas and in 15% to 30% of non–small cell lung carcinomas.

A number of other chromosome regions that may harbor tumor suppressor genes have been identified through deletion analyses; however, the relevant putative tumor suppressor genes have not been completely identified. For example, the short arm of chromosome 3 (3p) has been found to have several regions that could harbor tumor suppressor genes. Two candidates in this region are the *FHIT* gene at chromosome 3p14 and the *RASSF1A* gene at chromosome 3p21.3, both of which have been reported to suppress the tumor phenotype in model systems. Allelic changes are also frequently observed in the chromosome 9p21 region, and these changes are thought to affect expression of the *p16* gene, an important cyclin-dependent kinase inhibitor in the *Rb* pathway, and the *p19^{arf}* gene, thought to be important in regulating the *p53* pathway.

While tumor suppressor genes have traditionally been identified because of their association with deleted or mutated regions of the genome, it is now recognized that the expression of many tumor suppressor genes is reduced through a combination of genetic and epigenetic mechanisms, such as methylation of the gene's promoter. For example, the *p16* gene is an important regulator of the *Rb* pathway, which controls the cell cycle transition from G1 phase into S phase. While *p16* LOH is found in up to 40% of lung tumors and is frequently found in premalignant lung lesions, p16 protein expression is frequently lost in these lesions despite the presence of the remaining normal allele. This loss of protein expression is associated with methylation of the remaining allele's promoter, which results in blocking of gene expression. The list of lung-related tumor suppressor genes found to be inactivated through methylation is rapidly increasing and now includes members of several important regulatory pathways, including cell cycle regulation (e.g., *p16*), regulation of gene transcription (e.g., nuclear retinoic acid receptor beta), damage response genes (e.g., glutathione S transferase and methylguanine-DNA methyltransferase), and apoptosis (e.g., death-associated protein kinase).

Genes that Maintain Genomic Stability

A third type of genetic change associated with lung cancer development is alteration in genes that maintain the genomic stability of populations of cells. While these genetic changes may not directly result in a change in cell behavior that is characteristic of a tumor cell, they may be important in the accumulation of genetic errors that drive the tumorigenesis process. For example, evidence for microsatellite instability has been found in approximately 35% of small cell lung carcinomas and more than 20% of non–small cell lung carcinomas. Microsatellite instability in hereditary non-polyposis colon cancer has been demonstrated to be associated with mutations in mismatch repair genes, which are important because they participate in the recognition and repair of various types of genetic alterations due to extrinsic (e.g., carcinogen-induced DNA adducts) and intrinsic (e.g., errors in DNA replication) processes. Loss of function of such genes results in an increased rate of accumulation of genetic errors and thus augments the tumorigenesis process. While mutations in mismatch repair genes are infrequent events in lung cancer, downregulated expression of these genes has been reported.

Alterations in cell cycle regulatory genes, both positive and negative, can also lead to the accumulation of genetic changes over time and promote the tumorigenesis process. Examples of such alterations include overexpression of cyclins D1 and E (found in 40% to 50% of lung tumors) and altered expression of mitotic regulators, such as cdc25. Another mechanism for increasing the rate of accumulation of genetic alterations in lung tissue is alteration of genes that regulate cell turnover following carcinogenic insult. For example, genetic changes that alter the cell death signaling pathway after carcinogenic attack (e.g., loss of function of p53 or overexpression of Bcl-2) allow cells to survive that would normally die after being damaged. The effect of these changes is to allow the more damaged cells to survive and, ultimately, to increase the rate of accumulation of subsequent genetic changes.

New Technologies for Identification of Molecular Changes Associated with Lung Cancer Development

The technology for identifying genes important for lung cancer development is evolving quickly. The Human Genome Project has now succeeded in sequencing much of the human genome. This work provides the opportunity to place gene sequences onto chips for use in characterizing changes in gene copy number, gene sequence, or gene expression associated with individual lung tumors. It is hoped that these approaches will lead to identification of new genes important in lung tumor development and better understanding of the molecular basis of lung tumor development. Technologies for examining protein expression patterns in lung tumors (proteomics) are also evolving. On the basis of studies of other human tumors, it is expected that particular lung tumors will have repeated patterns of genetic changes, gene expression changes, and protein pattern changes that may allow better tumor classification and permit identification of new targets for preventive or therapeutic intervention. This technological evolution is in its early stages, and definitive findings are just beginning to be reported.

Molecular Pathways for Lung Cancer Development

Because lung cancers are thought to evolve over long periods, the number of genetic changes that can be found in any single case is enormous. It is therefore difficult to distinguish the genetic changes that have physiologic significance from those that simply occurred during tumor development and were carried along into the tumor. In addition, epigenetic changes may have occurred that are important in the tumorigenesis process, including changes in expression of genes encoding growth factor receptors (e.g., HER-2/*neu* and the epidermal growth factor receptor [EGFR], MET hepatocyte growth factor receptor, and insulin growth factor receptor genes); genes encoding growth factors (e.g., the transforming growth factor alpha, gastrin-releasing peptide, and insulin-like growth factor genes); BCL-2; and the telomerase gene. However, it appears that most of the relevant genetic and epigenetic changes found in tumors affect a limited number of necessary but not sufficient cellular pathways. This notion has recently been promoted in an enlightening paper by Hanahan and Weinberg in which the authors suggest that at least 6 major functional pathways must be affected during tumor development such that cells exhibit self-sufficiency in growth signals (e.g., alterations in growth factor receptors), insensitivity to antigrowth signals (e.g., defects in the *Rb* control pathway), evasion from apoptosis (e.g., alterations in *p53* or *Bcl*-2), limitless replicative potential (e.g., continued telomerase expression), sustained angiogenesis (e.g., upregulation of vascular endothelial growth factor), and tissue invasion and metastasis (e.g., alterations in integrin expression) (Hanahan and Weinberg, 2000). In addition, there might be other pathways that could enhance the development of genetic and epigenetic changes during the lung tumorigenesis process while not directly influencing a tumorigenic pathway (e.g., alterations in DNA repair genes).

It is important to recognize that lung tumorigenesis is a multistep process and that the order of acquisition of these functional alterations need not be fixed. However, it is possible that some of these changes have no detectable physiologic impact (e.g., histologic change or the development of metastatic capability) unless other genetic changes have already occurred. For example, it is possible that some of the changes important for metastatic development could occur early in the tumorigenesis process but might not become physiologically important (or be selected for) until other cellular changes have occurred (e.g., the ability to grow outside the normal lung environment). This notion could explain why some genetic changes are found more frequently in lesions thought to be early in the tumorigenesis process whereas other genetic changes are not usually detected until later in the tumorigenesis process.

IMPLICATIONS OF MOLECULAR CHANGES FOR RISK ESTIMATION, MONITORING OF RESPONSE TO CHEMOPREVENTIVE INTERVENTIONS, EARLY DETECTION, AND CHARACTERIZATION OF NEWLY DIAGNOSED LESIONS

The burden of lung cancer on the human population could be reduced through measures that interfere with factors that initiate and drive the lung tumorigenesis process (e.g., smoking cessation and chemoprevention). Another method proposed for reducing the burden of lung cancer is early detection of tumors, when the likelihood of definitive treatment may be greater. However, clinical studies to examine the impact of chemopreventive or early detection measures are hampered because of the difficulty of identifying individuals with a high lung cancer risk. For example, while chronic smoking significantly increases lung cancer risk, only approximately 10% of long-term smokers will develop lung cancer in their lifetime. As a result, chemoprevention trials using cancer incidence as a primary end point require tens of thousands of study participants and tens of years of follow-up for adequate statistical analysis. Similarly, even if physical tests such as spiral computed tomography (spiral CT) are one day proven effective in detecting early-stage lung lesions, tens of thousands of individuals would have to be screened to identify sufficient numbers of individuals with detectable (and relevant) lung lesions to permit examination of the value of early detection in decreasing the morbidity of lung cancer. Strategies are therefore needed to identify individuals at high risk for lung cancer, to evaluate the response of the lung to chemopreventive intervention, to improve the physical detection of early lesions, and to characterize the lung lesions identified by sensitive imaging techniques.

Risk Estimation

Since lung tumorigenesis is a multistep genetic process, one approach to estimating lung cancer risk is to examine lung tissue for molecular changes commonly associated with lung cancers. Theoretically, individuals with the highest number of molecular changes in their lung tissue would be at the highest risk for lung cancer development. Indeed, when normal and premalignant lesions in resected lung tumor specimens are molecularly characterized, clonal molecular changes are detected involving genes commonly altered in lung cancers (e.g., LOH at chromosomes 9p, 3p, and 17p and *p53* mutations), and the extent of such changes appears to be related to the degree of histologic change. Interestingly, normal and premalignant lesions adjacent to small cell lung cancers show higher frequencies of molecular changes than do normal and premalignant lesions adjacent to non–small cell lung tumors. These adjacent lesions represent regions at 100% risk for being in the field of a lung cancer, and it is known that individuals who suffer a first primary small cell lung cancer are at higher risk for developing a second primary lung tumor than are individuals with a first primary non–small cell lung cancer. Therefore, it is proposed that quantification of the extent of genetic damage in lung tissue may permit lung cancer risk estimates in individuals who do not yet have detectable lung cancer or who may be at risk for developing a second primary lung tumor.

One of the problems with assessing lung cancer risk in individuals known to be at increased risk for lung cancer (e.g., long-term chronic smokers, uranium miners, and individuals with chronic obstructive pulmonary disease) is that it is not possible to accurately predict the future cancer site within the lung. Moreover, while endobronchoscopy permits examination of the central component of the lung, it is difficult to gain access to the peripheral space, where many lung adenocarcinomas develop. Nevertheless, because of the field cancerization process, it is possible that molecular analyses of specimens obtained from random biopsies of lung tissue may provide useful information for determining lung cancer risk.

As part of several chemoprevention trials involving chronic smokers at M. D. Anderson and other institutions, pretreatment biopsies were obtained from 6 defined bronchial bifurcation sites and examined for both clonal and random genetic changes. In one study, Mao and colleagues examined polymorphic DNA loci of genes frequently altered in lung cancer in bronchial biopsy specimens from long-term smokers and found that nearly 76% of the cases showed evidence of LOH in at least 1 of 6 specimens obtained (Mao et al, 1997). Moreover, current smokers tended to show higher LOH levels than did former smokers. Similarly, Hittelman and colleagues used chromosome in situ hybridization techniques on tissue sections derived by bronchial biopsy to look for changes in chromosome copy numbers. Nearly all the bronchial biopsy specimens showed evidence of random chromosome gains and losses. The frequency of these random changes was higher in current smokers than in former smokers, was higher in lesions showing bronchial metaplasia, and increased with the number of packs smoked per day. Moreover, most specimens showed evidence of multiple spatial outgrowths of colonies of cells exhibiting chromosome changes. While there was a great deal of variation between individuals with similar smoking histories, the frequency of these clonal outgrowths was related to the extent of smoking history. Additionally, these clonal outgrowths were observed in multiple biopsy specimens taken from different lung sites, suggesting a global pattern of clonal outgrowths in the carcinogen-exposed lung.

Monitoring of Response to Chemopreventive Interventions

Current studies at M. D. Anderson are focusing on the questions whether the frequency of clonal outgrowths is related to the risk of developing lung cancer and whether effective chemopreventive strategies can reduce the size and frequency of clonal outgrowths in the lungs. The answers to these questions will be critical to the efficiency of future chemoprevention trials that attempt to identify potentially efficacious agents.

The use of validated, quantifiable, intermediate molecular end points may permit the identification of high-risk individuals who might best benefit from chemopreventive intervention. Focusing on the individuals at highest risk could reduce the number of participants and the duration of clinical follow-up required in chemoprevention trials. The use of molecular end points would also permit rapid determination of whether a particular chemopreventive approach is having a positive impact on the target tissue.

Early Detection

There is increasing interest being placed on detecting lung cancer at an early stage when the tumor burden is low. The finding that spiral CT examinations of the lung can detect very small abnormalities has led to the hope that this approach could provide a physical method for early detection. However, the clinical importance of these small lesions is uncertain since their natural history is poorly understood. In some cases, these visualized lesions, when biopsied, have turned out to be unrelated processes. In other cases, these lesions have proven to be cancerous, but it is not clear that the lesion would ever have progressed to a clinically important lesion in the individual's lifetime had the lesion not been removed. Comparisons of molecular changes in these specimens obtained following spiral CT to those found in specimens of later-stage disease might provide useful information regarding the expected natural history of these small lesions. In the long run, knowledge of the molecular changes associated with lung cancer development may lead to the development of reagents and targets for functional imaging studies that may predict the future behavior of small lung lesions without a requirement for biopsy.

Potential Noninvasive Methods of Assessing Molecular Changes

One of the problems with current molecular risk assessment and early detection technologies is the requirement for relatively invasive endobronchial or transthoracic biopsies to obtain lung tissue for molecular analysis. For this reason, there is increased interest in determining whether molecular assessment of exfoliated lung cells (e.g., in bronchial washings or sputum) or surrogate epithelial tissues (e.g., oral epithelial scrapings) might provide information about lung cancer risk.

The potential problem with analysis of exfoliated cells is that many of the molecular studies in use today involve bulk analyses that will not detect an event unless at least 10% to 60% of the cells harbor the same genetic change. Nevertheless, recent studies suggest that some molecular changes can be detected in specimens containing exfoliated cells. For example, Tockman and colleagues (1997) have provided evidence that detection of expression of a specific protein involved in the processing of heterogeneous RNA in sputum samples is associated with lung cancer risk. Other investigators are studying whether the presence of epigenetic changes (e.g., promoter methylation changes in lung cancer–associated tumor suppressor genes) in cells derived from bronchial washings of individuals known to have lung cancer can be used to estimate lung cancer risk in individuals who do not have lung cancer. Prospective studies are now ongoing at M. D. Anderson and other institutions to examine whether this approach will prove feasible for estimating lung cancer risk in specific individuals.

IMPLICATIONS OF MOLECULAR CHANGES FOR ESTIMATING PROGNOSIS AND PREDICTING RESPONSE TO THERAPY

With lung cancer, as with many other malignancies, the prognosis of an individual patient is difficult to assess solely on the basis of clinical and histologic parameters. While it is clear that advanced stage of disease is a poor prognostic factor, there is tremendous variation in outcome for patients with similar clinical characteristics. For example, for individuals with solitary lesions, local resection alone results in long-term survival in a high proportion of patients, but there is a significant fraction of patients at high risk for regional recurrences or metastases who might benefit from the addition of radiation therapy, chemotherapy, or both. One goal of molecular analyses is to identify changes that might provide prognostic information, either with regard to the natural history of the tumor or with regard to potential sensitivity or resistance to radiation therapy or particular chemotherapeutic approaches.

A number of specific molecular changes have been reported to be of significant prognostic value in lung cancer; however, the conclusions from different study groups regarding these changes have not been identical. For example, the presence of *p53* alterations in lung tumors has been suggested to be a poor prognostic factor by some groups and a good prognostic factor by other groups. One persistent trend is an inverse relationship between the number of molecular changes and positive outcome.

For most molecular markers, while there may be a statistically significant relationship between the presence or absence of a particular molecular change and outcome, the differences between the groups with and without this change are not sufficient to guide decisions regarding the need for adjuvant treatment in patients with early-stage disease or to guide the selection of a particular therapeutic regimen for patients with later-stage disease. Current studies at M.D. Anderson and other institutions are focused on the use of molecular chip and proteomic technologies to identify specific patterns in lung tumor specimens that are associated with specific clinical parameters, such as responsiveness to chemotherapy or radiation therapy or the likelihood of metastatic spread. The hope is that the discovery of such genetic or expression patterns would indicate which particular management strategy is most appropriate for a particular patient's tumor.

IMPLICATIONS OF MOLECULAR CHANGES FOR NEW THERAPEUTIC INTERVENTIONS

One problem with current preventive and therapeutic approaches to lung cancer is the side effects associated with the interventions. In the case of chemoprevention, since the individual does not yet have cancer and the efficacy of treatment is uncertain, treatment-associated side effects are a major issue. In the treatment of established lung cancer, significant efforts continue to identify new active cytotoxics, to examine the benefits of combinations of surgery, chemotherapy, and radiation therapy, and to develop strategies to protect normal tissues from side effects (e.g., use of amifostine and hematopoietic growth factor support).

The identification of specific molecular pathways important in lung cancer development has led to the idea of targeting these aberrant pathways as a strategy for treatment. The working assumption is that these pathways are selectively activated or inactivated in tumors such that interventions specifically targeting these pathways should have a limited impact on normal tissues.

Re-regulating Altered Signaling Pathways

One approach to molecularly targeted treatment of lung cancer is to re-regulate signaling pathways that have been altered. In the case of oncogenes, the idea would be to inhibit the activity of the oncogene by decreasing its expression, interfering with its signaling properties, or inhibiting its activity. For example, *ras* mutation, which results in constitutive activation, is a common molecular event in lung cancer. Since *ras* functions in mediating the growth factor–induced signaling pathway from the membrane to cytoplasmic intermediates to regulating gene transcription, many investigators are examining various aspects of this pathway for potential targets for intervention. For example, posttranslational farnesylation of mutant ras is necessary for activation of its transforming properties. Thus, investigators searched for peptides that can mimic the ras epitope targeted for farnesyltransferase, blocking ras farnesylation. Early clinical trials of farnesyltransferase inhibitors (FTIs), including phase I/II studies at M. D. Anderson, found that while these agents had clinical activity and minimal toxicity, *ras* mutation status did not correlate with FTI sensitivity or resistance. Thus it was possible that ras was not the only FTI target that might be important for the observed cell cycle arrest, apoptosis, and tumor response in both the preclinical and clinical settings. Other potential targets of FTIs include RhoB and centromere-binding proteins. A group at M. D. Anderson recently presented promising therapeutic results using the small-molecule farnesylation inhibitor SCH66336. These investigators showed evidence of antitumor activity in patients with advanced non–small cell lung cancer. Current studies are examining the use of this FTI in combination with taxanes in patients previously found to have disease unresponsive to taxanes alone.

Other purported oncogene products targeted for early clinical trials are EGFR and its family members, including HER-2/neu. Both EGFR and HER-2/neu have been found to be overexpressed in lung tumors. While EGFR was originally thought to primarily promote cell growth, more recent studies implicate the EGFR signaling pathway in other cancer-associated processes, such as cell motility, cell adhesion, invasion, angiogenesis, and survival after stress. Several approaches have been developed that target this important pathway, including monoclonal antibodies, immunotoxins, small peptide inhibitors of EGFR-associated tyrosine kinases, and agents that can downregulate EGFR expression. Many of these new approaches are now being studied in clinical trials at M. D. Anderson. Humanized anti-EGFR monoclonal antibodies (e.g., IMC-C225) have been shown to result in reduced tyrosine kinase activity of these membrane receptors and have been associated with some clinical activity. On the basis of preclinical studies demonstrating potential synergy with chemotherapeutic agents and radiation therapy, current clinical trials at M. D. Anderson are focusing on the use of anti-growth factor receptor monoclonal antibodies in combination with other modalities. For example, one clinical study is exploring the combination of trastuzumab (Herceptin; anti-HER-2/neu), cisplatin, and gemcitabine in patients with locally advanced or metastatic disease. Because of the high EGFR and HER-2/neu levels found in lung tumors, antibodies or growth factor ligands conjugated to toxins (e.g., ricin) or isotope emitters are also being explored to selectively deliver toxic molecules to lung tumors in relatively high concentrations while potentially averting normal tissue toxicity.

Another approach to targeting EGFR-associated activity in lung cancer involves the use of small peptide tyrosine kinase inhibitors, including ZD1839 (Iressa, an anilinoquinazoline-derived agent). This compound, which is given orally, is now being investigated in phase II and III trials, both alone and in combination with chemotherapy or radiation therapy. Finally, another EGFR-targeted approach being explored is downregulation of levels of EGFR on lung tumor cells. Preclinical studies have shown that nonselective retinoids can downregulate the transcriptional activation of EGFR and its associated ligand, transforming growth factor alpha, resulting in decreased cell proliferation. One such retinoid, LGD1069 (Targretin), a potent nuclear retinoid X receptor–selective retinoic acid agonist, has now been examined in combination with cisplatin and vinorelbine in a phase I/II trial at M. D. Anderson.

As more is discovered regarding the signaling pathways initiated by external factors, such as growth factors and cell-cell and cell-matrix interactions, additional molecules have been identified that are increasingly being explored as potential targets for new therapeutics. For example, the PI3K protein family of serine/threonine kinases has been found to be important in many types of signals that come from outside or inside the cell following stress reactions. The activity of PI3K is elevated in several tumors, including lung tumors, and elevated activity results in the phosphorylation of intermediate molecules that can decrease cell turnover. The antagonist to PI3K is PTEN, a phosphatase that counteracts PI3K activity by dephosphorylating the same targets and acts as a tumor suppressor gene. With the finding that rapamycin and its analogues show preclinical activity against several tumor models, there is now interest in exploring this pathway as a target for new therapeutics.

Replacing Defective Genes

Another approach to molecularly targeted treatment of lung cancer is to try to replace tumor suppressor gene function that has been lost during tumorigenesis. For example, loss of *p53* function is a common molecular change associated with lung cancer. Preclinical studies in vitro and in orthotopic murine lung tumor models showed antitumor activity following transfer of the *p53* gene into tumors using an adenovirus construct (Ad-p53). Interestingly, Ad-p53 gene transfer seemed to affect multiple tumor-associated pathways, including downregulation of vascular endothelial growth factor expression and subsequent inhibition of angiogenesis.

The first clinical trial using *p53* gene transfer in patients with non–small cell lung cancer at M. D. Anderson utilized a retroviral vector under the control of the actin promoter. This treatment showed some antitumor activity (e.g., induction of apoptosis in the tumor) without vector-associated side effects. However, these early retroviral vectors were limited in transduction efficiency, especially in nonproliferating lung cancer cells. For this reason, the Ad-p53 vector was modified by placing the *p53* expression cassette into a replication-defective adenovirus vector under the control of a more active cytomegalovirus promoter. A phase I trial showed that this vector could be administered in a multiple-dose regimen at high virus titer levels with low toxicity. While the treatment required intratumoral injections performed percutaneously using CT guidance or bronchoscopy, the incidence of pneumothoraces was low, *p53* transgene expression was detectable, and there was evidence of tumor shrinkage and disease stabilization in some patients.

At present, Ad-p53 delivery is being combined with radiation therapy or chemotherapy (e.g., cisplatin) or both because preclinical models showed enhanced antitumor activity with the addition of these treatment modalities. In one approach, intravenous cisplatin is administered on day 1 and Ad-p53 is injected intratumorally on day 4. Significant clinical activity (i.e., partial responses and some stable responses) and laboratory-detected activity (i.e., increased numbers of apoptotic cells) have been seen with this regimen, even in patients whose disease had progressed with platinum-based chemotherapy combinations. Ad-p53 administration is also being used in combination with radiation therapy to increase local control. In a phase II clinical trial at M. D. Anderson, patients with localized non–small cell lung cancer who were not candidates for surgery or chemoradiation were treated with intratumoral injections on days 1, 18, and 32 in conjunction with standard radiation therapy (60 Gy). Eight of 11 patients had pathologically negative biopsy specimens after treatment, and the 1-year progression-free survival rate was 45.5%, with most relapses consisting of metastatic progression rather than local recurrence (Swisher et al, 2000).

Similar strategies are being initiated that target other tumor suppressor genes whose function is commonly lost in lung tumors, including *p16*, *p21*, *bax* (a pro-apoptotic factor), *FHIT*, and some recently discovered genes in the region of deletion on chromosome 3p that exhibit antitumor activity when they are transduced into tumor cells.

Targeted Killing of Cells Lacking Tumor Suppressor Gene Function

Another approach currently being explored is the use of adenoviral vectors that will only reproduce in and kill cells that lack *p53* function. ONYX-015 is a replication-deficient adenovirus from which the adenoviral component that normally inactivates *p53* activity during productive infection has been deleted. In this way, the virus can reproductively replicate only in cells that lack *p53* functional activity, which in theory are lung cancer cells. Early clinical trials using ONYX-015 have shown interesting activity; however, some gastrointestinal and skin side effects have been observed.

While many of these gene and viral vector delivery strategies involve intratumoral injections, other routes of administration are also being explored. One appealing approach is to deliver the vectors by inhalation. This would allow a more global distribution of particles at high titers (since it is still a local delivery) and is especially attractive in the setting of lung cancer because of the adenoviral receptors found in lung tissue.

Other Investigational Approaches to Lung Cancer Treatment

As more is understood about the molecular events associated with the development, growth, and metastasis of human lung tumors, the number of potentially targetable gene products increases. For example, since loss of functional activity of the lung cancer tumor suppressor genes is associated with hypermethylation of their promoters, one approach being explored is the use of agents such as azacitidine analogues to reverse the hypermethylation patterns in proliferating cells. Similarly, since an important component of tumor establishment and growth is the ability to develop a vasculature (angiogenesis), molecules that interfere with vessel initiation and development are being explored as therapeutic agents in patients with lung cancer. Current trials ongoing at M. D. Anderson are exploring several potential antiangiogenic agents, including thalidomide, TNP-470, endostatin, an antibody to vascular endothelial growth factor receptor, interleukin-12, neovastat, and marimastat. These agents are thought to interfere with different components of the angiogenic pathway, including endothelial invasion, matrix remodeling, adhesion, and—by blocking growth factors and their receptors—proliferation.

Another important component of metastatic development is the ability of circulating lung tumor cells to find a suitable organ environment in which to attach and become established. This process has been shown to have some specificity with regard to "addressing" the tumor cell to a particular site and initiating interactive tumor/stromal/endothelial signaling. As the specificities of these interactions are better defined, small peptides will be developed that will serve to interfere with these interactions and thus decrease the risk of metastasis.

Chemoprevention Approaches

Common molecular pathways operate throughout the process of lung tumorigenesis. Thus, strategies used in the therapeutic management of lung cancer should also be applicable in the premalignant setting provided that the treatment is not unduly toxic. We and other investigators have identified various approaches that target molecular pathways important for lung tumor development and apparently have few ill effects on normal tissue. For example, in phase I and II clinical trials of the EGFR kinase inhibitor ZD1839, little normal tissue damage was identified. As a result, clinical trials using ZD1839 are being initiated that will examine the activity of this agent in the chemopreventive setting in chronic smokers. Similarly, since lung tumors are frequently found to exhibit increased cyclooxygenase-2 activity and since chronic administration of the cyclooxygenase-2 inhibitor celecoxib (Celebrex) has been shown to be well tolerated in patients with arthritis, chemoprevention trials at M. D. Anderson are being initiated that will explore the use of cyclooxygenase-2 inhibitors for chemoprevention.

KEY PRACTICE POINTS

- Lung cancer development involves a multistep process occurring throughout a field of tissue exposed to carcinogens. Molecular changes can be found throughout the exposed lung, and the extent of change may be associated with lung cancer risk.

- Individuals differ in their susceptibility to tobacco smoking because of individual differences in carcinogen activation, detoxification, DNA repair, and tissue response to chronic exposure to carcinogens.

- Smokers who quit continue to have an increased risk of lung cancer development. More than 50% of new lung cancer cases involve former smokers.

- Prevention and early detection provide the greatest chance for reducing the morbidity and mortality of lung cancer.

- The molecular characteristics of a patient's lung tumor have prognostic implications and may help to identify the most efficacious treatment approach.

- Molecular characterization of lung tumors has led to the identification of new targets for prevention and therapy. Clinical trials are ongoing involving the use of monoclonal antibodies against growth factor receptors and angiogenesis stimulators, the use of small peptide inhibitors of dysregulated signaling pathways, and gene replacement strategies.

- Targeted molecular therapies are now being combined with surgery, radiation therapy, and chemotherapy to augment and extend treatment response.

SUGGESTED READINGS

Fong KM, Sekido Y, Minna JD. Molecular pathogenesis of lung cancer. *J Thorac Cardiovasc Surg* 1999;118:1136–1152.

Gazdar AF, Minna JD. Targeted therapies for killing tumor cells. *Proc Natl Acad Sci U S A* 2001;98:10028–10030.

Hanahan D, Weinberg RA. The hallmarks of cancer. *Cell* 2000;100:57–70.

Hirsch FR, Franklin WA, Gazdar AF, et al. Early detection of lung cancer: clinical perspectives of recent advances in biology and radiology. *Clin Cancer Res* 2001;7:5–22.

Hittelman WN. Genetic instability assessments in the lung cancerization field. In: Brambilla C, Brambilla E, eds. *Lung Tumors: Fundamental Biology and Clinical Management.* New York, NY: Marcel Dekker; 1999:255–267.

Hittelman WN. Molecular cytogenetic evidence for multistep tumorigenesis: implications for risk assessment and early detection. In: Srivastava S, Hensen DE, Gazdar A, eds. *Molecular Pathology of Early Cancer.* Washington, DC: IOS Press; 1999:385–404.

Hong WK, Spitz MR, Lippman SM. Cancer chemoprevention in the 21st century: genetics, risk modeling, and molecular targets. *J Clin Oncol* 2000;18(21 suppl):9S–18S.

Khuri FR, Kurie JM. Antisense approaches enter the clinic. *Clin Cancer Res* 2000;6:1607–1610.

Kim ES, Hong WK, Khuri FR. Prevention of lung cancer. The new millennium. *Chest Surg Clin N Am* 2000;10:663–690.

Kurie JM. The biological basis for the use of retinoids in cancer prevention and treatment. *Curr Opin Oncol* 1999;11:497–502.

Kurie JM, Lippman SM, Hong WK. Chemoprevention trials: epithelial carcinogenesis and the biological basis of intervention. In: Bertino JR, ed. *Encyclopedia of Cancer.* Vol 1. San Diego, Calif: Academic Press; 1996;341–354.

Lippman SM, Spitz MR. Lung cancer chemoprevention: an integrated approach. *J Clin Oncol* 2001;19(18 suppl):74S-82S.

Mao L, Lee JS, Kurie JM, et al. Clonal genetic alterations in the lungs of current and former smokers. *J Natl Cancer Inst* 1997;89:857–862.

Saccomano G, Archer VE, Auerbach O, et al. Development of carcinoma of the lung as reflected in exfoliated cells. *Cancer* 1974;33:256–270.

Spitz MR, Wei Q, Li G, et al. Genetic susceptibility to tobacco carcinogenesis. *Cancer Invest* 1999;17:645–659.

Swisher SG, Roth JA. Gene therapy in lung cancer. *Curr Oncol Rep* 2000;2:64–70.

Swisher SG, Roth JA, Komaki R, et al. A phase II trial of adenoviral mediated p53 gene transfer (RPR/INGN 201) in conjunction with radiation therapy in patients with localized non–small cell lung cancer (NSCLC). *Proc Am Soc Clin Oncol* 2000;19:461.

Swisher SG, Roth JA, Nemunaitis J, et al. Adenovirus-mediated p53 gene transfer in advanced non-small-cell lung cancer. *J Natl Cancer Inst* 1999;91:763–771.

Tockman MS, Mulshine JL, Piantadosi S, et al. Prospective detection of preclinical lung cancer: results from two studies of heterogeneous nuclear ribonucleoprotein A2/B1 overexpression. *Clin Cancer Res* 1997;3(12 Pt 1):2237–2246.

Tong L, Spitz MR, Fueger JJ, et al. Lung carcinoma in former smokers. *Cancer* 1996;78:1004–1010.

Wistuba II, Gazdar AF, Minna JD. Molecular genetics of small cell lung carcinoma. *Semin Oncol* 2001;28(2 suppl 4):3–13.

INDEX

Acetaminophen, 245
N-Acetylcysteine, 269
Acinic cell carcinoma, 76
Ad-p53, 294-295
Addictions, assessment of, 223.
   See also Smoking
Adenocarcinoma
  atypical adenomatous
   hyperplasia progression to,
   67
  chest radiography of, 11-12
  CNS metastases, 28
  immunohistochemistry, 76-77
  k-*ras* mutations, 15
  mesotheliomas distinguished
   from, 77
  NSCLC classification as, 60
  p53 mutations, 78
  pathology, 73-74
  radiographic evaluations, 31
  WHO classification, 63
Adenoid cystic carcinoma, 76, 227
Adenoma, 47, 63
Adenosquamous carcinoma, 64,
  74
Adrenal glands, 6, 27, 30, 46
Adrenocorticotropic hormone, 29
Age
  cancer mortality rates, 4
  chemotherapy and, 162
  comorbid conditions and, 161
  lung cancer frequency, 7
  SCLC outcomes and, 188
Air leaks, prevention, 251-252
Air pollution, 6, 282

Airway compression, 228,
  235-236
Albumin levels, 29
Alcohol intake, 246
Alkaline phosphatase, 28, 46, 188,
  209
Alkylating agents, 210. *See also*
  entries for specific agents
Alpha-tocopherol. *See*
  α-Tocopherol
Altered mental status, 27, 29
Aluminum hydroxide, 245
Alveolar epithelial hyperplasia.
  See Atypical adenomatous
  hyperplasia
American Cancer Society (ACS),
  37
American College of Radiology
  Imaging Network Trial, 38
American College of Surgeons,
  107
American Joint Committee on
  Cancer (AJCC), 8, 102
American Society of Clinical
  Oncology (ASCO), 163-164
Amifostine, 21
Amputations, 225
Androgen receptor gene, 66
Anemia, 201, 250, 253
Anesthesiology, 92-93, 225
Angiogenesis, 287, 296
Anorexia, 7, 28, 223. *See also*
  Appetite; Cachexia;
  Weight loss
Anterior pituitary, 76-77